P9-ARO-171

NEUROSCIENCE
INTELLIGENCE
UNIT

MEASURING MOVEMENT AND LOCOMOTION: FROM INVERTEBRATES TO HUMANS

Klaus-Peter Ossenkopp, Ph.D.

Martin Kavaliers, Ph.D.

Neuroscience Program and Departments of Psychology,
Oral Biology and Pharmacology and Toxicology
University of Western Ontario
London, Ontario, Canada

Paul R. Sanberg, Ph.D.

Departments of Surgery, Neurology, Psychiatry, Psychology
and Pharmacology and Therapeutics
University of South Florida College of Medicine
Tampa, Florida, U.S.A.

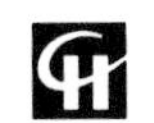

CHAPMAN & HALL
I(T)P An International Thomson Publishing Company

New York • Albany • Bonn • Boston • Cincinnati • Detroit • London • Madrid • Melbourne •
Mexico City • Pacific Grove • Paris • San Francisco • Singapore • Tokyo • Toronto • Washington

R.G. LANDES COMPANY
AUSTIN

NEUROSCIENCE INTELLIGENCE UNIT

MEASURING MOVEMENT AND LOCOMOTION:
FROM INVERTEBRATES TO HUMANS

R.G. LANDES COMPANY
Austin, Texas, U.S.A.

Printed in the U.S.A.

Please address all inquiries to the Publishers:
R.G. Landes Company, 909 Pine Street, Georgetown, Texas, U.S.A. 78626
Phone: 512/ 863 7762; FAX: 512/ 863 0081

North American distributor:
Chapman & Hall, 115 Fifth Avenue, New York, New York, U.S.A. 10003

U.S. and Canada ISBN: 0-412-10321-4

While the authors, editors and publisher believe that drug selection and dosage and the specifications and usage of equipment and devices, as set forth in this book, are in accord with current recommendations and practice at the time of publication, they make no warranty, expressed or implied, with respect to material described in this book. In view of the ongoing research, equipment development, changes in governmental regulations and the rapid accumulation of information relating to the biomedical sciences, the reader is urged to carefully review and evaluate the information provided herein.

Library of Congress Cataloging-in-Publication Data

Measuring movement and locomotion: from invertibrates to humans /
Klaus-Peter Ossenkopp, Martin Kavaliers, Paul Sanberg [editors].
p. cm. — (Neuroscience intelligence unit)
Includes bibliographical references and index.
ISBN 0-412-10321-4 (alk. paper)
1. Animal locomotion—Measurement. 2. Human locomotion—Measurement. I. Ossenkop, Klaus-Peter. II. Kavaliers, Martin. III. Sanberg, Paul.
[DNLM: 1. Movement—physiology. 2. Human locomotion—physiology.
3. Biomechanics. 4. Research Design. WE 103 M484 1996]
QP301.M3758 1996 591.1'852—dc20
DNLM/DLC 95-50025
for Library of Congress CIP

Publisher's Note

R.G. Landes Company publishes six book series: *Medical Intelligence Unit, Molecular Biology Intelligence Unit, Neuroscience Intelligence Unit, Tissue Engineering Intelligence Unit, Environmental Intelligence Unit* and *Biotechnology Intelligence Unit.* The authors of our books are acknowledged leaders in their fields and the topics are unique. Almost without exception, no other similar books exist on these topics.

Our goal is to publish books in important and rapidly changing areas of bioscience for sophisticated researchers and clinicians. To achieve this goal, we have accelerated our publishing program to conform to the fast pace in which information grows in bioscience. Most of our books are published within 90 to 120 days of receipt of the manuscript. We would like to thank our readers for their continuing interest and welcome any comments or suggestions they may have for future books.

Deborah Muir Molsberry
Publications Director
R.G. Landes Company

CONTENTS

EDITORS

Klaus-Peter Ossenkopp
Neuroscience Program and
Departments of Psychology, and Pharmacology and Toxicology
University of Western Ontario
London, Ontario, Canada
Chapters 1, 3, Appendix B

Martin Kavaliers
Neuroscience Program and
Departments of Psychology and Oral Biology
University of Western Ontario
London, Ontario, Canada
Chapters 1, 2, Appendix B

Paul R. Sanberg
Departments of Surgery, Neurology, Psychiatry, Psychology
and Pharmacology and Therapeutics
University of South Florida College of Medicine
Tampa, Florida, U.S.A.
Chapter 1

CONTRIBUTORS

V.J. Bolivar
Department of Psychology
Dalhousie University
Halifax, Nova Scotia, Canada
Chapter 6

K.M. Crofton
Neurotoxicology Division
Health Effects Research Laboratory
U.S. Environmental Protection Agency
Research Triangle Park, North Carolina, U.S.A.
Chapter 12

Warren O. Eaton
Department of Psychology
University of Manitoba
Winnipeg, Manitoba, Canada
Chapter 5, Appendix A

J.C. Fentress
Department of Psychology
Dalhousie University
Halifax, Nova Scotia, Canada
Chapter 6

CONTRIBUTORS

Frank E. Fish
Department of Biology
West Chester University
West Chester, Pennsylvania, U.S.A.
Chapter 9

Mark A. Geyer, Ph.D.
Professor of Psychiatry
Department of Psychiatry
School of Medicine
University of California, San Diego
La Jolla, California, U.S.A.
Chapters 13, 14

J.L. Howard
Pharmacology Division
Wellcome Research Laboratories
Research Triangle Park,
North Carolina, U.S.A.
Chapter 11

R.C. MacPhail
Neurotoxicology Division
Health Effects Research Laboratory
U.S. Environmental Protection
Agency
Research Triangle Park,
North Carolina, U.S.A.
Chapter 12

Nancy A. McKeen
Department of Psychology
University of Manitoba
Winnipeg, Manitoba, Canada
Chapter 5, Appendix A

Elena I. Miklyaeva
Department of Psychology
University of Lethbridge
Lethbridge, Alberta, Canada
Chapter 8

Martin P. Paulus, M.D.
Assistant Research Psychobiologist
Laboratory of Biological Dynamics
and Theoretical Medicine
Department of Psychiatry
School of Medicine
University of California, San Diego
La Jolla, California, U.S.A.
Chapters 13, 14

Sergio M. Pellis, Ph.D.
Department of Psychology
University of Lethbridge
Lethbridge, Alberta, Canada
Chapter 7

T. S. Perrot-Sinal
Neuroscience Program
Division of Oral Biology
Faculty of Dentistry and
Department of Psychology
University of Western Ontario
London, Ontario, Canada
Chapter 2

G.T. Pollard
Pharmacology Division
Wellcome Research Laboratories
Research Triangle Park,
North Carolina, U.S.A.
Chapter 11

Deborah C. Rice, Ph.D.
Toxicology Research Division
Bureau of Chemical Safety
Health Protection Branch
Department of Health
Ottawa, Ontario, Canada
Chapter 4

CONTRIBUTORS

Kimberly J. Saudino
Department of Psychology
Boston University
Boston, Massachusetts, U.S.A.
Chapter 5, Appendix A

Henk C. Schamhardt, Ph.D.
Equine Biomechanics
Research Group
Faculty of Veterinary Medicine
University of Utrecht
Utrecht, The Netherlands
Chapter 10

Ian Q. Whishaw
Department of Psychology
University of Lethbridge
Lethbridge, Alberta, Canada
Chapter 8

PREFACE

This book provides an overview of the methodology and data analysis procedures for measuring movement and locomotion. Following an overview and perspective of the book in an introductory chapter by the editors, K.-P. Ossenkopp, M. Kavaliers and P.R. Sanberg, four chapters examine the various methods for measuring activity levels. M. Kavaliers and T.S. Perrot-Sinal discuss the measurement of activity in invertebrates and lower vertebrates. K.-P. Ossenkopp and M. Kavaliers cover the measurement of spontaneous locomotor activity in small mammals, such as rats, mice, gerbils and voles. Assessment of locomotor behavior in nonhuman primates is provided by D.C. Rice and for humans W.O. Eaton, N.A. McKeen and K.J. Saudino discuss the measurement of individual differences in general motor activity.

Part II deals with the measurement of other types of movement and consists of five chapters. J.C. Fentress and V.J. Bolivar describe the developmental aspects of movement sequences in mammals. Next, the righting reflex and the modular organization of motor programs is discussed by S.M. Pellis. An interesting descriptive and quantitative analysis of reaching and grasping behavior in rats is provided by I.Q. Whishaw and E.I. Miklyaeva. F.E. Fish presents a fascinating methodology for measuring and analyzing swimming kinematics in small mammals followed by a discussion of some methods developed to quantitatively analyze equine locomotion by H.C. Schamhardt.

The last part of the book examines issues dealing with experimental design and data analysis and consists of 4 chapters. A technique which describes the use of single-subject designs for measuring locomotor activity is provided by G.T. Pollard and J.L. Howard. K.M. Crofton and R.C. MacPhail discuss the very important issue of the reliability of motor activity assessments. Multivariate approaches to the analysis of locomotor and investigatory behavior in rodents are discussed by M.A. Geyer and M.P. Paulus, followed by a new perspective on the assessment of motor behavior by the application of nonlinear techniques based on the behavior of complex physical systems, presented by M.P. Paulus and M.A. Geyer. At the end of the book (Appendix B) can be found a list of equipment manufactures which provide commercially available behavioral measurement technology, much of it discussed in the various chapters in the book.

BIOGRAPHICAL SKETCHES

KLAUS-PETER OSSENKOPP, PhD

Dr. Klaus-Peter Ossenkopp is full professor in the Department of Psychology and a faculty member in the Neuroscience Program at the University of Western Ontario, teaching courses on statistical methods, behavioral neuroscience, behavioral pharmacology and sociobiology. Dr. Ossenkopp received his BA (Hons) and MA in Psychology from the University of Manitoba and his PhD in Biopsychology from York University in Toronto, Canada. He previously held both a Natural Sciences and Engineering Research Council (NSERC) of Canada Postdoctoral Fellowship as well as a NSERC University Research Fellowship in the Department of Psychology at the University of Western Ontario. Dr. Ossenkopp is currently on the editorial boards of the journals, *Brain Research Bulletin, Electro- and Magnetobiology and Physiology and Behavior.*

He is currently doing research in behavioral neuroscience. This research encompasses investigations of regulatory behaviors, behavioral toxicology, brain mechanisms of ingestive behavior, and hormonal and neuropeptide influences on conditioned changes in ingestive behavior and other learning paradigms.

MARTIN KAVALIERS, PhD

Dr. Martin Kavaliers is a full professor in Psychology and Oral Biology at the University of Western Ontario teaching courses on neurosciences, pharmacology and behavior. Dr. Kavaliers earned his BSc at Sir George Williams University in Biology and his PhD at The University of Alberta. He has taught at The University of Alberta. Dr. Kavaliers is currently on the editorial board of the journal, *Life Sciences.*

He is doing research in neuropeptides and behavior and the ethopharmacology of aggression. This research encompasses investigations of sex differences in animal behavior and the impact of reproductive status. His more current research deals with the impact of parasitism on animal behavior.

PAUL R. SANBERG, PhD

Dr. Paul R. Sanberg is professor of Surgery, Neurology, Psychiatry, Psychology, Pharmacology and Therapeutics and Research Director of Neurological Surgery at the University of South Florida College of Medicine. Dr. Sanberg earned his BSc (Hons) at York University (Canada) in Biopsychology. He earned his MSc at the Autstralian National University. He was a Postdoctoral Fellow in Neuroscience at the Johns Hopkins University School of Medicine, followed by academic positions at Ohio University, the University of Cincinnati and Brown University prior to his current position. He was also Scientific Director for CytoTherapeutics, Inc., Providence, Rhode Island. Dr. Sanberg is Editor in

Chief of Cell Transplantation (Elsevier Science, Inc. Publisher). He is the author of more than 200 scientific articles and has published the books *Over the Counter Drugs: Harmless or Hazardous* (Chelsea House Publishers), *Prescription Narcotics: The Addictive Painkiller* (Chelsea House Publishers), and *Cell Transplantation for Huntington's Disease* (R.G. Landes Publishers) among others.

Dr. Sanberg is currently doing research in the areas of animal models of neurodegenerative disorders and studying experimental therapeutics such as neural tissue transplantation for Parkinson's and Huntington's diseases. He is also Principal Investigator of an NIH-funded clinical study looking at the effects of transdermal nicotine in Tourette's Syndrome.

CHAPTER 1

Measuring Movement and Locomotion: Perspective and Overview

Klaus-Peter Ossenkopp, Martin Kavaliers and Paul R. Sanberg

PERSPECTIVE

The measurement of movement and locomotion is central to obtaining qualitative and quantitative information about an animal's general behavior. Changes in an animal's spatial location and/or changes in the spatial relationship of the animal's limbs and body have consequences for the expression and measurement of all aspects of behavior. Spontaneous locomotor activity, along with various class-common and species-specific behaviors, as well as learned or conditioned behaviors, are all heavily interwoven with movement and locomotion.[1] Our attempts to characterize behavior can range from description of the effects of a single muscle on movement to more global descriptions of the movement of parts of limbs, the whole limbs, or the entire animal. This can include the interrelationships of these various components with each other. As a consequence the measurement of movement and locomotion is essential in our examination of such adaptations as finding food, avoiding predators, attracting a mate, caring for the young, or finding a suitable dwelling place.

Much of our measurement of behavior relies on direct observation and classification of sequences of movement into functional units.[2-4] However, recent technological advances have led to the development of automated procedures that provide simultaneous measurements of a number of behavioral variables[5-7] and allow for a more objective and complete approach to the description and quantification of behavior. Some of these approaches include automatic tracking of an animal's

Measuring Movement and Locomotion: From Invertebrates to Humans, edited by Klaus-Peter Ossenkopp, Martin Kavaliers and Paul R. Sanberg.

spatial position, automatic tracking of limb position or spatial relationship to the rest of the organism or the environment, and video recording of movement sequences with subsequent analysis in "slow-motion." In addition to decisions about the measurement method, the researcher also needs to address the issues of *reliability* and *validity* of the variables quantified.[4] Data analysis is dependent on an understanding of the qualities of the measurements in terms of the preceding two characteristics. Finally, an appreciation of the influences of a large variety of organismic and environmental factors, that can affect the expression and interpretation of the behavioral measures, is necessary to understand overall behavioral adaptations.

In attempting to capture the richness of behavior, often obtained in subjective clinical observation of a behavioral phenomenon but much more difficult to extract objectively in a quantitative manner, it has been suggested that multiple, simultaneous behavioral measures (multivariate) be obtained in the same situation.[8-10] This multivariate approach presents additional problems in terms of statistical inference and interpretation of behavioral complexity.[9] A variety of common statistical procedures, such as principal component and factor analysis, are available to deal with multiple measures.[11] More problematic are approaches to the analysis of sequential and spatial patterns of behavior, with very few statistical methods available to examine these components. Multivariate analysis, both methodological and analytical, thus represents attempts to promote "phenomenon realism" by providing more adequate characterization of general behavior processes. It also allows for a better match between subjective clinical impression and objective quantitative measurement.

Behavioral measurement can serve two different purposes in the investigation of brain-behavior relationships. Behavioral variables can be used as indices of activity in the neural systems of interest, especially following exposure to toxic substances, therapeutic medications, damage to specific brain structures, or other manipulations.[12] On the other hand, an analysis of behavior itself might be of primary interest. This latter approach tries to understand the functions of specific neural systems and the relationships among these systems in the initiation or modulation of behavior.[13] In many studies both types of approaches may be required. It should also be recognized that the measurement of motor activity levels generally involves procedures which produce very little, or no invasiveness of the organism. Direct observation, in both field and laboratory studies, and automated laboratory procedures used for measuring activity, are essentially noninvasive procedures. In terms of animal welfare concerns, these methodologies are ideally suited to have either no or minimal impact on the well-being of the subjects being studied. This can be very important, not only from an ethical perspective, but also for the experimental use of subjects that may be either rare, in short supply, or to be used in further studies.

OVERVIEW

Measuring Movement and Locomotion is organized into three main sections. Part I deals with the methodology of measuring activity levels, whether spontaneous or induced, in a range of different animal species. The emphasis is on techniques which quantify the various components of general activity, especially those which are automated and allow for multivariate assessment. These methodologies range from simple direct observation to automated techniques which use infrared photobeam technology or video-image analysis to monitor and quantify a number of different activity variables simultaneously. Part II emphasizes descriptive approaches to basic movement patterns from a developmental and species-specific perspective. The applications of rigorous descriptive methodologies, such as movement notation and kinematic analysis, allow for a better appreciation of behavior patterns, their organization and development. Special emphasis is given to the analysis and measurement of such behaviors as reaching, grooming, swimming and locomotion. The fluid and fine-grained characteristics of these behaviors are the targets of these analytical approaches. The last part of the book focuses on issues of experimental design and statistical analysis. The chapters in this section deal with such issues as single-subject designs, reliability of measurement procedures, and multivariate statistical approaches to locomotor activity analysis. The emphasis in this last section is on the interpretation of data and new approaches to understanding the complexities of motor activity, especially in a quantitative multivariate fashion.

The first part, on measuring activity levels, starts with an overview of the measurement of activity and locomotion in invertebrates and lower vertebrates. Following a description of the basic forms of locomotion from a phylogenetic perspective, chapter 2 examines a number of factors that can influence the expression and measurement of locomotor activity. Physical factors, such as environmental temperature and light, as well as biological factors, such as species, age, sex, health and social environment, and methodological and procedural factors, such as housing conditions and stress and anxiety levels induced by the testing procedure, are listed and discussed. Next, this chapter examines activity measurement methodology in selected invertebrates and lower vertebrates. These include direct observational methods, actographic procedures, such as activity wheels, fine trip wires, or displacement of small flexible rods, infrared photobeam activation and computer-automated video tracking systems. These techniques are described for the measurement of activity in such invertebrates as snails, small flies, crayfish, crabs and spiders. Similar discussion of activity measurement is provided for fish, frogs and tadpoles.

Chapter 3 deals with the measurement of locomotor activity in small mammals. Following a discussion of the historical interpretations of activity measures, an overview of various laboratory measurement techniques is provided. Direct observation of locomotor activity in an open-field apparatus is described and the variables quantified are defined. Descriptions of the apparatus and testing procedures are given and discussed. Next, a variety of automated procedures are reviewed, including stabilimeters, running wheels, and automated open-field systems using photobeam activation and video tracking. The measurement issues of reliability and validity are discussed for open-field variables and the principle of aggregation is discussed in the context of reliability. A number of studies on the effects of variable aggregation on the reliability of locomotor activity variables are described and it is suggested that score aggregation is a very useful procedure to improve reliability. The major emphasis of this chapter is on automated procedures which provide multivariate approaches to quantifying locomotor activity. By trying to capture the complexity of this behavior with the measurement of multiple variables, the richness of the phenomenon is preserved, both at a descriptive and quantitative level. These principles are then featured in some examples of research with an automated open-field activity monitoring system.

Chapters 4 and 5 deal with the measurement of activity levels in primates. Chapter 4 discusses the various methodologies available to measure activity levels in nonhuman primates. These range from direct observation procedures, typically used in field research (and some laboratory work) on social behavior, to automated procedures used in pharmacological and behavioral toxicological studies, and the analysis of gait patterns in comparative studies. This chapter discusses the type of equipment used, such as apparatus based on photocell activation or microswitch (attached to perches) activation, or kinematic analysis from video records. Various forms of observational scoring are also described, including bout sampling, continuous sampling and subjective rating systems. Chapter 5 describes in detail a methodology used to measure activity levels in humans by means of actometers. Following a brief historical overview of activity measurement in humans, this chapter describes an actometer made from a modified wrist watch. This technique is objective, technologically simple, yet easily used in both field and laboratory settings. This apparatus allows for recording over prolonged time periods and has been used in infants, preschoolers, school-aged children, adolescents and adults. Details on the use, collection and scoring of data, as well as interpretation of the results, are provided. Validity and reliability checks of the apparatus are described and the data presented.

Part II, on measuring other types of movement, contains chapters that provide a sharper focus on the more dynamic aspects of basic movement patterns, from both an organizational and developmental perspective. Chapter 6 examines behavioral pattern formation expressed across various levels of organization. The methodological approach in this chapter is to isolate individual action properties of movement and determine how these are combined in space and time. Of special interest are the dynamic systems, properties of movement and development and the fluid and fine-grained examination of movement characteristics. Grooming behavior is used to illustrate the features of sequential and hierarchical rules of organization. Of special interest in this chapter is the discussion of Golani's[14] application of movement choreography, a system of movement notation analysis developed from the Eshkol-Wachmann movement notation system (EWMNS).[15] This system uses a polar coordinate framework to describe posture, limb segment kinematics and constellations of movement across limb segments in time. This methodology is then used to describe ontogeny of movement in such behaviors as swimming and grooming. A particular example of how this approach can be used to study genetic influences on the development of movement is provided using the mutant weaver mouse.

The next chapter also emphasizes organization and development. The righting reflex, a behavior fundamental to the performance of standing and locomotion, is shown to be composed of a cluster of relatively independent sensorimotor patterns. These patterns are then combined to produce a flexible, adaptive response. The EWMNS is used to isolate the modular components of righting and to show that these are selected and then organized into suitable responses. This conceptual approach has implications for our understanding of righting behavior in such motor disorders as Parkinson's disease. It also has implications for the study of righting deficits following either exposures to putative neurotoxins or other types of damage to the central nervous system. It is suggested that each type of righting program needs to be examined in order to understand the neural damage contributing to the observed deficits.

Reaching in the rat is presented in chapter 8 as an example of a skilled movement which can be used to assess the effects of brain damage that may spare coordinated limb movement used for walking, grooming and other basic complex behaviors, but may affect the learned behavior. The methodology consists of video recording to capture a record of the behavior, followed by slow-motion analysis. This technique examines limb transport and withdrawal, as well as hand and digit movements. Following a discussion of the skeletal, muscular and sensory basis of reaching, this behavior is then examined both in the capturing and eating of an insect prey and in a skilled reaching task developed for use in the laboratory. The EWMNS is used in this analysis as well, and the asymmetries in limb use, end point measures, and kinematics of reaching are described and discussed. This technique is presented as a methodology that can examine the neural control of reaching along with examination of loss, recovery and restoration of function following brain damage. Throughout this chapter the authors emphasize the utility of multiple measures to capture the "richness of movement."

The next two chapters focus on the kinematics of different forms of locomotion. Chapter 9 uses kinematic analysis to examine swimming in semiaquatic and terrestrial mammals. The study of swimming is promoted as ideal for examination of motor response and development because it requires coordinated trunk and limb movements that are mechanically less stressful than other types of locomotion. Details are presented in the use of various types of swim and flow tanks to allow video recording of the behavior. Then the various kinematic variables are described and defined. A two-dimensional approach to quantification is used since the paddling stroke is confined to the vertical plane. Kinematic analysis of equine locomotion is presented in the last chapter of Part II. Following a short historical discussion of the use of kinematic analysis in studying equine locomotion, the qualitative and quantitative aspects of gait analysis are examined. It is noted that each type of analysis has both advantages and disadvantages. The high speed, computer-assisted kinematic analysis system, described in this chapter, produces 3-dimensional coordinates for markers located at strategic points on the surface of the limbs. With the aid of a rigid and portable scanner, which serves as a frame of reference, kinematic data for stride variables can be readily derived by tracking markers applied to the skin covering palpable skeletal landmarks. Both the derivation and the presentation of kinematic data are discussed. Data from studies using treadmills, force transduction plates, and electromyography are presented and discussed. Of special interest are the measurement and analysis of strain forces, both of bones and of tendons. These are important in any attempt to produce models of the equine locomotor system as well as in clinical investigation and interpretation.

The last section of the book, on experimental design and data analysis, deals with some specialized designs and statistical approaches used in the interpretation of the data obtained in studies of locomotion and movement. Chapter 11 presents a discussion of the utility of single subject designs in the study of motor activity levels. The rationale and relative advantages of single subject, as opposed to group designs, are presented. In these designs, long-term measurements of activity levels in a subject are then contrasted with the short term effects of some experimental manipulation, such as a drug injection. This approach emphasizes the reduction of response variability by the use of repeated measures in a single subject. Some experimental data, from a study of the effects of three standard drugs on motor activity levels, are presented and analyzed. It is demonstrated that this approach seems to work as well for studying unconditioned motor activity levels as it does in the study of operantly conditioned behavior.

The next chapter addresses the reliability of motor activity assessment by examination of within laboratory sources of variability and between laboratory variability. Reliability is discussed in terms of reproducibility of data over time and the control of within experiment variability. Important organismic and procedural variables, that can influence motor activity, are listed and discussed. Both intra- and inter-laboratory reliability is examined for control group motor activity measures and found to be fairly reliable. Other measures related to motor activity, such as habituation rates and the effective doses of various drugs (ED50), are also shown to be reliable across laboratories.

Chapter 13 provides a masterful examination of the utility of multivariate analyses in the measurement of motor activity. Theoretical issues, such as the influence of response competition, and the distinction between activation of locomotor activity versus exploration, are discussed and methodological approaches suggested to deal with these issues. An in-depth description of an automated apparatus, designed to measure both activity and exploration concurrently, is given and the application of this approach to the study of drug effects on activity is illustrated. The utility of examining the patterns of locomotion in animals as they explore the test chamber, both in terms of spatial and perseverative patterns, is elaborated. A measure of spatial behavioral sequence changes (Spatial Coefficient of Variation), defined by transitions between five areas in the test chamber, is presented and applications of this measure in drug studies on motor activity are provided.

The last chapter of Part III focuses on the assessment of the organization of locomotor activity by examination of the sequential aspects of this behavior, an approach not commonly found in the current literature. This chapter uses simple and extended scaling measures to extract information about the average spatial, temporal, or sequential organization of movements in activity analysis. These approaches, borrowed from nonlinear dynamics, the physics of complex systems, and the ergotic theory of dynamical systems, provide a framework for a quantitative analysis of locomotor organization. The behavioral state is described quantitatively by measures which are analogous to thermodynamic potentials. Thus, the behavior of an organism is treated as a complex system of interacting elements and the quantitative analysis of behavioral organization rests on the assessment of the interdependencies among the behavioral elements. The complexity of behavior is quantified with a measure analogous to the concept of entropy in thermodynamics. This chapter also deals with the development of scaling measures, describing both the geometric structure of movement patterns and the temporal durations of behavioral elements, to characterize the hierarchical aspects of behavioral organization. All of these concepts are illustrated with examples from studies on the effects of various drugs on locomotor activity.

Measuring Movement and Locomotion focuses on methodology and data analysis in the study of motor activity from a broad perspective. It is not intended to provide an exhaustive review of the various topics, but to present enough information on methodology and design to help investigators make appropriate choices. Another aim of this volume is to stimulate further interest in the questions and procedures related to the measurement of locomotor activity and its application in understanding behavior in health and disease. To the extent that this volume contributes to the study of brain-behavior relationships, we will have achieved our purpose.

ACKNOWLEDGMENTS

We would like to acknowledge support from the Natural Sciences and Engineering Research Council of Canada (KPO and MK), as well as partial support from the Smokeless Tobacco Research Council and the National Institute of Neurological Disease and Stroke (PRS), in the preparation of this volume. We also thank the many graduate students, postdoctoral fellows, and colleagues who have participated in research and discussions from which this volume has benefited.

REFERENCES

1. Kolb B, Whishaw IQ. Problems and principles underlying interspecies comparisons. In: Robinson TE, ed. Behavioral Approaches to Brain Research. New York:Oxford University Press, 1983:237-263.
2. Hutt SJ, Hutt C. Direct Observation and Measurement of Behavior. Springfield, IL:Thomas Pub, 1970.
3. Hutt SJ, Hutt C. Why measure behavior? In: Robinson TE, ed. Behavioral Approaches to Brain Research. New York:Oxford University Press, 1983:14-26.
4. Martin P, Bateson P. Measuring behaviour: an introductory guide. 2nd ed. Cambridge:Cambridge University Press, 1993.
5. Schwarting RKW, Fornaguera J, Huston JP. Automated video-image analysis of behavioral asymmetries. In: Sanberg PR, Ossenkopp K-P, Kavaliers M, eds. Motor Activity and Movement Disorders:Research Issues and Applications Totowa NJ:Humana Press, 1996:141-174.
6. Sanberg PR, ed. Locomotor Behavior:New Approaches in Animal Research. Proceedings of a Satellite Symposium to the 14th Annual Meeting of the Society for Neuroscience. Neurobehav Toxicol Teratol 1985; 7:70-100.
7. Sanberg PR, ed. Locomotor Behavior: Neuropharmacological Substrates of Motor Activation. Proceedings of a Satellite Symposium to the 15th Annual Meeting of the Society for Neuroscience. Pharmacol Biochem Behav 1986; 25:229-300.
8. Robbins TW. A critique of the methods available for the measurement of spontaneous motor activity. In: Iversen L, Iversen S, Snyder S., eds. Handbook of Psychopharmacology, Vol 7. Principles of Behavioral Pharmacology. New York:Plenum Press, 1977:37-82.
9. Ossenkopp K-P, Mazmanian DS. The measurement and integration of behavioral variables:Aggregation and complexity as important issues. Neurobehav Toxicol Teratol 1985; 7:95-100.

10. Sanberg PR, Henault MA, Hagenmeyer-Houser SH et al. The topography of amphetamine and scopolamine-induced hyperactivity:Toward an activity print. Behav Neurosci 1987; 101:131-133.
11. Frey DF, Pimentel RA. Principal component analysis and factor analysis. In: Colgan PW, ed. Quantitative Ethology. New York:John Wiley & Sons, 1978:219-245.
12. Sanberg PR, Ossenkopp K-P, Kavaliers M, eds. Motor Activity and Movement Disorders:Research Issues and Applications. Totowa NJ:Humana Press, 1996.
13. Robinson TE, ed. Behavioral Approaches to Brain Research. New York:Oxford University Press, 1983.
14. Golani I. A mobility gradient in the organization of vertebrate movement: the perception of movement through symbolic language. Behav Brain Sci 1992; 15:249-308.
15. Eshkol N, Wachmann A. Movement Notation. London:Weidenfeld & Nicholson, 1958.

PART I

Measuring Activity Levels

CHAPTER 2

Measuring Activity in Invertebrates and Lower Vertebrates

Martin Kavaliers and T. S. Perrot-Sinal

INTRODUCTION

Locomotion is a fundamental property of animals. The ability to move from one location to another is an important feature in the life and behavior of all but a few sessile animals. Almost all animals travel locally to obtain necessary resources and avoid adverse conditions. The mode of locomotion of an animal is, however, constrained by its biological and physical environment, size, architecture or morphology, and phylogenetic history.

Through phylogeny, from single-celled stages to multicellularity and bilaterality, body size tends to dramatically increase. This increase in body size, coupled with directed movement, is accompanied by the evolution of a variety of support structures and associated locomotor mechanisms. This has resulted in several basic locomotor patterns in animals: ameboid movement, ciliary and flagellar movement, hydrostatic propulsion, lateral and vertical trunk movements and appendage limb movements.[1-5] In association, there are three fundamental kinds of architectural support systems: structural endoskeletons, structural exoskeletons and hydrostatic endoskeletons.

Each animal utilizes the mode of locomotion best suited to its basic architecture, physical and biological environment and neurobiology. A simple list of different types of locomotion includes:

1. Movement of pseudopods, cilia, or flagella in protozoans
2. Pumping actions and other jet-propulsive techniques used by cnidarians, scallops and cephalopods

Measuring Movement and Locomotion: From Invertebrates to Humans, edited by Klaus-Peter Ossenkopp, Martin Kavaliers and Paul R. Sanberg.

3. Paddling, flipper and rowing motions for swimming
4. Undulatory movements such as swimming by fish and leeches or the terrestrial movements of animals such as snakes
5. Tunneling, burrowing, digging, peristalsis-like motions, and other underground movements evident in many worms, amphibians, reptiles and some mammals
6. Gliding, friction, and extension type of movements shown by flatworms, gastropods, earthworms and snakes
7. Crawling as evident in insect larvae
8. Walking
9. Galloping used by crocodilians
10. Jumping
11. Running, trotting, pacing and cantering
12. Climbing and related movements in trees and on other vertical surfaces
13. Various kinds of flight and gliding.

Locomotion reflects a variety of processes and is inherent in many behavioral patterns such as exploration, migration, territoriality, reproduction, foraging and predator avoidance. Thus, locomotor activity and its patterns potentially contain a range of information about the ecological, physiological, hormonal and neural state of an animal.

Many studies have described and quantified physical components of locomotion, including the anatomical basis of locomotion, biophysics of locomotion, locomotory neurophysiology and energetics.[3-8] Comparative studies of locomotion have attempted to relate morphological and ecological variables to differences in locomotor performance. Studies of natural locomotor behavior have examined foraging behavior, home range sizes, migration distances and activity patterns. The field methods typically used to measure locomotory behavior have ranged from estimates of distances by eye and using a stopwatch to record elapsed time to sophisticated telemetry techniques. The quantitative analysis of locomotory activity in the laboratory as an integrated whole is, however, relatively new, coming into fruition with the advent of the computer and automated video systems. This chapter outlines a number of automated methods available for the quantitative measurement and analysis of the locomotor activity of selected invertebrates and lower (i.e. ectothermic) vertebrates. This is preceded by a general consideration of the problems and limitations associated with the measurement and interpretation of movement and locomotor activity in the laboratory.

FACTORS AFFECTING THE EXPRESSION AND MEASUREMENT OF LOCOMOTOR ACTIVITY

Behavior, viewed as coordinated movement, is the major output of an animal's nervous system. Each species' behavior, including movement and locomotory patterns, and nervous system have evolved in the context of its natural habitat. Thus, one cannot achieve a proper understanding of either the nervous system or locomotor behavior without addressing the inter-relationship of these two against the background of the species' natural habitat. This encompasses a suite of physical and biological environmental factors, some of which are briefly addressed here.

Physical Factors

Various physical factors that can affect activity are listed in Table 2.1. Clearly, to deal with the influences of each of these factors on behavioral activity in detail is not possible here. Rather, a brief consideration of several of the more prominent of these factors is provided. Detailed characteristics of environmental physics and chemistry are available in various biophysical ecology texts (e.g. refs. 9, 10).

Invertebrates and lower vertebrates are ectothermic (poikilothermic), with their activity markedly affected by environmental temperature. The energy status of aquatic organisms is strongly coupled to the ambient temperature of their environment by means of the thermal conductivity of the water. Terrestrial organisms are more loosely coupled by conduction and convection because of the very poor thermal conductance of the air. However, all ectotherms must acquire and assimilate resources, obtain mates and avoid predation while simultaneously regulating body temperature so as to maintain appropriate levels of physiological performance for each of these activities.[11] Ectotherms can control body temperature by behavioral selection of appropriate activity times and thermal microclimates, bodily posturing and orientation, core-shell heat conductance changes, and evaporative cooling. Decreased short-term physiological performance can arise from excessively high or low body temperature. This translates into a direct effect of ambient temperature on the levels and patterns of activity in both the field and the laboratory. This effect of temperature on activity indicates the need to consider the interactions between locomotory and thermoregulatory behaviors. It raises the possibility that apparent alterations in locomotor activity may arise from, or be secondary to, thermoregulatory responses.

Table 2.1. Environmental factors affecting locomotor activity

Temperature
Light
Humidity
Soil and Terrestrial Surface Conditions
Water Conditions
Air and Atmospheric Conditions
Sound
Gravity
Magnetic and Electric Fields

in suites of traits such as sensory responses, behavior and physiology evolving in concert, thus producing populations and, eventually, species that differ in multiple characteristic ways. Initially, this may involve adaptation or acclimatization to specific environmental conditions.

Traditionally, adaptation is thought of as genetic changes in a population occurring in response to either natural or artificial selection. However, adaptation also refers to changes that occur within an individual in response to changes in the environment, and that helps the organism function better under those changed conditions. Nongenetic changes in physiology occurring during the lifetime of an organism are termed acclimation or acclimatization. Acclimation refers to changes that occur in response to changes in any component of the environment in the wild. Acclimatization refers to the same, but takes place in the laboratory. Changes as a result of acclimation or acclimatization are generally reversible and may be considered as examples of phenotypic plasticity.[15,16]

The age of an individual, along with its developmental stage or form and the habitat utilized, can affect the nature and type of locomotor activity displayed. For example, there are marked differences in the movement and locomotor patterns displayed by larval and adult forms of insects.[18] Adults can also vary in their activity patterns. In many species of animals, adults display both sex and reproductive status related activity behavioral differences. Sex differences in locomotor activity have been reported in reproductive adults of a range of species of vertebrates and invertebrates, with females generally displaying lower levels of activity than males.[19] In vertebrates attempts have been made to relate these sex differences to mating systems and reproductive patterns.

Intra- and interspecific interactions also influence activity levels and patterns. Competitive, agonistic, aggressive, social and sexual interactions can markedly affect the extent and nature of activity displayed.[20-22] In group living animals the activity of a solitary individual may be substantially different from that of the group (e.g. shoaling fish[23]). In addition, interspecific interactions and competition can result in shifts in activity levels and their temporal patterning.[24]

Various aspects of behavior are also affected by predation and resource availability. For example, predators often have strong impacts on prey activity rates, which can influence feeding and growth rates, competitive ability and related behaviors. In the presence of predators, prey individuals might increase, decrease or not alter their movement rates and patterns.[22] In turn, the presence of prey and food items can significantly influence the activity of the foraging individuals. The behavior and activity levels of both predators and prey are also related to hunger levels and nutritional status. For example, in fish hunger levels can affect the activity levels and times spent feeding in the vicinity of a potential predator.[20]

Another factor shaping behavior in much the same manner as predation and resource availability are external and internal parasites and parasitoids. Parasites can alter the behavior of infected hosts in a variety of ways.[25-27] Some altered behaviors, such as those that facilitate transmission of the parasite from one host to another, have a dramatic fitness cost to the host. More often, the alteration in host behavior is more subtle, a sequela to parasite-induced changes is host physiology and neurobiology.[28] Changes in host activity are among the more evident behavioral alterations. In some cases activity is reduced, in others, increased, while in other situations activity patterns are modified to facilitate parasite transmission.[25-27] Alterations in activity can also be associated with either avoidance, repulsion or removal of parasites.[29]

The effects of parasites are related to the overall health and immune status of the individual. Disease and poor health can significantly influence the activity levels and patterns of an individual. Various components of the immune system can also influence behavior and activity, there being substantial evidence for a bidirectional communication between the nervous and immune systems.[30] Stress (e.g. confinement, dominance relationships, etc.), infection and disease related modifications of immune activity could, thus, potentially impact on locomotory activity levels and patterns.

Animals also display temporal adaptations and responses to their environments. Many organisms display distinct rhythms (e.g. diurnal, nocturnal, crepuscular activity patterns) in their locomotor activity and related behaviors. These responses are not merely exogenous reactions to the environment but in most cases involve biological timers capable of correction to local time.[31,32] In terms of adaptive responses of animals to time-oriented signals, four major periodicities of animal rhythms are known: daily, tidal, semi-lunar and annual. For each of these periodicities a biological pacemaker has been demonstrated or is strongly suspected. There are also ultradian (e.g. 0.5-4.0 h) cycles in many physiological and behavioral functions, with their exact origins remaining to be defined.[33]

Methodological and Procedural Variables

This section draws attention to the importance of the methodological and procedural factors used when measuring locomotor activity (Table 2.3). The majority of these factors are related to the biology of the animal being studied and their influences on activity (Table 2.2). This reinforces the need for ethological and ecological considerations in the design of studies examining and recording locomotor activity, as well as in the subsequent interpretation of activity data.

The experimental manipulations used and pretreatments of animals (including capture, prior conditions in captivity, transport, etc.) can impact on the behavioral repertoires and activity levels displayed in the laboratory. The stress and "anxiety" associated with confinement and the novel laboratory situation (including cage/housing cleaning and human contact) may substantially limit or modify activity (e.g. induction of stereotypic behaviors). These behavioral effects may, in part, be related to the type of housing used and modifications in: (i) the physical environment (e.g. temperature, relative humidity, air and water exchange and quality, noise and vibration, olfactory cues including pheromones, substrate and its texture, etc.), including the absence of appropriate natural microhabitats; (ii) the social environment, including the presence/absence of same or opposite sex conspecifics, population density (individual vs group housing), reproductive and early developmental conditions; and (iii) the nutritional environment, including modifications in diet, food availability and feeding schedules.[34,35]

Potential complications arising from acclimatization and other environmental effects can be dealt with by acclimating animals in the laboratory to standard conditions before measuring behavioral and physiological responses. However, not all environmental effects on physiological, morphological, or behavioral traits are reversible, particularly if they occur during early or critical periods of development.

Additional behavioral modifications can result from the recording procedures used and stress associated with accompanying changes in the laboratory environment. This can often involve marked changes in the space provided to the animals, the availability of cover and refuges and dramatic increases in light levels and changes in the social environment. In this regard, the length and timing of the activity recording sessions and their relations to the natural activity periods (e.g. diurnal, nocturnal, crepuscular) and laboratory feeding schedules are particularly important.[32]

MEASUREMENT OF LOCOMOTOR ACTIVITY

This section describes a number of techniques used for measuring locomotor activity in selected invertebrates and lower vertebrates.

Table 2.3. Methodological and procedural factors affecting locomotor activity

Experimental Manipulations (handling) and Pretreatments
Stress and Anxiety Levels and Responses
Housing Equipment (type, material, dimensions)
Prior Handling
Prior Stress (acquisition and delivery/transport)
Acclimation
Prior Experience with Apparatus
Environmental Conditions During Activity Measurements
Food and Water Intakes and Schedules
Time of Day and Endogenous Rhythms

Emphasis is placed on automated procedures that have been used with molluscs, arthropods and fishes.

Observational methods have been extensively used to observe mollusc activity.[36] Actographic procedures, such as activity wheels were among the first automated methods used to measure locomotion and activity rhythms in molluscs. For example, locomotion of individual pulmonate slugs, *Limax maximus*, caused rotations of small wheels that were recorded with an event recorder.[37,38] Activity of the nudibranch sea hare, *Aplysia californica*, was monitored using protruding rods or finer nylon lines attached to microswitches which were tripped when the animals moved.[39,40]

Time-lapse photographic and video techniques have also been used to record the rhythmic behaviors of various species of molluscs. These studies examined day-night, circadian, tidal and ultradian activity rhythms and their modulation by temperature, photoperiod, tidal cycles and season.[41-45] An ultrasonic technique was used to measure circadian and ultradian activity rhythms of the freshwater pulmonate gastropod, *Helisoma trivolis*.[46] This system detected small water displacements and alterations in standing wave ultrasound patterns created by the fine localized movements of individual animals.

Field studies have utilized telemetric procedures to record mollusc locomotor activity levels and their day-night patterns. This technique provided high resolution determinations of the positions, depth and jet respiratory pressures of the cephalopod, *Nautilus*.[47] These types of telemetric studies are not particularly amenable to the laboratory situation. They do, however, serve to validate laboratory findings in the field.

The majority of laboratory studies with molluscs have provided qualitative rather than quantitative measures of locomotor activity. Quantitative data are difficult to obtain using the techniques commonly employed in the assessment of mollusc activity. Various automated techniques have, however, been developed and utilized for the multivariate assessment of spontaneous locomotor activity. One system which is specifically designed to examine quantitative as well as qualitative aspects of spontaneous locomotor activity, is the Digiscan automated activity monitoring system.[48-51]

The Digiscan system is an automated open field capable of assessing a large number of activity measures simultaneously and is described in detail by Ossenkopp and Kavaliers in this volume. It consists of activity monitors that are provided with a grid of infrared beams connected to a microcomputer. During operation the patterns of beam interruptions are recorded and analyzed for a system-differentiated multivariate assessment of activity. A variety of activity variables either calculated directly or derived from the measured variables is available (e.g. total distance [horizontal or vertical] traveled; number of movements; average distance per movement; average speed; time per movement; etc.).

Along with providing detailed information on many aspects of behavior, the Digiscan system is also appropriate for studying behavioral activity over extended time periods. Although the Digiscan system has been primarily used to examine the activity patterns of rodents,[48-51] it is applicable to other species. Various measures of the spontaneous locomotor activity of the land snail, *Cepaea nemoralis*, that were obtained with the Digiscan system are shown in Figure 2.1. Multivariate studies of the activity of terrestrial snails and slugs with automated systems such as the Digiscan can contribute to a more accurate characterization of locomotor behavior patterns and the influences of various biological and physical factors.

A variety of procedures have been used to monitor the locomotor activity of arthropods. With relatively large species of insects, such as crickets or cockroaches, rhythmic locomotor activity has been measured using rocking or tilt actographs and running wheels.[52-54] With smaller insects, other devices such as phototransistors using infrared light, or intensifiers of flight noise have been used to measure activity rhythms.[52,55,56] Actographs have also been extensively used to record activity rhythms of marine and intertidal species. For example, the locomotor activity of the shore crab, *Carcinus maenas*, has been monitored with activity being recorded as interruptions of infrared beams.[57,58]

The activity of aquatic insect larvae has been quantified by means of an impedance conversion technique.[59] In this procedure fine electrodes carrying alternating current were placed in a tank with the insect larva and the surrounding water functioning as the dielectrium of a capacitor. Any movement of the larva leads to a change in the dielectrium and consequently to a change of the impedance of the capacitor, which is converted into signals registering activity. These techniques have been used to examine the impact of pollutants on the activity of various species of stream-dwelling insect larvae.[59,60] Similar capacitance techniques have also been used to measure the jump and escape responses of flies.[61] Telemetry procedures also incorporating electric potential changes have been employed with tethered and free flying insects. Using this procedure electrical signals generated by muscles of free flying locusts, *Schistocerca gregaria*, were transmitted providing a record of flight activity.[62]

Recently, a variety of video techniques have been used to measure and analyze the locomotor activity of insects and other invertebrates. Computer-automated video tracking systems have been used to measure the behavior of zooplankers such as the copepod, *Centropages hamatus*,[63] kinematics of crawling in small larval flies,[64] free flight behavior of small flies in vertical flight chambers,[65] the locomotor patterns and behavior of crayfish and ghost crabs,[66,67] and wolf spider locomotion.[68] In the latter study a detailed multivariate assessment of the spontaneous locomotor activity of wolf spiders revealed significant

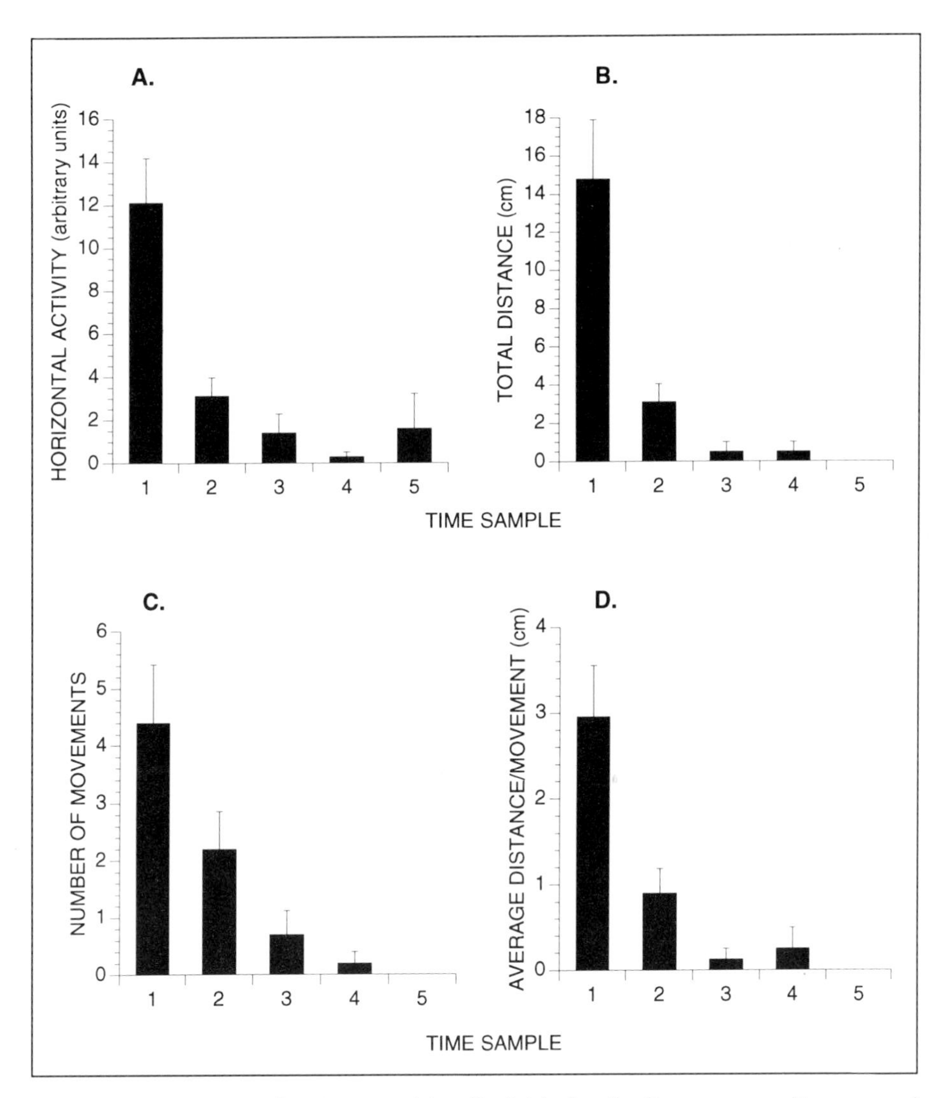

Fig. 2.1 A-D. Spontaneous locomotor activity of individual snails, Cepaea nemoralis, *measured with the Digiscan automated animal activity monitoring system. Snails were individually placed in sealed 40 x 40 cm clear Plexiglas boxes, maintained at a high relative humidity, that were provided with a grid infrared beams mounted horizontally every 2.5 cm. Two tiers of beams were mounted 2 and 13.5 cm above the floor. A barrier of toothpaste prevented the snails from reaching and crawling on the top cover of the chamber. The activity monitors were connected to a Digiscan Analyzer that transmitted the activity data to a microcomputer. The (A) total horizontal activity, (B) total distance moved, (C) number of movements made, and (D) average distance per movement of individual snails (n = 6) over 5 minute time intervals is shown.*

sex differences in locomotor activity, with adult male spiders displaying greater activity than adult females. Video-tracking systems have also been used to examine the orientation and locomotor responses of insects to pheromones,[69,70] as well as the responses of insect parasitoids to various host odors.[71,72]

Computer video-image analyzing systems have also been employed in the analysis of the activity of invertebrates such as protozoans,[73-75] rotifers[76] and insects.[77-80] Similar systems have also been used in studies of rodent and fish activity.[81-83] All of these systems permit the description of the locomotory parameters of the studied individual by computerized reconstitution and analysis of its trajectories. This allows a detailed assessment of a range of locomotor parameters of individual as well as groups of animals. Image analysis has been used to measure the spatial and temporal patterns of activity inside ant nests,[78,80] as well as the exploratory behavior of honey bees.[79] Video-image analysis was also was used to study behavioral circadian rhythms in insect parasitoids.[77] In this study both the automatic detection of the insect and the calculation of several activity variables (e.g., linear and angular speed, locomotor levels etc.) were carried out in real time, permitting long-term studies without any experimenter intervention. In this system the camera was sequentially displaced by robotics allowing the simultaneous study of many individuals.

A variety of actographic procedures have been used to measure the locomotor activity of fish and other lower vertebrates.[84-86] For example the activity of the eel, *Anguilla anguilla,* was measured using flexible metal rods dipping vertically into an aquarium. When these rods were displaced by a swimming fish, an electrical circuit was closed and activity registered.[87] In lizards and alligators activity rhythms have been measured using tilt actometers, with movements of the animals deflecting microswitches and registering movement.[88,89]

The activity of aquatic vertebrates has also been monitored using either single or multiple arrays of infrared photodetectors.[90-95] This technique is, however, subject to error caused by flexion of the body (e.g. tail beats of fish) of relatively stationary animals, or incomplete disruption of photobeams by the fish. This procedure also requires relatively clean water and is not appropriate to species living in turbid environments. Fish activity has also been recorded using ultrasonic beam interruptions.[96-99] Ultrasonic techniques have been used to examine circadian and ultradian locomotory activity rhythms, the effects of various feeding regimes, as well as various light and temperature conditions on the activity of a variety of species of fish. This technique is, however, limited to experimental situations with relatively gentle or slow water flows. Activity has also been recorded in systems monitoring voltage changes as a result of muscular activity, though again this is limited to relatively stationary water.[100] A magnetic activity-detection procedure has also been described. In this technique movements of magnetically tagged fish were recorded as fluctuations in the voltage output of sensor coils that were placed in the water.[101] This procedure is limited by the need to tag the fish, as well as the possible effects of the magnetic fields on the behavior of the fish.[14]

Video-tracking systems have also been used to record the activity of fish and other aquatic vertebrates such as bullfrog and green frog tadpoles.[102-107] This technique has been used to asses the preference and avoidance responses of fish such as the fathead minnow, *Pimephales promelas*, to discrete plumes of toxicants in a multiple choice test arena.[108] It has also been used to examine the development of swimming and activity rhythms in larval fish.[109,110]

Recently, computerized video-image analysis systems have been used to measure the spontaneous locomotor activity of fish. This technique has been used to examine the effects of anoxia on locomotor activity of crucian carp, *Carassius carassius*,[111] the relations between brain serotonergic activity and the spontaneous locomotor activity of dominant and subordinate arctic charr, *Salvenius alpinus*,[112] and the locomotor responses of male goldfish, *Carassius auratus*, to sex pheromones.[113] These video-image analysis techniques permitted a much more detailed and precise quantification of spontaneous locomotor activity than provided by earlier methods.

Acknowledgment

Preparation of this chapter was supported by a Natural Sciences and Engineering Research Council of Canada grant to M.K.

References

1. Alexander RM. Locomotion of Animals. Cambridge: Cambridge University Press, 1982.
2. Childress S. Mechanics of Swimming and Flying. Cambridge: Cambridge University Press, 1981.
3. Eilam D. Comparative morphology of locomotion in vertebrates. J Mot Behav 1995; 27:100-111.
4. Alexander RM. Optimization and gaits in the locomotion of vertebrates. Physiol Rev 1989; 69:1199-1227.
5. Schmidt-Nielsen K. Locomotion:Energy cost of swimming, flying and running. Science 1972; 177:418-419.
6. Adolph SC, Porter WR. Temperature, activity, and lizard life histories. Am Nat 1993; 142:273-295.
7. Camhi JM. Neural mechanisms of behavior. Curr Op Neurobiol 1993; 3:1011-1019.
8. Sibly RM, Calow DM eds. Physiological Ecology of Animals:An Evolutionary Approach. Oxford: Blackwell, 1986.
9. Dusenbery DB. Sensory Ecology. New York, W. H. Freeman Co, 1992.
10. Gates DM. Biophysical Ecology. New York: Springer Verlag, 1980.

11. Magnuson JJ, Crowder LB, Medvick PA. Temperature as an ecological resource. Am Zool 1979; 19:331-343.
12. Hailman JP. Optical Signals:Animal Communication and Light. Bloomington, Indiana: Indiana University Press, 1977.
13. Endler JA. On the measurement and classification of colour in studies of animal colour patterns. Biol Jour Linn Soc 1990; 41:315-352.
14. Kavaliers M, Ossenkopp KP. Effects of magnetic and electric fields in invertebrates and lower vertebrates. In: Carpenter DO, ed. Biological Effects of Electric and Magnetic Fields. Volume 1. San Diego: Academic Press, 1994:205-240.
15. Rollo CD. Phenotypes:Their Epigenetics, Ecology and Evolution. New York: Chapman and Hall, 1995.
16. Garland T Jr, Adolph SC. Physiological differentiation of vertebrate populations. Ann Rev Ecol Syst 1991; 22:193-228.
17. Kavaliers M. Opioid systems, behavioral thermoregulation and shell polymorphism in the land snail, *Cepaea nemoralis*. J Comp Physiol B 1992, 162:172-178.
18. Willmer PG. Microclimate and the environmental physiology of insects. Adv Insect Physiol 1982; 16:1-57.
19. Gaulin SJC, Fitzgerald RW. Sex differences in spatial ability:an evolutionary hypotheis and test. Am Nat 1986; 127:74-88.
20. Milinski M, Parker JA. Competition for resources. In: Krebs JR, Davies NB, eds. Behavioural Ecology:an Evolutionary Approach. Boston: Blackwell Scientific, 1991:137-168.
21. Endler JA. Interactions between predators and prey. In: Krebs JR, Davies NB, eds. Behavioural Ecology:an Evolutionary Approach. Boston: Blackwell Scientific, 1991:169-202.
22. Lima SL, Dill LM. Behavioral decisions made under the risk of predation:a review and prospectus. Can J Zool 1990; 68:619-640.
23. Kavaliers M. Social groups and circadian activity of the killifish (*Fundulus heteroclitus*). Biol Bull 1980; 158:69-76.
24. Wooster D, Sih A. A review of the drift and activity responses of stream prey to predator presence. Oikos 1995; 73:3-8.
25. Holmes JC, Zohar S. Pathology and host behavior. In: Barnard CJ, Behnke JE, eds. Parasitism and Host Behaviour. London: Taylor and Francis, 1990:34-63.
26. Moore JN, Gotelli NJ. A phylogenetic perspective on the evolution of altered host behaviours:a critical look at the manipulation hypothesis. In: Barnard CJ, Behnke JE, eds. Parasitism and Host Behaviour. London: Taylor and Francis, 1990:193-223.
27. Moore J. Parasites and the behavior of biting flies. J Parasitol 1993; 79:1-16.
28. Thompson SN, Kavaliers M. Physiological bases for parasite-induced alterations of host behaviour. Parasitology 1994; 109:S119-S138.
29. Hart BL. Behavioural defense against parasites:interaction with parasite invasiveness. Parasitology 1994; 109:S139-S151.

30. Carr DJJ, Blalock JE. Neuropeptide hormones and receptors common to the immune and neuroendocrine systems:Bidirectional pathways of intersystem communication. In: Ader R, Cohen N, Feltens, eds. Psychoneuroimmunology. 2nd Ed. New York: Academic Press, 1991:573-588.
31. Moore-Ede MC, Sulzman FM, Fuller CA. The Clocks that Time Us. Cambridge MA: Harvard University Press, 1982.
32. Mistelberger RE. Circadian pitfalls in experimental designs employing food restriction. Psychobiology 1990; 18:23-29.
33. Lloyd D, Stupfel M. The occurrence and functions of ultradian rhythms. Biol Rev 1991; 66:275-299.
34. Claassen V. Neglected Factors in Pharmacology and Neuroscience Research, Techniques in the Behavioral and Neural Sciences. Vol 12. New York: Elsevier, 1994
35. Clough G. Environmental effects on animals used in biomedical research. Biol Rev 1982; 57:487-523.
36. South A. Terrestrial Slugs:Biology, Ecology and Control. New York: Chapman and Hall, 1992.
37. Sokolove PG, Beiswanger CM. Prior DJ et al. A circadian rhythm in the locomotor behavior of the giant garden slug, *Limax maximus*. J Exp Biol 1977; 66:47-64.
38. Hess SD, Prior DJ. Locomotor activity of the terrestrial slug, *Limax maximus*:response to progressive dehydration. J Exp Biol 1985; 116:323-330.
39. Lickey MJ, Wozniak J, Block G et al The consequences of eye removal for the circadian rhythm of behavioral activity in *Aplysia*. J Comp Physiol 1977; 118:121-143.
40. Jacklet J. Neural organization and cellular mechanisms of circadian pacemakers. Int Rev Cytol 1984; 89:251-294.
41. Beeston DC, Morgan E. A crepuscular rhythm of locomotor activity in the freshwater prosobranch, *Melanoides tuberculata*. Anim Behav 1979; 27:284-291.
42. Bailey, SER. Circannual and circadian rhythms in the snail *Helix aspersa* and the photoperiodic control of annual activity and reproduction. J Comp Physiol A 1981; 142:89-94.
43. Ford DJG, Cook A. The effects of temperature and light on the circadian activity of the pulmonate slug, *Limax pseudoflavus*. Anim Behav 1987; 35:1754-1765.
44. Ford DJG, Cook A. The modulation of rhythmic behaviour in the pulmonate slug *Limax pseudoflavus* by season and photoperiod. J Zool Lond 1994; 232:419-434.
45. Blanc A. Ultradian and circadian rhythmicity of behavioral activities in the young snail *Helix aspersa maxima* (Gastropoda, Helicidae). Can J Zool 1993; 71:1506-1510.
46. Kavaliers M. Circadian and ultradian activity rhythms of a freshwater gastropod, *Helisoma trivolis*:the effects of social factors and eye removal. Behav Neural Biol 1981; 32:350-363.

47. O'Dor RK, Forsythe J, Webber DM et al. Activity level of *Nautilus* in the wild. Nature 1993; 362:626-628.
48. Sanberg PR, Hagenmeyer SH, Henault MA. Automated measurement of multivariate locomotor behavior in rodents. Neurobehav Toxicol Teratol 1985; 7:87-94.
49. Ossenkopp K-P, MacRae LK, Teskey GC. Automated multivariate measurement of spontaneous activity in mice:Time course and reliabilities of the behavioral measures. Pharmacol Biochem Behav 1987; 27:565-568.
50. Mead LA, Hargreaves EL, Galea LAM. Sex differences in rodent spontaneous activity levels. In: Sanberg PR, Ossenkopp K-P, Kavaliers M, eds. New Jersey: Humana Press, 1996:111-139.
51. Mead LA, Hargreaves EL, Ossenkopp KP et al. A multivariate assessment of spontaneous locomotor activity in the mongolian gerbil (*Meriones unguiculatus*):Influences of age and sex. Physiol Behav 1995; 57:893-899.
52. Saunders DS. Insect Clocks. 2nd ed. Oxford: Permagon Press, 1982.
53. Nowosielski JW, Patton RL. Studies on circadian rhythms of the house cricket, *Gryllus domesticus* L. J Insect Physiol 1963; 9:401-410.
54. Page TL. Circadian organization in the cockroach:Effect of temperature cycles on locomotor activity. J Insect Physiol 1985; 31:235-242.
55. Page TL. Circadian rhythms of locomotor activity in cockroach nymphs:Free running and entrainment. J Biol Rhyth 1990; 4:273-289.
56. Kenny NAP, Saunders DS. Adult locomotor rhythmicity as "hands" of the maternal photoperiodic clock regulating larval diapause in the blowfly, *Calliphora vicina*. J Biol Rhythm 1990; 6:217-233.
57. Reid DG, Bolt SRL, Davies A et al. A combined tidal stimulator and actograph for marine animals. J Exp Mar Biol Ecol 1989; 125:137-144.
58. Reid DG, Naylor E. Entrainment of bimodal circatidal rhythms in the shore crab, *Carcinus maenas*. J Biol Rhyth 1990; 4:333-347.
59. Heinis F. Swain WR. Impedance conversion as a method of research for assessing behavioral responses of aquatic invertebrates. Hydrobiol Bull 1986; 19:183-192.
60. van der Zant PTJ, Heinis F, Kikkert A. Effects of narcotic industrial pollutants on behavior of midge larvae (*Chironomus riparius* (Meigen), Diptera):a quantitative structure-activity relationship. Aquat Toxicol 1994; 28:209-221.
61. Snowball MF, Holmqvist MH. An electronic device for monitoring escape behaviour in *Musca* and *Drosophila*. J Neurosci Methds 1994; 51:91-94.
62. Kutsch W, Schwarz G, Fischer H et al. Wireless transmission of muscle potentials during free flight of a locust. J Exp Biol 1993; 185:367-373.
63. Hwang J-S, Turner JT, Costello JH et al. A cinematographic comparison of behavior by the calanoid copepod *Centropages hamatus* Lilljeborg:tethered versus free-swimming animals. J Exp Mar Biol Ecol 1993; 167:277-288.
64. Berrigan D, Pepin DJ. How maggots move:Allometry and kinematics of crawling in larval diptera. J Insect Physiol 1995; 41:329-337.

65. Blackmer JL, Byrne DN. Flight behaviour of *Bemisia tabaci* in a vertical flight chamber:effect of time of day, sex, age and host quality. Physiol Entomol 1993; 18:223-232.
66. Weinstein RB. Locomotor behavior of nocturnal ghost crabs on the beach:focal animal sampling and instantaneous velocity from three-dimensional motion analysis. J Exp Biol 1995; 198:989-999.
67. Jamon M, Clarac F. Locomotor patterns in freely moving crayfish (*Procambarus clarkiii*). J Exp Biol 1995; 198:683-700.
68. Baatrup E, Bayley M. Quantitative analysis of spider locomotion employing computer-automated video tracking. Physiol Behav 1993; 54:83-90.
69. Kaiser L, Pham-Delegue MH, Kerguelen V. Quantitative analysis of the foraging behavior of honeybees on oilseed rape genotypes. Ethol Ecol Evol 1992; 4:411-412.
70. Sheehan W, Wackers FL, Lewis WJ. Discrimination of previously searched, host-free sites by *Microplitis croceipes* (Hymenoptera:Braconidae). J Insect Behav. 1993; 6:323-331.
71. Noldus LPJJ, Lewis WJ, Tumlinson JH. Beneficial arthropod behavior mediated by airborne semiochemicals. IX. Differential responses of *Trichogramma pretiosum*, an egg parasitoid of *Helithois zea*, to various olfactory cues. J Chem Ecol 1990; 16:3531-3544.
72. Noldus LPJJ, van Lenteren JC, Lewis WJ. How *Trichogramma* parasitoids use moth sex pheromones as kairomones:orientation behaviour in a wind tunnel. Physiol Entomol. 1991; 16:313-327.
73. Gualtieri P, Colombetti G, Lenci F. Automatic analysis of the motion of microorganisms. J Microscop 1985; 139:57-62.
74. Hasegawa K, Tanakadate A, Ishikawa H. A method for tracking the locomotion of an isolated microorganism in real time. Physiol Behav 1988; 42:397-400.
75. Hader D-P, Vogel K. Simultaneous tracking of flagellates in real time by image analysis. J Math Biol 1991; 30:63-72.
76. Coulon PY, Charras JP, Chasse JL et al. An experimental system for the automatic tracking and analysis of rotifer swimming behavior. Hydrobiologia 1983; 104:197-202.
77. Allemand R, Pompanon F, Fleury F et al. Behavioural circadian rhythms in real-time by automatic image analysis:applications in parasitoid insects. Physiol. Entomol. 1994; 19:1-8.
78. Strickland TR, Franks NR. Computer image analysis provided new observations of ant behaviour patterns. Proc R Soc Lond B 1994; 257:279-286.
79. Bachine-Huber E, Marion-Poll F, Pham-Delegue MH et al. Real-time detection and analysis of the exploratory behavior of small animals. An application to the study of the olfactory behavior of honeybees in a four-choice device. Naturwissenschaften 1992; 79:39-42.
80. Cole BJ. Short-term activity cycles in ants:generation of periodicity by worker interaction. Amer Nat 1991; 137:244-259.

81. Spruijt BM, Holt T, Roussseau J. Approach, avoidance, and contact behavior of individually recognized animals automatically quantified with an imaging technique. Physiol Behav 1992; 51:747-752.
82. Bonatz AE, Steiner H, Huston JP. Video image analysis of behavior by microcomputer:categorization of turning and locomotion after 6-OHDA injection into the substantia nigra. J Neurosci Methd 1987; 22:13-26.
83. Schwarting RKW, Fornaguera, Houston JP. Automated video image analysis of behavioral asymmetries. In: Sandberg PR, Ossenkopp K-P, Kavaliers M, ed. Motor Activity and Movement Disorders:Research Issues and Applications. New Jersey: Humana Press, 1996:141-174.
84. Schwassmann HO. Biological rhythms. In: Hoar WS, Randall DJ, eds. Fish Physiology. Vol. 6. New York:Academic Press, 1971:371-428.
85. Spencer WP. An icthyometer. Science 1929; 70:557-558.
86. Underwood H. Endogenous rhythms. In: Gans C, ed. Biology of the Reptilia. Vol. 18. Physiology and Hormones, Brain and Behavior. Chicago: University of Chicago Press, 1992:229-297.
87. Genot G, Conan GY, Barthelemy L et al. Effects of 5-HT on spontaneous locomotor activity of eels. Comp Biochem Physiol 1984; 79C:189-192.
88. Underwood H. Circadian pacemaker in lizards:phase-response curves and effects of pinealectomy. Am J Physiol 1983; 244:R857-R867.
89. Kavaliers M, Ralph CL. Circadian organization of an animal lacking a pineal organ:the young American alligator (*Alligator mississippiensis*). J Comp Physiol 1980; 139:287-292.
90. Kleerkoper H. Olfaction in Fishes. Bloomington:Indiana University Press, 1969.
91. Chibia A, Kikuchi M, Aoki K. Entrainment of the circadian locomotor activity rhythm in the Japanese newt by melatonin injections. J Comp Physiol A 1995; 176:473-477.
92. Naruse M, Oishi T. Effects of light and food as zeitgebers on locomotor activity rhythms in the loach, *Misgurnus anguillicaudatus*. Zool Sci 1994; 11:113-119.
93. Kirkpatrick T, Schneider CW, Pavloski R. A computerized infrared monitor for following movement in aquatic animals. Behav Res Methd Instr Cmpt 1991; 23:16-22.
94. Tabata M, Minh-Nyo M, Oguri M. Involvement of retinal and extraretinal photoreceptors in the mediation of nocturnal locomotor activity rhythms in the catfish *Silurus asotus*. Exp Biol 1988; 47:219-225.
95. Morgan E, Cordiner A. Entrainment of a circa-tidal rhythm in the rock-pool benny *Lopophrys pholis* by simulated wave action. Anim Behav 1994; 47:663-669.
96. Kavaliers M, Ross DM. Twilight and day length affects the seasonality of entrainment and endogenous circadian rhythms in a fish, *Couesius plumbeus*. Can J Zool 1981; 59:1326-1334.
97. Spieler RE, Clougherty JJ. Free-running locomotor rhythms of feeding-entrained goldfish. Zool Sci 1989; 6:813-816.

98. Scherer E, Van der Veen B. A ultrasonic beam actograph for laboratory and field use. 1982; Can Tech Rep Fish Aquat Sci 1982; 1137:1-15.
99. Scherer E, Harrison SE. Exogenous control of diel locomotor activity in the whitefish *Coregonus clupeaformis*:effects of light and temperature. Oecologia 1988; 76:254-260.
100. Spoor WA, Neiheisel TW, Drummond RA. An electrode chamber for recording respiratory and other movements of free-swimming animals. Trans Am Fish Soc 1971; 100:22-28.
101. Krum HN, Sheehan RJ. Development of a magnetic activity-detection system. Anim Behav 1992; 43:688-690.
102. Scarfe AD, Steele CW, Rieke GK. Quantitative chemobehavior of fish:An improved methodology. Enviro Biol Fish 1985; 13:183-194.
103. Steele CW, Owens DW, Scarfe AD et al Behavioral assessment of the sublethal effects of aquatic pollutants. Mar Poll Bull 1985; 16:221-224.
104. Korver RM, Sprague JB. Zinc avoidance by fathead minnows (*Pimephales promelas*):computerized tracking and greater ecological relevance. Can J Fish Aquat Sci 1989; 46:494-502.
105. Boisclair D. Relationship between feeding and activity rates for actively foraging juvenile brook trout (*Salvenius fontinalis*). Can J Fish Aquat Sci 1992; 49:2566-2573.
106. Steele CW, Stricker-Shaw S, Taylor DH. Behavior of tadpoles of the bullfrog, *Rana catesbeiana*, in response to sublethal lead exposure. Aquat Toxicol 1989; 14:331-344.
107. Taylor DH, Steele CW, Stricker-Shaw, S. Responses of green frog (*Rana clamitans*) tadpoles to lead-polluted water. Enviro Toxicol Chem 1990; 9:87-93.
108. Farr AJ, Chabot CC, Taylor DH. Behavioral avoidance of fluoranthese by fathead minnows (*Pimephales promelas*). Neurotoxicol Teratl 1995; 17:265-271.
109. Massicotte B, Dodson JJ. Endogenous activity rhythms in tomcod (*Microgadus tomcod*) post-yolk sac larvae. Can J Zool 1991; 69:1010-1016.
110. Coughlin DJ, Strickler JR, Sanderson B. Swimming and search behaviour in the clownfish, *Amphipiron perideraion*, larvae. Anim Behav 1992; 44:427-440.
111. Nilsson GE, Rosen P, Johansson D. Anoxic depression of spontaneous locomotor activity in crucian carp quantified by a computerized imaging technique. J Exp Biol 1993; 180:153-162.
112. Winberg S, Nilsson GE, Sprujit BM et al. Spontaneous locomotor activity in arctic charr measured by a computerized imaging technique:role of brain serotonergic activity. J Exp Biol 1993; 179:213-232.
113. Bjerselius R, Olsen KH, Zheng W. Behavioural and physiological responses of mature male goldfish to the sex pheromone 17-,20-dihydroxy-4-pregnen-3-one in the water. J Exp Biol 1995; 198:747-754.

CHAPTER 3

Measuring Spontaneous Locomotor Activity in Small Mammals

Klaus-Peter Ossenkopp and Martin Kavaliers

INTRODUCTION

The measurement of locomotor activity is central to obtaining information about an animal's general behavior. Changes in locomotor activity have consequences for the measurement of all aspects of behavior, from spontaneous and species specific behavioral patterns to learned or conditioned behaviors. Measurement of locomotor activity, in both natural and laboratory settings, has ranged from simple direct observations to sophisticated automated procedures.

The measurement of locomotor activity is of importance for many areas of both basic animal and biomedical human directed research. The theoretical importance of measuring motor activity lies in the classic view that spontaneous activity represents a state of arousal[1] or "nonspecific excitability level"[2] in the animal. Despite the desire to use particular measures of motor activity as indices of arousal or general activity levels, the various measures of activity commonly used, such as those obtained in photocell cages, the open-field apparatus, stabilimeter cages, or running wheels, show low intercorrelations.[3,4] The failure to obtain moderately large and consistent correlations among these measures suggests that they cannot be used indiscriminately as indices of arousal or general activity since they assess different aspects of behavior. Another problem that has been recognized in this research area is that of reliability.[5,6] For example, of the many measures of motor activity obtained in the open-field test only two, ambulation and rearing responses, have been found to be reliable measures,[5,7] when the variables are not aggregated appropriately.[6]

Measuring Movement and Locomotion: From Invertebrates to Humans, edited by Klaus-Peter Ossenkopp, Martin Kavaliers and Paul R. Sanberg.

The present chapter will provide an overview of the different methods of laboratory measurement of locomotor activity in rodents. This chapter is not intended as an exhaustive review. A number of previous publications have reviewed various procedures used to measure motor activity in general psychobiological research[8,9] or in psychopharmacological investigations.[10-12] Rather, we will discuss the various procedures in general terms and focus on specific laboratory techniques which allow multivariate assessments of locomotor activity in rodents. Although the emphasis will be on methodology, we will also deal with the issues of reliability and validity of the measures, as well as the principle of aggregation and the issue of behavioral complexity. In this context, we will present some data from our laboratory that has been obtained both with the traditional open-field apparatus and with an automated technique of obtaining multivariate assessments of locomotor activity.

METHODS OF MEASURING LOCOMOTOR ACTIVITY

THE OPEN-FIELD TEST (DIRECT OBSERVATION)

Since its development by Hall[13,14] the open-field test has attained the status of one of the most widely used instruments in the laboratory analysis of animal behavior (see reviews in refs. 8 and 15). Typically, the open-field apparatus consists of a novel open space from which escape is prevented by either a surrounding wall or by elevation of the field above the floor. A subject, usually a small rodent, such as a rat, mouse, gerbil or vole, is placed in this apparatus for some fixed time interval. While in this open space the incidence (and if applicable, latency or duration) of certain behaviors is recorded. Although the number of activity variables quantified in the open-field test has increased substantially over time (see Table 3.1), the most common and reliable measures used are ambulation and rearing.[5] The key to the continuing popularity of the open-field test is the simplicity of the procedure, which requires only simple visual observation and the recording of data with paper and pencil.

Open-Field Apparatus and Test Procedure

The shape of the open-field apparatus can be circular, square, or rectangular. Circular open-fields[16,17] have been most popular because many rodents display thigmotaxis, i.e., the "prepared" fear reactions[18,19] of small animals consisting of avoidance of open areas and a strong tendency to stay near walls or protected areas to reduce exposure to predators. This thigmotactic behavior can increase the tendency of test subjects to stay in the corners of a square or rectangular open-field, since the presence of two walls (i.e., a corner) may afford greater protection. The circular open-field avoids this "corner" problem and allows for greater symmetry in the distribution of behaviors in the open-field space.

The size of the open-field apparatus can vary enormously.[8] The typical sizes used for mice, rats, gerbils and voles are about 0.5 to 1 m in diameter of a circular field, or length of a side in a square field. Materials used to construct the open-field apparatus can also vary widely. Wood, metal sheeting and plastic are most common, but alternatively, one can simply place a "wall" on a washable floor, or even use the floor of a small room as the open-field. Traditionally, the open field has been painted a neutral color, such as all black, grey, or white, with the floor usually marked off into equal sized subdivisions to aid in the scoring of ambulation and measures of location. Figure 3.1A shows a picture of a circular open-field apparatus and Figure 3.1B provides an example of the floor markings used in such an open field.

The test environment can strongly influence the results obtained in the open-field test. A number of the environmental factors (listed in chapter 2) have been examined in open-field testing situations.[8]

Table 3.1. Some common open-field (direct observation) measures of activity

A.	**Activity related variables**		
1.	*ambulation*	frequency	number of floor segments entered in a given time period
2.	*ambulation*	time	total time spent ambulating
3.	*ambulation*	latency	latency to leave the first floor segment
4.	*rearing*	frequency	number of times animal rears up on its hind legs and extends its body
5.	*rearing*	time	total time spent rearing
6.	*rearing*	latency	latency to first rearing response
7.	*immobility*	time	total time spent immobile
8.	*grooming*	frequency	number of grooming bouts
9.	*grooming*	time	total time spent grooming
10.	*grooming*	latency	latency to first grooming bout
11.	*jumps*	frequency	number of jumping responses
B.	**Activity distribution variables**		
12.	*center*	ambulation	number of nonmargin floor segments entered
13.	*center*	time	total time spent in the non-margin floor area
14.	*margin*	ambulation	number of margin (adjacent to wall) floor segments entered
15.	*margin*	time	total time spent in the margin (adjacent to wall) floor area
16.	*thigmotaxis*	ratio	margin ambulation (or time) divided by total [margin + center] ambulation (or time)

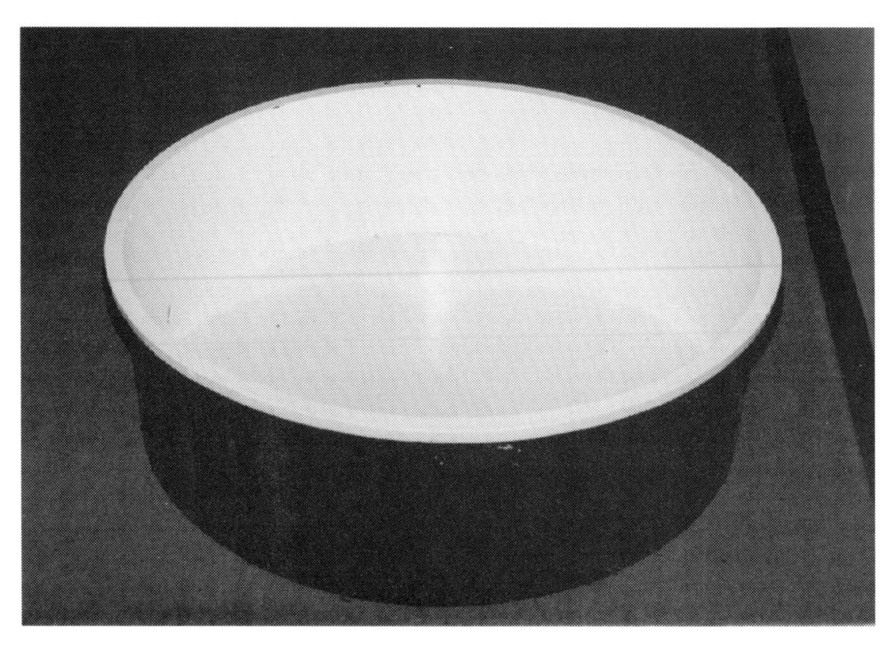

Fig. 3.1A. Photograph of a circular open field apparatus. This open field is 90 cm in diameter with 30 cm high walls.

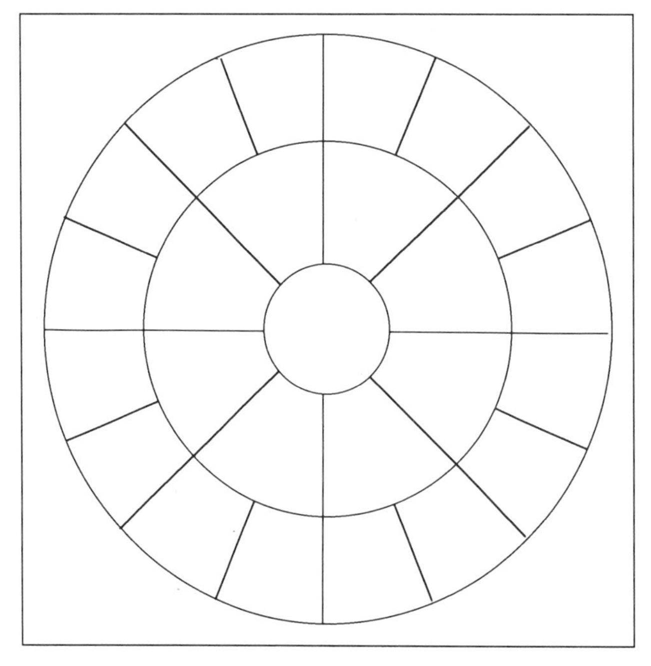

Fig. 3.1B. A diagram of the markings used to divide the floor of the circular open field into 25 equal area segments.

Lighting level and background noise level are two of the more important environmental features that have been examined. In general, high levels of illumination are associated with reduced levels of motor output and increased thigmotaxis.[20] Increasing the overall background noise level with the addition of "white noise" to mask any other unusual or sudden noises, can influence ambulation and other behaviors.[8] More importantly, the presence of the observer can have pronounced effects on the behavior of the test subject. The observer's presence may also introduce subtle bias, even though the subjects appear to be well habituated to the situation. Suarez and Gallup[21,22] have suggested, and provided supporting data, that open-field testing contains elements of both a predatory encounter (i.e., the presence of the experimenter) and of social separation from conspecifics. As such, open-field behaviors are interpreted as responses designed to either minimize detectability (predator evasion), or to reinstate contact with familiar conspecifics. Reducing the visibility of the experimenter, by placing a curtain around the open-field apparatus[23,24] and having the observer stand outside of this curtain, is a partial solution to this problem. A better solution involves the use of automated testing and appropriate habituation procedures. These can largely eliminate the influence of the observer. Individual housing of the test subjects may also be useful, since such animals are less likely to attempt to reinstate social contact with conspecifics. However, it should also be noted that isolation may induce behavioral modifications that can influence behavioral activity (see review in ref. 25).

A number of biological factors (see chapter 2) can also strongly influence the behaviors obtained in open-field testing. For example, genetic background,[25] age,[26,27] sex[28] and day-night differences in activity levels[29] have been observed in a variety of different studies. These factors can influence how subjects are affected by drugs[30,31] or to what degree they display abnormalities following brain lesions.[32]

The presence of conspecifics or predators, or their odors,[33] can also influence activity levels. Methodologically, it is important to avoid the presence of odors from conspecifics (unless these are of experimental interest). The test apparatus and the floor of the open-field apparatus should be rinsed with water or a weak vinegar solution after each subject has been tested.[23,24]

Automated Procedures

Stabilimeters

One method of recording the general activity of an animal housed in a cage is to measure the energy produced by the animal's movement which is transferred to the cage. The cage can be spring-suspended, or designed in such a fashion that movement of the cage can occur and be readily measured. A simple method of measuring the displacement of the floor of the cage is to attach a magnet to the bottom of the cage, with the magnet suspended inside a "fixed" coil. Movement of the magnet inside the coil produces an electrical current which can be displayed directly, or which can activate a voltage sensitive relay. Several commercially available activity monitoring systems use this approach (e.g., LaFayette animal activity monitor; see ref. 34). By altering the sensitivity of the voltage-sensitive relay, adjustments can be made for variations in body weight, size of movement to be detected, etc.

Other methods of transducing the movement of the cage into a quantifiable signal have been described. For example, the use of an inexpensive phonograph type crystal pick-up to sense the vibrations of a cage resting on a foam rubber cushion provides an inexpensive and simple way to detect movement of the animal in the cage.[35] This method allows measurement of movement in the home cage and does not require the animal to be placed in a special test chamber.

There are several drawbacks to this method of measuring activity. The data generated by these devices are relative values in arbitrary units. Furthermore, these devices do not discriminate between different types of movement, but rather determine the overall motoric output and provide a global measure of "general" motor activity. That is, walking, grooming, rearing, and other behaviors cannot be measured separately.

Running Wheels

Activity or running wheels are a means of allowing the animal to produce a great deal of locomotor behavior in a small restricted space. By having the animal run on a "runway" attached to the inside of a wheel that is rotating about a central axis, the animal can engage in vigorous locomotor behavior in a continuous fashion, and the device also allows for easy quantification of the behavior (see descriptions in refs. 36, 37). Almost all publications employing this device describe the apparatus which can be built in most workshops, or be obtained from a variety of commercial suppliers.

Running wheels have been especially popular in examining temporal changes in degree or pattern of locomotor behavior, either driven by the daily changes in the light-dark cycle or reflecting an innate pattern controlled by an endogenous biological "clock."[29] In these devices wheel revolutions are detected by a switch closure which can activate a counter or serve as input to a computer. With the appropriate computer software, wheel revolutions can be displayed continuously or aggregated over convenient, brief time periods and then graphically displayed over consecutive 24-hour time periods. These programs also calculate values for statistical variables which describe characteristics of the temporal changes in locomotor activity, such as the period (duration of a daily cycle) and variability of the period.[29] However, usually an adaptation period is required before stable levels of wheel running are obtained, and there are often large individual differences in levels of activity.

Interpretation of the wheel running measure has been problematic and Mather[38] has suggested that the usual interpretation of wheel running, as a measure of general activity or arousal, is incorrect. Rather, she has suggested that wheel running is a specific measure of "exploratory migration." Exploratory migration can be viewed as a measure analogous to that of migratory restlessness quantified in caged migratory birds (Zugunruhe[39]) and to reflect activity designed to gain information about resource location in the environment. However, since the running takes place in a wheel in the laboratory and a goal is not attainable, long "distances" are often covered under these conditions.

Telemetry Systems

Various biotelemetry systems have been developed to allow monitoring of freely moving small animals.[40,41] One commercially available and popular wireless telemetry system (Mini-Mitter Co., Sunriver, OR) monitors heart rate, core temperature, and gross locomotor activity in freely behaving rodents during various tasks.[42] The gross locomotor activity is derived from changes in the orientation of the implanted transmitter with respect to the receiver, arising from change in spatial location (movement) of the subject. The resulting change in signal strength is detected by the receiver and increments the activity count. The drawback to this approach is the inability of the system to differentiate various types of movement and locomotor behaviors.

The Automated Open-Field System (Photobeam)

In an effort to avoid some of the problems associated with direct visual observation of behavior in the open-field test[44] and simplify data processing and analysis, several automated "open-field" instruments have been designed and tested.[44-46] These instruments use arrays of infrared photobeams. Beam interruptions are processed by computer software to simultaneously reveal many aspects of the spontaneous activity of the test animal in the apparatus. The Digiscan Animal Activity Monitor (Omnitech Electronics, Inc., Columbus, OH) is one such automated computer-based system which we have used in our laboratory. Several other models are marketed by other companies (see Appendix B).

The Digiscan monitor consists of clear Plexiglas boxes (40 x 40 x 30.5 cm) with infrared monitoring beams (light sources and sensors) mounted every 2.54 cm along the perimeter (i.e., 16 beams along each side). This array of beams can be set at various distances from the floor of the box; heights are adjusted for the particular species of small mammal being tested. A second series of infrared photobeams are located above the bottom array, and these are used to detect vertical movements of the animal (such as rearing responses or jumps). The beam interruptions are analyzed by a Digiscan Analyzer (e.g., Omnitech Model DCM) which in turn transmits the data to a personal computer.

The Digiscan System permits the derivation of a large number of variables, based on the interpretation of the photobeam interruptions by the Digiscan Analyzer and computer software. Table 3.2 provides a list of these variables and their definitions. This system also allows for flexibility of data collection over time. Time bins, during which data are cumulated, can be preset over a large range (minutes, hours and days) and this allows the experimenter to choose the level of detail at which the activity variables are examined. The automated procedure also removes the observer from the experimental environment, thus, greatly reducing subtle biases that may be introduced by the observers presence. As well, automation removes such factors as fatigue, observation error, and extended time periods of tedious observation and data recording and analysis.[44] Finally, the attachment of multiple recording devices (monitoring boxes) to the same computer, allows for the simultaneous collection of data from many subjects by a single experimenter. This would of course not be possible with the direct observation procedure.

Automated Open Field System (Video-recording)

The automated analysis of video images generally relies on images obtained with a video camera positioned above the animal testing environment, such as an open field. The video image is then converted into digitized data which are transferred to a computer where the data are analyzed further with appropriate computer software.[47] Detection of the subject in the testing environment depends on the degree of contrast between the background and the test subject.[48] For example, an albino rat placed in a black open field or a black-hooded rat or dark brown vole tested in a white apparatus give the required degree of contrast.

Many of the same variables, as those obtained with the infrared photobeam automated open field monitors, can be obtained with this approach. The most common measures are distance travelled or time spent moving[49,50] and resting time[51] or immobility. Spatial distribution measures include central and peripheral activity or distance travelled[50,52] and these can be converted to a thigmotaxis ratio. With the addition of a second camera, providing a simultaneous horizontal view of the subject, additional behaviors, such as rearing, standing, sitting, lying and grooming, can be measured as well.[48,53,54]

An additional advantage with this type of monitoring system is the ability to analyze video images obtained in a wide variety of experimental situations. In the Morris water-maze the swimming behavior of a variety of small mammals can be quantified in terms of distance travelled and directional changes made.[55-57] Movement in other

Table 3.2. Variables that can be measured or computed in the Digiscan Animal Activity Monitoring System

1.	*Horizontal Activity:*	Total number of beam interruptions in the lower set of photobeams.
2.	*Total Distance:*	Distance travelled by the animal.
3.	*Number of Movements:*	This parameter is incremented by 1 each time the animal's ambulatory activity stops for more than 1 sec.
4.	*Movement Time:*	Total time that animal is ambulating.
5.	*Rest Time:*	Total time that animal is not ambulating.
6.	*Vertical Activity:*	Total number of beam interruptions in the upper set of photobeams.
7.	*Number of Vertical Movements:*	Each time the animal goes below the upper sensors for more than 1 sec and then breaks the upper sensors again, this parameter is incremented.
8.	*Vertical Time:*	Total time upper sensors are activated.
9.	*Average Speed:*	Total distance divided by total movement time.
10.	*Average Distance per Movement:*	Total distance divided by number of movements.
11.	*Average Time per Vertical Movement:*	Vertical time divided by number of vertical movements.
12.	*Clockwise Revolutions:*	Number of times the animal runs in a clockwise circle of at least 5.08 cm.
13.	*Anti-clockwise Revolutions:*	Number of anti-clockwise runs in a circle.
14.	*Margin Distance:*	Distance animal travels while within 6.35 cm from a wall of the box.
15.	*Margin Time:*	Time spent by the animal while within 6.35 cm from a wall of the box.
16.	*Center Distance:*	Distance travelled while in the center of the box (i.e., not in a margin).
17.	*Center Time:*	Time spent in the center of the box (i.e., not in a margin).
18.	*Corner Time:*	Time spent in two different margins (i.e., near two walls) simultaneously.
19.	*Number of Stereotypic Movements:*	Number of times the animal repeatedly breaks the same photobeam, with a break of 1 sec separating individual counts.
20.	*Stereotypy Time:*	Time spent in stereotypic movements.
21.	*Zone Times:*	Time spent in on any one of nine different zones within the test box.

types of dry and wet mazes (such as the radial-arm maze, T- or Y-maze, or more complex mazes) also can be analyzed in this manner. As well, social interaction measures can be obtained for several subjects monitored in the same test apparatus. By placing special markers on the dorsal surface of the animals, the system can "identify" each subject and provide analyses of relative position and frequency of behavioral interaction for two or more animals.[58]

Turning behavior and behavioral asymmetries also can be quantified with a modified video-image analysis system.[59] The Video-Image Analyzing System (VIAS) developed for this purpose can measure turning, discriminate between different diameters of turning, detect partial and full turns, and also measure the usual variables, such as distance travelled.[59-61] More recently a new measure called "thigmotactic scanning" has been added to this list of quantifiable variables. This measure is defined as locomotion along the wall of the experimental enclosure so that the vibrissae of one side can have contact with the wall.[59]

A number of commercially available automated video-image analysis systems are on the market. These include Videomex-V; SMART, The Observer, Etho Vision; Poly-Track, and Video Tracking Activity System (see Appendix B).

Other Automated Open-field Systems

Several other measurement approaches or variations on systems described above have been described in the literature. For example, some devices use capacitance-sensing plates to monitor the position of a subject. One such device requires the subject to be placed in a special chamber and the monitoring system is able to differentiate fine movements, gross movements and rearing responses.[62]

Another device uses photodetectors to monitor locomotion of rodents on a grid walking system and quantifies such measures as the number of footfalls, times and position of footfalls, and fore- or hind-limb footfalls, along with the usual measures of distance traversed and time taken for locomotion.[45] A validity check of this computerized system against a videotaped record of these behaviors provided high correlations. This automated system is designed to monitor fine locomotory deficits and appears to be very useful in quantifying neurological dysfunction.

A rather novel and inexpensive device requires subjects to wear a plastic collar which is then attached to a tether line. This system then monitors the behavior of the subjects in a open-field arena.[63] By attaching the tether line to a joy-stick connected to the appropriate port on a personal computer this monitoring system is able to record horizontal and vertical positions of the animal with a resolution of 1 cm. Appropriate software can differentiate gross locomotor activity and rearing, along with the structural characteristics of movement patterns (fractal dimension). The major drawback to this system would seem to be the requirement for tethering the subject. Not all rodents will readily allow themselves to be tethered, especially when a collar or similar mechanism is required.

MEASUREMENT ISSUES

Reliability and Validity of Variables

The two most important characteristics of the variables used to quantify locomotor activity or movement are their reliability and validity.[64] *Reliability* refers to the consistency with which the procedure produces a measurement of the variable of interest. *Validity* refers to the degree to which the procedure produces a measure that can be interpreted as being, or representing, the variable or construct that we are interested in measuring.

Of these two characteristics, reliability is the easier to determine. Typically, we test the same subjects, under experimental conditions that are as similar as possible, at two different points in time, and quantify the variable of interest. We then calculate a correlation coefficient between the two data sets. If the correlation is sufficiently large (for e.g., $r > .60$) then we are willing to suggest that the measurement procedure is reliable. The weaker the relationship between the scores obtained on two different occasions under similar conditions, the more likely we are to suspect that the scores are being influenced by chance factors, and thus, not very reliable. Table 3.3 provides some reliability estimates for ambulation and rearing responses from several different studies with rats tested in an open-field apparatus and measured by direct observation.

Reliability also can be discussed in terms of intra-observer, inter-observer or even inter-laboratory levels of reliability.[64] That is, to what degree is the observation or measurement consistent for the same observer, across observers in the same laboratory or across laboratories (see chapter 12). These features of reliability are perhaps most relevant to direct observation procedures. However, even with automated monitoring devices the issue of inter-laboratory reliability remains. Intra- and inter-observer reliabilities can be most easily assessed by having the same individual (at two different points in time), or two different individuals, measure behavior obtained from a particular video record and then calculate correlation coefficients for the variables recorded.

The issue of measurement validity is more difficult to deal with. Measurements made from visual observations (or videotaped recordings) are valid to the extent that there is agreement about the label used to describe a certain behavior. More problematic are the measures obtained from automated procedures, such as the Digiscan Monitoring System. These procedures use precisely defined algorithms to generate the values for the variables being measured. However, in all cases it is desirable to validate the automated measures against those based on visual observations of the behaviors being quantified. For example, the Digiscan Monitoring System quantifies Number of Vertical Movements (see Table 3.2), a measure of rearing behavior, by incrementing this measure each time the animal goes below the upper bank of photobeams for at least 1 sec and then activates this upper series of photobeams again. An observer watching the animal, and quantifying rearing behavior, may not use the same criteria as the one used by the computer program. Thus, a discrepancy between the automated procedure and visual monitoring can easily arise. To check the validity of the automated measurement procedure the behavior of

Table 3.3. Some reliability coefficients for open-field ambulation and rearing responses in rats (direct observation)

Variable	Reliability Coefficient	Comparison	Sample Size	Reference
Ambulation	0.57	Day 1:2	96	86
	0.66	Day 3:4		
	0.70		45	5
	0.58		43	
	0.77	Session 1	30	7
	0.89	Session 2		
	0.43	Mins	26	24
	0.62	Days		
	0.87	Days 1+3: 2+4		
	0.30	Day 1:2	80	106
	0.57	Day 3:4		
	0.51	Days 1+2: 3+4		
Rearing	0.62		45	5
	0.70		43	
	0.70	Session 1	30	7
	0.83	Session 2		
	0.60	Mins	26	24
	0.76	Days		
	0.92	Days 1+3: 2+4		
	0.39	Day 1:2	80	106
	0.52	Day 3:4		
	0.56	Days 1+2: 3+4		

the animal should be videotaped simultaneously and a correlation coefficient calculated between the automated measure and the visually obtained measure. This type of validation has been carried out for rearing,[65] stereotypic movements,[66] and thigmotactic behavior[67] in the Digiscan Monitoring System. Horizontal activity variables in the Digiscan have been validated against running wheel data.[68]

THE PRINCIPLE OF AGGREGATION

The "principle of aggregation" has received renewed interest in psychological measurement.[69-72] It is based on the notion that the sum of a set of multiple measurements is a more stable and unbiased estimator than any single measurement from the set. Since any measurement has an error component associated with it,[73] the combining of several measurements tends to average out these error components, providing a better estimate of the true value of the parameter in the population of interest. Perhaps the best known example of this principle is the common rule that the larger the sample size of a set of measurements, the more representative the sample mean is of the population mean.

In behavioral neuroscience research, as in psychological measurement, the principle of aggregation can be used to obtain better estimates of the true values of various behavioral, physiological, or neurochemical parameters. Few people would consider an experiment with one subject per experimental condition as adequate. Yet multiple sampling with regard to stimuli, occasions, or time, is much less common. Epstein[70] identified four forms of aggregation: aggregation over subjects, aggregation over time, aggregation over stimulus situations, and aggregation over modes of measurement.

Aggregation over subjects requires little comment since it is a type of aggregation that is commonly applied to behavioral neuroscience research. However, it can be used as an instructive example.[70,73] It is well known that the larger the size of a sample drawn from a population of measurements, the more representative the sample mean is of the population mean. The random errors associated with each measurement tend to average out and the resultant sample statistic will more closely approximate the population parameter.[73] Increasing sample size also has the effect of increasing generalizability from the sample to the population. This is illustrated by an early example.[74] Subjects were asked to rank a series of weights, the ranks were averaged over different number of subjects, and the average ranks were correlated with the true ranks. The obtained correlations, when 1, 5, and 50 subject scores were averaged, were 0.41, 0.68, and 0.94, respectively. This example illustrates that reliability (and therefore validity) increases when a greater averaging of error of measurements occurs. This principle is also commonly applied in the practice of averaging the decisions of several judges to obtain relative rankings of subjective qualities of people in competitions, such as those related to physical beauty, artistic ability, or athletic ability.

Aggregation over trials and/or occasions cancels out the uniqueness of particular trials and/or occasions and thus, increases temporal reliability, or replicability.[70] However, data derived from the first time encounter of a stimulus situation may differ considerably from data obtained in subsequent tests, and experiments which rely on single occasion testing may not be generalizable to multiple occasion situations. In many studies the correlations obtained for data from the first encounter with a situation differ considerably from those of subsequent encounters[24] and the experimenter needs to take this issue into account in the experimental design. Aggregation over stimulus situations cancels out the unique effects associated with particular stimulus situations and thus, allows generalization to a larger domain of stimuli. This is especially true when measuring spontaneous locomotor activity in small mammals.[6]

As already mentioned "behavioral profiles"[12,75] are viewed by many investigators as more useful than single measures. Aggregating over variables achieves much the same effect as obtaining a behavioral profile, i.e., combines several variables, but at the same time allows for the reduction in method variance relative to true variance,[70] as long as the various measures are related (such as with measures of spontaneous locomotor activity).

Aggregation and the Measurement of Locomotor Activity

We have examined the effects of score aggregation over trials and/or over test days on measures of reliability of frequently used measures of activity, both in the conventional open-field test (see Table 3.3) with rats[24] and with the automated Digiscan Activity Monitor with mice and rats.[76,77]

Activity measures in the open-field test with direct observation were obtained for male rats given 4 open-field trials (4 min duration) at 48 hr intervals. In all cases the reliability correlations for 2 day aggregates (days 1 + 3:2 + 4) were substantially larger than for the less aggregated scores. This effect of aggregation is especially pronounced when minute by minute correlations (for the 4 minutes of each test session) were compared to the total scores.

Aggregation also substantially increased correlations between variables. For example, the mean correlation between ambulation and rearing scores calculated on a minute by minute basis was 0.39, for daily totals, 0.62 and for the 4 day total scores, 0.81. This represents an increase in the coefficient of determination of 50% when comparing the total scores to the minute scores.

Increases in the reliabilities of variables aggregated over time were also observed in mice tested in the Digiscan Monitoring System. Table 3.4

lists some effects of aggregation on the reliability of several measures obtained with male CF-1 mice tested for 1hr, on two different days of the week, for 3 consecutive weeks.[76] When scores were combined into weekly aggregates the reliability values were substantially larger than those obtained for scores aggregated over individual test sessions. In this study it also was observed that Session 1 scores had substantially lower correlations with the other 5 test sessions than the mean correlations among Sessions 2 to 6. This further illustrates the importance of the "first-time encounter" effect.

It should be noted that aggregation fails to increase the magnitude of correlations for variables which are not related. Indeed, aggregation should not create artificial correlations for unrelated measures, and aggregation of random numbers fails to produce increases in correlation magnitude.[24]

COMPLEXITY OF BEHAVIOR AND INTERPRETATION OF FUNCTION

Recognition that "single variable" approaches to the study of behavior are often inadequate to describe a behavioral phenomenon[78,79] has led to multivariate descriptions. For example, one solution has been to use behavioral profiles[12] or an activity print[75] consisting of quantification of a number of behavioral variables at the same time. However, there are problems associated with studying several variables independently since their interrelationships are not taken into account.[80] A variety of multivariate analytical methods, such as principal component and factor analysis, are available to deal with multiple measures. These procedures tend to promote "phenomenon realism" by more adequate characterization of general behavioral processes.

Factor analysis is a generic term which refers to a collection of statistical techniques whose purpose is the reduction or simplification of data.[81,82] These procedures allow one to reduce a large number of variables or observed relationships to a smaller set of more complex, hypothetical variables. Thus, the original set of variables is reduced to

Table 3.4. The effects of score aggregation on reliability of open-field (automated) activity measures in mice

Variables	Type of Aggregation	
	Test Sessions	Weekly
Total Distance	0.56	0.68
Number of Movements	0.49	0.58
Movement Time	0.59	0.73
Average Distance	0.56	0.70
Average Speed	0.49	0.66

a smaller, more complex set of variables called factors. These factors acquire meaning because of structural properties that may exist within the set of relationships among the variables.[83] Essentially this involves a process of subjective reduction of larger sets of variables, describing complex phenomena, to a smaller set which gives a broader interpretation to a particular behavioral process. Whishaw et al[79] describe this process of subjective reductionism when they suggest that "clinical" impressions about the "normality of behavior" often are better discriminators between normal and brain-damaged subjects than any single variable approach. Factor analytic procedures attempt to achieve the same result with the application of appropriate statistical procedures.

Factor analytic procedures have been used to examine open-field behaviors (see review in ref. 84). Whimbey and Denenberg[85,86] provided the first studies which proposed two factors to describe open-field behavior in rats: 'exploration' and 'emotional reactivity.' Ambulation, rearing, thigmotaxis, and habituation measures have been shown to be related to these broader factors of exploration and emotional reactivity in subsequent studies as well.[23,84,87] These factors can provide factor scores for subjects used in experiments and the relationships of these factor scores to other variables (such as physiological measures) have been examined.[23]

SOME RESEARCH APPLICATIONS OF THE AUTOMATED OPEN FIELD (DIGISCAN)

In our laboratory we have used the Digiscan System to examine the effects of a variety of experimental manipulations on the spontaneous locomotor activity of rats, mice, gerbils, and voles.

Role of the Vestibular System in Locomotor Activity

The vestibular system detects the position and motion of the head in space and, together with information from visual, proprioceptive, and other somatosensory receptors, provides a multimodal integrated system that vertebrates can use for spatial orientation.[88,89] Vestibular dysfunction has been found to have pronounced and long-lasting effects on behavior.[89] We investigated the effects of chemical labyrinthectomy on spontaneous activity in rats[90] and meadow voles.[91] Animals were chemically labyrinthectomized by intratympanic injections of sodium arsanilate and then tested for presence of the air-righting and contact-righting reflexes.

Rats with bilateral vestibular dysfunction exhibited increased ambulation and decreased rearing responses in a standard open-field test. When tested in the Digiscan Monitoring System, vertical activity, especially Time per Vertical Movement, was substantially reduced in labyrinthectomized animals.[90] Meadow voles exhibited very pronounced hyperambulation but, similar to the rats, decreased vertical activity. Stereotypic movements also were increased in the labyrinthectomized voles and when their movements in the Digiscan Monitor were plotted in real time, clear differences in ambulatory patterns were noted. The meadow voles with a dysfunctional vestibular system exhibited more horizontal (ambulatory) activity, especially a characteristic circling behavior.[91]

When rats were subjected to horizontal rotation, strongly stimulating the vestibular system, spontaneous activity was markedly reduced following the treatment.[92] Both ambulatory and rearing responses were depressed, but only in rats with an intact vestibular system. When labyrinthectomized rats were subjected to the rotation treatment, no significant changes in activity were obtained. These studies demonstrate the profound effects of overstimulation, or loss of, the vestibular system on spontaneous activity.

Sex Differences and Day-Night Effects

Sex differences in spontaneous activity levels have important implications for the measurement of the effects of a variety of experimental manipulations. These can include drug and toxin effects, CNS stimulation and lesion effects, as well as developmental, housing and diet effects, among many others. In addition, sex differences in activity levels can also provide insight into the evolutionary effects of sexual selection.[93,28]

Rats tested in the Digiscan Monitoring System exhibited sex differences in Total Distance, Average Distance and Average Speed variables, with female rats traveling longer distances at greater speeds. However, no differences were obtained for Horizontal Movements, Vertical Movements, Total Movement Time or Time per Movement. Thus, the sex differences reflected longer distances traveled at faster speeds by females, but not a greater number of movements. Interestingly, these differences were most pronounced on the first test day with much reduced differences by the fourth test day.[94,95] These differences were interpreted as reflecting sex differences in exploratory activity. It was suggested that these sex differences in activity are influenced by both the novelty and the exploratory demands of the test situation.[28]

Examination of adult meadow vole activity levels in the Digiscan Monitoring System in our laboratory[96] has also demonstrated sex differences in activity levels, with males showing greater levels. Total Distance and Movement Time were significantly greater for males, with no significant difference in Average Speed. These sex differences were obtained only when male-female pairs were housed together under reproductively stimulatory long-day, light dark cycles.[28,97] No sex differences in activity were observed in either pairs exposed to a short-day, light dark cycle, or when housed individually.

This multivariate approach with the Digiscan Monitoring System, confirmed previous findings of sex differences in the activity levels of both rats and voles, with greater levels in female relative to male rats, but a reversal of this pattern in meadow voles, i.e., greater levels in male relative to female voles. The latter is also consistent with the activity patterns of meadow voles in the wild.[28] Data on the field activity of the rat ancestors of the laboratory subjects are lacking however. The multivariate approach also showed that only certain variables exhibited sex differences (such as Total Distance) while other variables failed to differentiate between the sexes. Furthermore, a variety of factors, such as housing conditions and reproductive status (c.f. meadow voles) can influence these observed sex differences.

The Digiscan Monitoring System has also been used to examine changes in rat activity levels during the light and dark components of the day-night lighting cycle.[98] In this study male rats were housed individually in the Digiscan Monitoring Apparatus for 5 days under a 14 hr light: 10 hr dark cycle with free access to food and water. Following one day of habituation, the activity of each rat was monitored by summing activity variable data into 15 min time bins over the next 4 days. Results of the data analyses revealed day-night differences with pronounced light-dark and dark-light transition effects for the number and time of Horizontal and Vertical Movements (see Fig. 3.2 for an example). In contrast, Average Speed and Average Distance variables showed minimal transition effects. Thus, the Digiscan Monitoring System can also be used to examine rhythmic changes in spontaneous activity levels in a multivariate fashion.

Effects of Exposure to a Predator Odor

The threat of predation decreases nondefensive behaviors and increases defensive behaviors in many species of rodents.[99,100] One class of behavior that is strongly influenced by exposure to a predator or predator odor, is activity level.[99-102] In microtine rodents exposure to predator odor can be used to simulate threat of predation, and this has been shown to cause field voles and Orkney voles to avoid traps tainted with either weasel or red fox anal gland and fecal odors. As well, bank voles avoided tubes containing a red fox odor and reduced their activity levels. The principal component of fox feces, 2, 5-dihydro-2, 4, 5-trimethyl thiazoline[103] has been shown to elevate corticosterone levels and decrease open-field activity in laboratory rats.[104]

We exposed meadow voles to a variety of odors, including red fox odor, and then measured their activity levels in the Digiscan Monitoring System.[33] Exposure to butyric acid, extract of orange or no novel odor, had no differential effect on activity levels in male and female meadow voles. In contrast, exposure to the main component of red fox fecal odor significantly suppressed locomotor activity in male voles, but not female voles (Fig. 3.3). As indicated earlier, reproductive meadow voles exhibit a sexual dimorphism in their activity levels in the Digiscan Monitoring System,[28] with males exhibiting greater levels of activity than females. When exposed to the red fox odor, males immediately decreased their activity levels to those normally displayed by the female voles (see Fig. 3.3) and these levels gradually increased to normal male levels by the end of the 60 min test session. Following exposure to the other odors, or no novel odor, the males still exhibited greater levels of activity than females over the entire test session. These laboratory findings are consistent with field studies[105] showing that adult male, but not adult female, bank voles show significantly reduced home range sizes in responses to weasel predation.

SUMMARY AND CONCLUSIONS

There exists a variety of procedures that can be used to measure various aspects of spontaneous locomotor activity in small mammals.

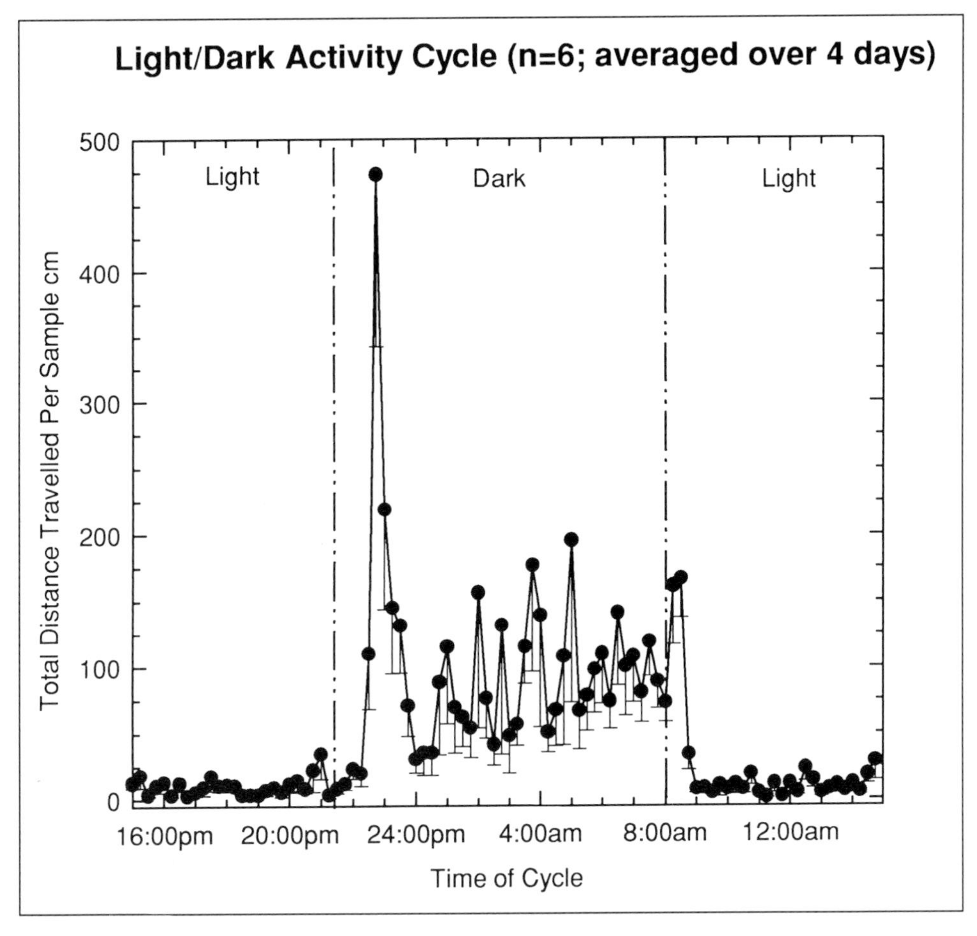

Fig. 3.2. Mean (4 days) 15 min total horizontal activity in adult male rats over a 24 hr period. Note the clear changes in activity levels for the light-dark and dark-light transitions periods (vertical broken lines). Error bars are standard errors of the mean.

These procedures range from simple direct observation of subjects in an open-field situation to more complex and sophisticated approaches involving measurement with infrared photobeam sensors or video-tracking methods. The automatic tracking methods (both photobeam and video camera) can differentiate a large number of movement variables, such as total distance travelled, total time spent moving, number of movements made in the horizontal or vertical planes, average speed of movements, circling or turning behaviors, plus many more. Additional advantages of the automated procedures are the removal of the observer (and any related biases) from the experimental situation, reduction of systematic errors across observers, and increased ease and speed of data acquisition and analysis.

The statistical issue of score aggregation was shown to be an important issue with regards to the reliability of variables. As well, aggregation of variables directly, or indirectly with factor analytic procedures, was shown to be useful in the more complex description of behavior in a phenomenological sense and to increase the ease of interpretation of multivariate data. The ability to easily quantify many different aspects of locomotor activity in an experimental session requires statistical approaches which can deal with the interrelationships of the variables used. Principle component and factor analysis are some of the statistical procedures which can be applied to such data.

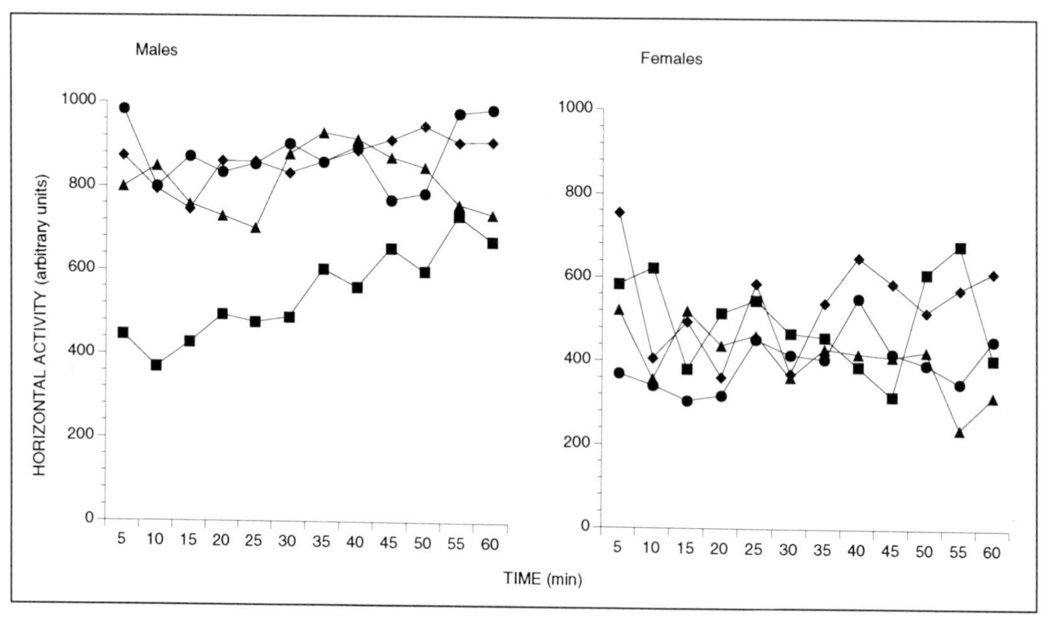

Fig. 3.3. Mean horizontal activity (5 min time bins) in the Digiscan Monitoring System following exposure to fox odor (squares), extract of orange odor (circles), butyric acid odor (triangles), and a control condition (diamonds). Data are for male (n = 10) and female (n = 9) adult meadow voles.

We anticipate that improvements in technology and computer software will increase our ability to monitor an animal's ongoing behavior, both in terms of complexity and detail. This in turn will require more sophisticated methods of data analysis and interpretation. This form of behavioral research will continue to play a key role in our further understanding of brain-behavior relationships, in both normal animals and the many different types of animal models of human neural and behavioral pathology.

Acknowledgments

Our research and the preparation of this chapter was supported by individual operating grants from the Natural Sciences and Engineering Research Council of Canada. We thank Drs. Ricki Ladowsky, Dwight Mazmanian, Campbell Teskey, Eric Hargreaves, Liisa Galea, Duncan Innes and Lisa Eckel for their participation in various phases of the research projects and for their helpful discussion. We also thank the many faculty and graduate students who helped with various aspects of the research. Special thanks go to John Orphan for construction of some of the experimental apparatus and to Omnitech Inc. for their technical help and valued discussion about methodology and interpretation.

References

1. Miezejeski C, Lamon S, Collier G et al. Partitioning of behavioral arousal. Physiol Behav 1976; 17:581-586.
2. Lat J. The relationship of the individual differences in the regulation of food intake, growth, and excitability of the central nervous system. Physiol Bohemoslov 1956; 5:38-42.
3. Anderson E. The interrelationship of drives in the albino rat: II. Intercorrelations between 47 measures of drives and learning. Comp Psychol Monogr 1938; 14: No. 72.
4. Tapp JT, Zimmerman RS, D'Encarnacao PS. Intercorrelational analysis of some common measures of rat activity. Psychol Rept 1968; 23:1047-1050.
5. Ivinskis A. The reliability of behavioral measures obtained in the open-field. Austr J Psychol 1968; 20:173-177.
6. Ossenkopp K-P, Mazmanian DS. The measurement and integration of behavioral variables: Aggregation and complexity as important issues. Neurobehav Toxicol Teratol 1985; 7:95-100.
7. Goma M, Tobeña A. Reliability of various measures obtained in open-field tests. Psych Rept 1978; 43:1123-1128.
8. Walsh RN, Cummins RA. The open-field test: A critical review. Psychol Bull 1976; 83:482-504.
9. Finger FW. Measuring behavioral activity. In: Myers RD, ed. Methods in Psychobiology, vol 2. London: Academic Press, 1972:1-19.
10. Irwin S. The action of drugs on psychomotor activity. Rev Can Biol 1961; 29:239-250.

11. Kinnard WJ, Watzman N. Techniques utilized in the evaluation of psychotropic drugs on animal activity. J Pharm Sci 1966; 55:995-1012.
12. Robbins TW. A critique of the methods available for the measurement of spontaneous motor activity. In:Iversen L, Iversen S, Snyder S,eds. Handbook of Psychopharmacology. Vol. 7. Principles of Behavioral Pharmacology. New York: Plenum Press, 1977:37-82.
13. Hall CS. Emotional behavior in the rat: I. Defecation and urination as measures of individual differences in emotionality. J Comp Psychol 1934; 18:385-403.
14. Hall CS. Emotional behavior in the rat: III. The relationship between emotionality and ambulatory activity. J Comp Psychol 1936; 22:345-352.
15. Archer J. Tests for emotionality in rats and mice: A review. Anim Behav 1973; 21:205-235.
16. Broadhurst PL.Determinants of emotionality in the rat: I. Situational factors. Br J Psychol 1957; 48:1-12.
17. Broadhurst PL, Eysenck HJ. Interpretations of exploratory behavior in the rat. In: H. J. Eysenck HJ, ed. Experiments in Motivation. Elmsford, New York: Pergamon Press, 1964:285-291.
18. Treit D, Fundytus M. Thigmotaxis as a test for anxiolytic activity in rats. Pharm Biochem Behav 1989; 31:959-962.
19. Kvist SBM, Selander RK. Open-field thigmitaxis during various phases of the reproductive cycle. Scand J Psychol 1994; 35:220-229
20. Valle FP. Effects of strain, sex, and illumination on open-field behavior of rats. Am J Psychol 1970; 83:103-111.
21. Suarez SD, Gallup GG. An ethological analysis of open-field behavior in rats and mice. Learn Motiv 1981; 12:342-363.
22. Suarez SD, Gallup GG. Open-field behavior in guinea pigs: developmental and adaptive considerations. Behav Proc 1982; 7:267-274.
23. Ossenkopp K-P, Mazmanian DS. Some behavioral factors related to the effects of cold-restraint stress in rats: A factor analytic - multiple regression approach. Physiol Behav 1985; 34:935-941.
24. Ossenkopp K-P, Mazmanian DS. The principle of aggregation in psychobiological correlational research: An example from the open-field test. Anim Learn Behav 1985; 13:339-344.
25. Classan V. Neglected Factors in Pharmacology and Neuroscience Research. Vol 12. Techniques in the Behavioral and Neural Sciences. New York: Elsevier, 1994.
26. Bronstein PM. Open field behavior of the rat as a function of age: Cross sectional and longitudinal investigations. J Comp Physiol Psychol 1972; 80:335-341.
27. Kenrick DC. Open-field behaviour, growth rate and life span in the black-hooded rat. Mech Age Develop 1984; 26:265-275.
28. Meade LA, Hargreaves EL, Galea LAM. Sex differences in rodent spontaneous activity levels. In: Sanberg PR, Ossenkopp K-P, Kavaliers M, eds. Motor Activity and Movement Disorders: Research Issues and Applications. Totowa NJ: Humana Press Inc, 1996:111-139.

29. Mistlberger RE. Circadian organization of locomotor activity in mammals. In: Sanberg PR, Ossenkopp K-P, Kavaliers M, eds. Motor Activity and Movement Disorders: Research Issues and Applications. Totowa NJ: Humana Press Inc, 1996; 81-109.
30. Martin-Iverson MT, Iversen SD. Day and night locomotor activity effects during administration of (+)-amphetamine. Pharmacol Biochem Behav 1989; 34:465-471.
31. Meng ID, Drugan RC. Sex differences in open-field behavior in response to the β-Carboline FG 7142 in rats. Physiol Behav 1993; 54:701-705.
32. Sanberg PR, Johnson DA, Moran TH et al. Investigating locomotor abnormalities in animal models of extrapyramidal disorders: A commentary. Physiol Psychol 1984; 12:48-50.
33. Perrot-Sinal TS, Heale VR, Ossenkopp K-P et al. Sexually dimorphic aspects of spontaneous locomotor activity in meadow voles (*Microtus pennsylvanicus*): effects of exposure to fox odour. Behav Neurosci 1995; submitted.
34. Ossenkopp K-P, Sutherland C, Ladowsky RL. Motor activity changes and conditioned taste aversions induced by administration of scopolamine in rats: Role of the area postrema. Pharmacol Biochem Behav 1986; 25:269-276.
35. Thiel V, Barnes DS, Mrosovsky N. A simple method for recording activity patterns of small animals. Physiol Behav 1972; 8:549-551.
36. Richter CP. Biological Clocks in Medicine and Psychiatry. Springfield, IL: CC Thomas, 1965.
37. Rusak B, Zucker I. Biological rhythms and animal behavior. Annu Rev Physiol 1975; 27:137-171.
38. Mather JG. Wheel-running activity: a new interpretation. Mammal Rev 1981; 11:41-51.
39. Gwinner E, Czeschlik D. On the significance of spring migratory restlesness in caged birds. Oikos 1978; 30:364-372.
40. Diamant M, De Wied D. Autonomic and behavioral effects of centrally administered corticotrophin-releasing factor in rats. Endocrinology 1991; 129:446-454.
41. Schlatter J, Elsner J, Zbinden G. Correlation of telemetered heart rate and locomotor behavior in cyclazocine treated rats. Neurobehav Toxicol Teratol 1983; 5:413-419.
42. Diamant M, van Wolfswinkel L, Altorffer B, de Wied D. Biotelemetry: Adjustment of a telemetry system for simultaneous measurement of acute heart rate changes and behavioral events in unrestrained rats. Physiol Behav 1993; 53:1121-1126.
43. Beninger RJ, Cooper TA, Mazurski EJ. Automating the measurement of locomotor activity. Neurobehav Toxicol Teratol 1985; 7:79-85.
44. Sanberg PR, Hagenmeyer SH, Henault MA. Automated measurement of multivariate locomotor behavior in rodents. Neurobehav Toxicol Teratol 1985; 7:87-94.

45. Prakriya M, McCabe PM, Holets VR. A computerized grid walking system for evaluating the accuracy of locomotion in rats. J Neurosci Meth 1993; 48:15-25.
46. Young MS, Li YC, Lin MT. A modularized infrared light matrix system with high resolution for measuring animal behaviors. Physiol Behav 1993; 53:545-551.
47. Livesey PJ, Leppard K. A TV monitored system for recording open-field activity in the rat. Behav Res Meth Instrum 1981; 13:331-333.
48. Spruijt BM, Gispen WH. Prolonged animal observation by use of digitized videodisplays. Pharmacol Biochem Behav 1983; 19:765-769.
49. Renner MJ, Pierre PJ, Schlicher PJ. Contrast-based digital tracking versus human observers in studies of animal locomotion. Bull Psychon Soc 1990; 28:77-79.
50. Vorhees CV, Acuff-Smith KD, Minck DR et al. A method for measuring locomotor behavior in rodents: contrast-sensitive computer-controlled video tracking activity assessments in rats. Neurotoxicol Teratol 1992; 14:43-49.
51. Ye S, Bell WJ. A simple video position-digitizer for studying animal movement patterns. J Neurosci Meth 1991; 37:215-225.
52. Tanger HJ, Vanwersch RAP, Wolthuis OL. Automated TV-based system for open field studies: effects of methamphetamine. Pharmacol Biochem Behav 1978; 9:555-557
53. Kernan WJ, Mullenix PJ, Hopper DL. Pattern recognition of rat behavior. Pharmacol Biochem Behav 1987; 27:559-564.
54. Hopper DL, Kernan, WJ, Wright JR. Computer pattern recognition: an automated method for evaluating motor activity and testing neurotoxicity. Neurotoxicol Teratol 1990; 12:419-428.
55. Cain DP, Saucier D, Hall J et al. Detailed behavioral analysis of water maze acquisition under APV or CNQX: contributions of sensorimotor disturbances to drug-induced acquisition deficits. Behav Neurosci 1995; in press.
56. Spruijt BM, Pitsikas N, Algeri S et al. Org2766 improves performance of rats with unilateral lesions in the fimbria fornix in a spatial learning task. Brain Res 1990; 527:192-197.
57. Spooner RIW, Thomson A, Hall J et al. The Atlantis platform: a new design and further developments of Buresova's on-demand platform for the water maze. Learn Memory 1994; 1:203-211.
58. Crawley JN, Szara S, Pryor GT et al. Development and evaluation of a computer-automated color TV tracking system for automatic recording of the social and exploratory behavior of small animals. J Neurosci Meth 1985; 5:235-247.
59. Schwarting RKW, Fornaguera J, Huston JP. Automated video-image analysis of behavioral asymmetries. In: Sanberg PR, Ossenkopp K-P, Kavaliers M., eds. Motor Activity and Movement Disorders: Research Issues and Applications. Totowa NJ: Humana Press, 1996, 141-174.
60. Bonatz AE, Steiner H, Huston JP. Video image analysis of behavior by microcomputer: categories of turning and locomotion after 6-OHDA injection into the substantia nigra. J Neurosci Meth 1987; 22:13-26.

61. Schwarting RKW, Goldenberg R, Steiner H et al. A video-image analyzing system for open-field behavior in the rat focusing on behavioral asymmetries. J Neurosci Meth 1993; 49:199-210.
62. Stoff DM, Stauderman K, Wyatt RJ. The time and space machine: Continuous measurement of drug-induced behavior patterns in the rat. Psychopharm 1983; 80:319-324.
63. Brodkin J, Nash JF. A novel apparatus for measuring rat locomotor behavior. J Neurosci Meth 1995; 57:171-176.
64. Martin P, Bateson P. Measuring Behaviour: An Introductory Guide. 2nd ed. Cambridge: Cambridge Univ Press, 1993.
65. Sanberg PR, Moran TH, Kubos KL et al. Automated measurement of rearing behavior in adult and neonatal rats. Behav Neurosci 1984; 98:743-746.
66. Sanberg PR, Moran TH, Kubos KL et al. Automated measurement of stereotypic behavior in rats. Behav Neurosci 1983; 97:830-832.
67. Sanberg PR, Zoloty SA, Willis R et al. Digiscan activity: automated measurement of thigmotactic and stereotypic behavior in rats. Pharmacol Biochem Behav 1987; 27:569-572.
68. Moran TH, Sanberg PR, Kubos KL et al. Asymmetrical effects of unilateral cortical suction lesions: Behavioral characterization. Behav Neurosci 1984; 98:747-752.
69. Epstein S. The stability of behavior: I. On predicting most of the people much of the time. J Person Soc Psychol 1979; 37:1097-1126.
70. Epstein S. The stability of behavior: II. Implications for psychological research. Amer Psychol 1980; 35:790-806.
71. Rushton JP, Brainerd CJ, Pressley M. Behavioral development and construct validity: The principle of aggregation. Psychol Bull 1983; 94:18-38.
72. Paunonen SV. On the accuracy of ratings of personality by strangers. J Person Soc Psychol 1991; 62:447-456.
73. Gulliksen H. Theory of Mental Tests. New York: Wiley & Sons, 1950.
74. Gordon K. Group judgements in the field of lifted weights. J Exp Psychol 1924; 7:398-400.
75. Sanberg PR, Henault MA, Hagenmeyer-Houser SH et al. The topography of amphetamine and scopolamine-induced hyperactivity: Toward an activity print. Behav Neurosci 1987; 101:131-133.
76. Ossenkopp K-P, MacRae LK, Teskey GC. Automated multivariate measurement of spontaneous motor activity in mice: Time course and reliabilities of the behavioral measures. Pharmacol Biochem Behav 1987; 27:565-568.
77. Teskey GC, Ossenkopp K-P, MacRae LK. Automated multivariate measurements of spontaneous activity in rats and mice: Comparison of the time course, reliabilities, and intercorrelations of the measures. Soc Neurosci Abstr 1987; 13:1544.
78. Hinde RA. Animal Behaviour: A Synthesis of Ethology and Comparative Psychology. 2nd ed. New York: McGraw-Hill, 1970.

79. Whishaw IQ, Kolb BE, Sutherland RJ. The analysis of behavior in the laboratory rat. In: Robinson TE, ed. Behavioral Approaches to Brain Research. New York: Oxford University Press, 1983:141-211.
80. Frey DF, Pimentel RA. Principal component analysis and factor analysis. In: Colgan PW, ed. Quantitative Ethology. New York:John Wiley & Sons, 1978:219-245.
81. Cattell RB. The three basic factor-analytic research designs: Their interpretations and derivatives. Psychol Bull 1952; 49:499-520.
82. Nunally J. Psychometric Theory. 2nd ed. New York: McGraw-Hill, 1978.
83. Harris RJ. A Primer of Multivariate Statistics. New York: Academic Press, 1975.
84. Royce JR. On the construct validity of open-field measures. Psychol Bull 1977; 84:1098-1106.
85. Whimbey AE, Denenberg VH. Experimental programming of life histories: The factor structure underlying experimentally created individual differences. Behaviour 1967; 29:296-314.
86. Whimbey AE, Denenberg VH. Two independent behavioral dimensions in open field performance. J Comp Physiol Psychol 1967; 63:500-504.
87. Maier SEE, Vandenhoff P, Crosne DP. Multivariate analysis of putative measures of activity, exploration, emotionality, and spatial behavior in the hooded rat (*Rattus norvegicus*). J Comp Psychol 1988; 102:378-387.
88. McNaughton BL, Chen LL, Markus EJ. "Dead reckoning," landmark learning and the sense of direction: a neurophysiological and computational hypothesis. J Cogn Neurosci 1991; 3:190-202.
89. Parker PE. The vestibular apparatus. Sci Amer 1980; 243:118-135
90. Ossenkopp K-P, Prkacin A, Hargreaves EL. Sodium arsanilate-induced vestibular dysfunction in rats: Effects on open-field behavior and spontaneous activity in the automated Digiscan monitoring system. Pharmacol Biochem Behav 1990; 36:875-881.
91. Ossenkopp K-P, Eckel LA, Hargreaves EL et al. Sodium arsanilate-induced vestibular dysfunction in meadow voles (*Microtus pennsylvanicus*): Effects on posture, spontaneous locomotor activity and swimming behavior. Behav Brain Res 1992; 47:13-22.
92. Ossenkopp K-P, Rabi YJ, Eckel LA et al. Reductions in body temperature and spontaneous activity in rats exposed to horizontal rotation: Abolition following chemical labyrinthectomy. Physiol Behav 1994; 56:319-324.
93. Gaulin SJC, FitzGerald RW, Wartell MS. Sex differences in spatial ability and activity in two vole species (*Microtus ochrogaster* and *M. pennsylvanicus*). J Comp Psychol 1990; 104:88-93.
94. Hargreaves EL, Tysdale DM, Cain DP et al. Sex differences in the spontaneous locomotor activity of the laboratory rat: multivariate and temporal patterns. Soc Neurosci Abstr 1990; 16:742.
95. Hargreaves EL, Cain DP. Speed of movements and not number of movements characterize sexually dimorphic open-field behavior of adult rats. Can Psychol Assoc Abstr 1990; 31(2a):359.

96. Tysdale DM, Hargreaves EL, Kavaliers M et al. Sex differences in the spontaneous locomotor activity of the meadow vole (Microtinae): Reversal of the usual laboratory rodent pattern. Soc Neurosci Abstr 1990; 16:742
97. Splinter AL, Galea LAM, Kavaliers M et al. Effects of live-trap restraint on motor activity levels and scentmarking in meadow voles. Can Soc Brain Behav Cognit Sci Abstr 1993; 71.
98. Hargreaves EL, Ossenkopp K-P, Kavaliers M et al. Day-night rhythms of spontaneous locomotor activity of male rats: A multivariate approach using an automated open-field. Abstr 3rd IBRO World Cong Neurosci 1991;254.
99. Blanchard DC, Shepherd JK, Carobrez AD et al. Sex effects in defensive behavior: baseline differences and drug interactions. Neurosci Biobehav Rev 1991; 15:461-468.
100. Blanchard DC, Shepherd JK, Rogers RJ et al. Evidence for differential effects of 8-OH-DPAT on male and female rats in the anxiety/defense test battery. Psychopharm 1992; 106:531-539.
101. Kavaliers M, Colwell DD. Sex differences in opioid and nonopioid mediated predator-induced analgesia in mice. Brain Res 1991; 568:173-177.
102. Kavaliers M, Innes D, Ossenkopp K-P. Predator-odor analgesia in deer mice: neuromodulatory mechanisms and sex differences. In: Doty RL, ed. Chemical Signals in Vertebrates VI. New York: Plenum Press, 1992: 529-535.
103. Sullivan TP, Crump DR, Sullivan DS. Use of predator odors as repellents to reduce feeding damage by herbivores. III. Montane and meadow voles (*Microtus montanus* and *Microtus pennsylvanicus*). J Chem Ecol 1988; 14:363-377.
104. Vernet-Maury E, Polak EH, Demael A. Structure-activity relationship of stress-inducing odorants in the rat. J Chem Ecol 1984; 10:1007-1018.
105. Jedrzejewski W, Jedrzejewski B. Effect of a predator's visit on the spatial distribution of bank voles: experiments with weasels. Can J Zool 1990; 68:660-666.
106. Tachibana T. Higher reliability and closer relationship between open-field test measures on aggregation data. Anim Learn Behav 1985; 13:345-348.

CHAPTER 4

METHODS FOR ASSESSMENT OF LOCOMOTOR BEHAVIOR IN PRIMATES

Deborah C. Rice

OVERVIEW

Methodology currently used to assess locomotor behavior in primates may be divided into several categories. The use of automated equipment such as photocells or acoustic sensing devices has the advantage of obviating the need for observation of the animal(s), providing the possibility of monitoring locomotor behavior over long periods of time. The disadvantage of such a strategy is that the behaviors in which the animal(s) is actually engaged are unknown. There are a number of established procedures in the literature for observational scoring of locomotor and other behaviors. Such procedures have been used extensively in field research, and to a more limited extent in the laboratory. This methodology allows different types of locomotor and postural behaviors to be collated separately, along with other behaviors. It has the disadvantage of being labor intensive, necessitating that behavior be sampled over a relatively short amount of time, which may result in sampling bias. A third area of exploration, analysis of gait pattern, includes determination of footfall sequences under various conditions, parameters determining gait transitions, and biomechanics of propulsion, among other variables. Primate locomotor patterns exhibit more plasticity than those of nonprimate species, and differ from them in fundamental ways. Locomotor behaviors of primate species therefore may be more easily disrupted than those of nonprimate species, particularly during development. Such analyses have the significant drawback of being extremely labor-intensive, but may

Measuring Movement and Locomotion: From Invertebrates to Humans, edited by Klaus-Peter Ossenkopp, Martin Kavaliers and Paul R. Sanberg.

nonetheless provide a fruitful avenue of research in the fields of developmental physiology and pharmacology/toxicology. Such diverse approaches, intended for different purposes, are obviously measuring very different aspects of locomotor activity in primates. This chapter reviews these general approaches, drawing examples from the current literature.

AUTOMATED EQUIPMENT

"Activity" is typically assessed by photocell or microswitch counts, or by ultrasonic devices. In general, a laboratory computer is used to tally the output of the measuring device, often sequentially over short time periods. The assessment period may be short, for example when determining effects of short-acting drugs, or extended over hours or days, as when studying the effects of chronic exposure to a neurotoxicant. Assessment may be made in the home cage, a familiar environment, or a novel environment, any of which may vary considerably in size between studies. Clearly, such differences in apparatus and experimental design mean that different behavioral end points are being studied. This may be legitimate or even desirable given that different species of different sizes and locomotor patterns are studied, and that the experimental question being asked may differ across studies. It must be pointed out, however, that there has been no apparent attempt to standardize procedures, or even to identify relevant variables, as has been attempted to a limited extent in the rodent toxicological and pharmacological literature.

A method of monitoring locomotor activity used routinely with rodents and adapted for use with primates is the use of a series of photocells. Photocells may be mounted at various points around the enclosure; crossing a beam results in a count of movement. For primates these should be placed to include the volume of the space; monkeys should be provided the opportunity to climb if appropriate for the species being assessed. Typically, counts are cumulated over a series of relatively short time intervals; the total test time depends on the experimental question. Equipment may be configured so that counts are recorded separately from different parts of the cage (e.g. floor vs. perch, middle vs. walls), or to eliminate counts in which one photocell beam is broken a number of times sequentially, but this is rarely done. Another methodology adapted from research with rodents is measurement of the force exerted against the floor of the cage or perch, usually by means of a microswitch closure. These two methodologies obviously may be measuring different aspects of motor behavior, although data from such studies are often discussed as if a unitary behavior is being studied.

In studies on the effects of dopaminergic drugs on the behavior of normal marmosets or those rendered Parkinsonian[1-3] or squirrel monkeys,[4] activity was measured in small cages equipped with photocells mounted at various vertical levels. Data were accumulated in short intervals for two-six hours after drug treatment, with no differentiation of cage position. A similar technique was used to study movement in rhesus monkeys exposed developmentally to PCBs.[5,6] In these studies, two photobeams were mounted in cages about the size of the home cage. Monkeys were assessed for 90 min a day for 16 days, with the data recorded in 15 min increments. There were differential effects over the course of the 16 daily sessions between control and PCB-treated monkeys, which would not have been apparent if monkeys had been tested for only a few days. In another study on the effects of developmental lead exposure on locomotor activity,[7] monkeys were housed in pairs in large exercise cages 23 hours a day for three weeks, with sets of photocells dividing the cage horizontally and vertically. Activity counts were recorded separately from each vertical level. Monkeys registered the most activity across the top of the cage and at a perch about three feet off the floor. Most of the daily activity occurred during the first two hours after being reintroduced into the cage; there was little activity during the dark period.

Detection of movement off or onto a perch by means of a microswitch was used to study the effects of drugs on circadian rhythms in singly caged squirrel monkeys.[8] Counts were monitored continuously by a microcomputer. The onset of the active period was defined as the first 10 min interval in which activity was above average after 4 hours of below average activity, as defined for each individual. Changes in phase or period of activity rhythms were calculated by least squares regression. Such a method may be more sensitive than the more standard approach used in toxicological research of simply comparing counts at different time periods.

A number of recent pharmacological and toxicological studies have used acoustic sensing devices. In a series of studies in baboons,[9-11] animals wore an "activity-monitoring" device around their necks. Although the supplier was stated, in two of the papers there were no details concerning what was actually being recorded, beyond the statement that the response frequency was 0.5-10 Hz. The third paper,[11] not referenced in the other two, states that "the monitor is sensitive to accelerations exceeding 1/10 of a g force." While it may be assumed that duration of movement was not monitored, the manner in which the sensor recorded the complex movements made by living organisms was not described. Similarly, an inadequate description of methodology for assessment of activity was provided in a study on circadian rhythm in owl monkeys.[12] An electroacoustic device was used to transduce the vibrations produced by the wire mesh cage as the animals moved into square wave signals that activated an event recorder. Although samples of the event records are provided, the parameter(s) being measured are not clear. It is unclear, for example, whether each vibration resulted in a "count," or whether the recorder pen was deflected for the duration of a single movement. While the overall impression of "activity" provided by the graphic representations was apparently used to determine phase shifts in circadian rhythms (Fig. 4.1), it is nevertheless necessary to define the dependent variable being measured. In contrast, in an experiment using a similar electroacoustic device,[13] the authors state explicitly that a TTL DC signal was generated as long as the animal was in motion, and that the length of the signal was stored by computer. The hardware and software system are adequately described, and the dependent variables explicitly defined, which included large (longer than 1 sec) and small movements, and time spent in each type of movement, plus totals (Fig. 4.2).

The effects of drugs on nocturnal activity of rhesus monkeys was studied by a device of which the complete description in one paper is "an ultrasonic device";[14] in a second paper from the same laboratory[15] it is stated that "an ultrasound field was generated in each cage so that each movement interrupting this ultrasound field could be detected by a receiving transducer." There is no other description of hardware, software, or dependent variables. In one paper the data are

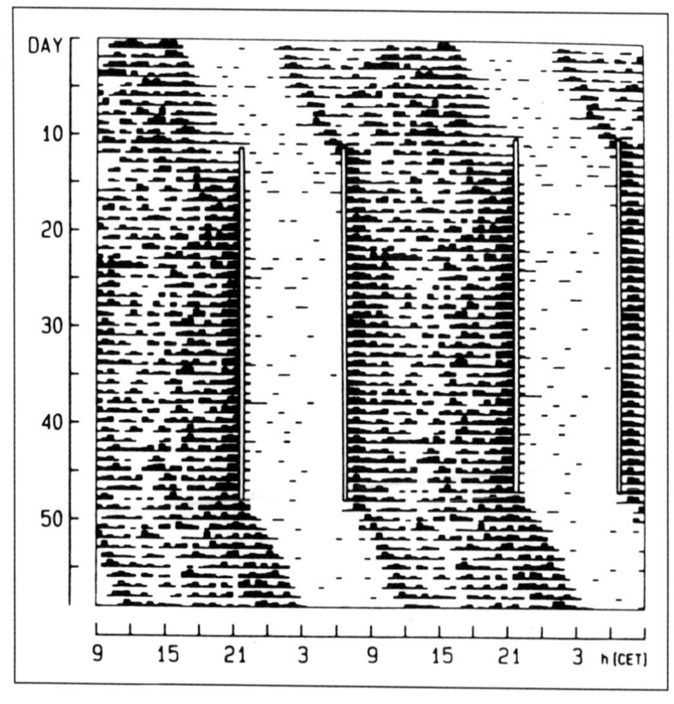

*Fig. 4.1. Activity measures across 60 days for a singly caged owl monkey, and the effects of two 30-minute exposures to light at specific intervals on entrainment of circadian rhythm. Cage vibrations were translated into square waves on an event recorder in an undefined manner. Reprinted with permission from Rauth-Widmann B, Thiemann-Jager A, Erkert HG. Significance of nonparametric light effects in entrainment of circadian rhythms in owl monkeys (*Aotus lemurinus Griseimembra*) by light-dark cycles. Chronobiol Internat 1991; 8:251-266.*

presented graphically with a label of minutes; in the other paper the units of measurement are not given at all. It is in fact impossible to determine what was being measured.

In another study on the effects of developmental lead exposure on activity,[16] monkeys were tested in groups of two or three in large exercise cages, as well as singly in the home cage. Activity was recorded by a "piezoceramic plate" mounted under the cage or perch; output was fed into a microcomputer and summed in one-hour intervals. The authors state that "even fine locomotor movements in any direction everywhere in the cage could be detected." Whether this device was a force transducer or a piezoelectric acoustic transducer (as suggested by the above statement) is unstated, nor is there an indication of what the dependent variable actually was (Fig. 4.3).

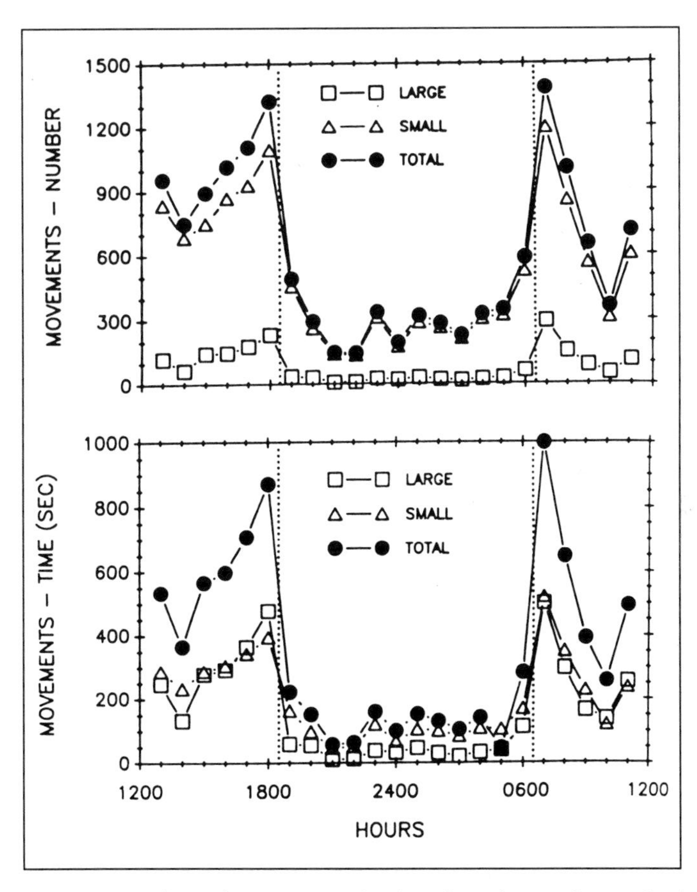

Fig. 4.2. Number of movements (top) and total time (bottom) of diurnal spontaneous activity of squirrel monkeys, measured in the home cage, and divided into small (< 1 sec), large and total movements. Lights were off between dotted vertical lines. Reprinted with permission from Holtzman SG, Young CW. Motor activity of squirrel monkeys measured with an ultrasonic motion detector. Pharmacol Biochem Behav 1991; 38:633-637.

There are a number of issues that are apparent from this sampling of the current literature. A number of different techniques are in current use, which may be measuring very different aspects of activity. It is doubtful that activity counts from photocells are measuring the same behaviors as microswitches mounted under cages. The former system is measuring mostly locomotion, particularly if repeated counts from one sensor are eliminated. It is not measuring other behaviors, however, such as grooming or stereotypy. Rarely are counts from single photocells or sets of photocells recorded separately, obviating the possibility of analyzing changes in distribution of activity, e.g., activity at the top vs. bottom of a cage. A number of studies used photocells to record from the home cage, where there is little opportunity for actual locomotor behavior. Microswitches or force plates, on the other hand, record any gross movement, without differentiating between types. The recent use of off-the-shelf acoustic systems has in general resulted

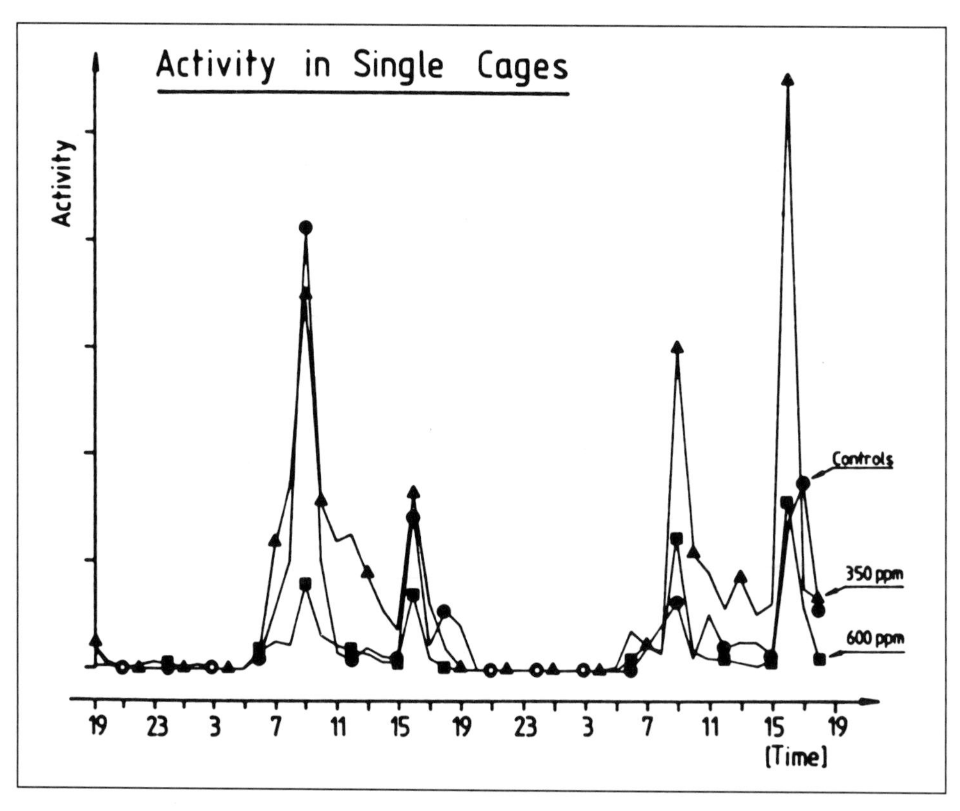

Fig. 4.3. "Activity" in the home cage over a 48-hour period of monkeys exposed in utero and postnatally to 0, 350, or 600 ppm of lead in the diet. Peaks in activity represent feeding times at 9 AM and 4 PM. The dependent variable is not defined. Reprinted with permission from Lilienthal H, Winneke G, Brockhaus A et al. Pre- and postnatal lead exposure in monkeys: Effects on activity and learning set formation. Neurobehav Toxicol Teratol 1986; 8:265-272.

in experimenters not knowing (or not describing) either the measurement system or the dependent variable(s). Perhaps even more surprisingly, reviewers of such manuscripts submitted for publication are not requiring an adequate description of the methodology.

The issue of different types of devices measuring different behaviors has plagued the rodent literature, where reviewers of specific literature have often reported contradictory results without apparent recognition of the importance of identifying the dependent variable(s) actually being measured in each study. As well, variables such as length of period of assessment, how often data are collated during assessment, whether assessment is performed in home cage or a novel environment, whether assessment is performed only once or over a number of days, and at what point in the diurnal cycle assessment is performed may have a profound effect on study results.

OBSERVATIONAL SCORING SYSTEMS

Observational scoring systems enjoy a long history in primatology, having been used extensively in field research into primate social behavior. A number of techniques for scoring various behavioral categories are in use. In instantaneous sampling, data are only recorded for a brief period at specified time points.[17] Locomotor bout sampling[18] or focal-animal sampling[17] records all instances of locomotor behavior, and may or may not include the distance traveled in each bout.[19] In continuous sampling,[20] particular locomotor behaviors are sampled (along with other behaviors) for a specified period of time at regular intervals. Results and conclusions may be heavily dependent upon the sampling method chosen. For example, in a field study in chimpanzees, different sampling methods were directly compared.[19] It was found that locomotor bout sampling (no distance) greatly overestimated the frequency of behaviors occurring frequently but for short distances, as well as skewing the proportion of various types of locomotor activity, compared to either instantaneous sampling or locomotor bout sampling with distance (Fig. 4.4).

A novel playroom environment was used to assess the effects of developmental exposure to neurotoxicants in rhesus monkeys (Fig. 4.5).[21-23] Monkeys exposed to lead were tested individually, while in another study monkeys exposed to 2, 3, 7, 8-tetrachlorodibenzo-p-dioxin(TCDD) were tested in peer groups. A focal-animal scoring technique was used. Operationally defined behaviors were entered into a personal computer in real time. These categories were apparently not highly correlated, since effects were often observed on one variable but not others. For example, lead affected duration of inactivity but not duration of locomotion, while TCDD affected play behaviors but not locomotion. Lead did, however, affect the number of sectors entered, again suggesting that distance traveled is an important variable in the assessment of locomotion (see above)

(Fig. 4.6). In a concurrent study, the same lead-exposed monkeys[24] were tested in their home cages on the same behaviors assessed in the open field. Under these conditions, there were no differences between lead-treated and control monkeys; further, the pattern of activities of both groups differed between the home cage and playroom environment. The authors suggest that the novelty of the playroom was responsible for the lack of treatment-related effect in the home cage in contrast to the playroom, although there were in fact a

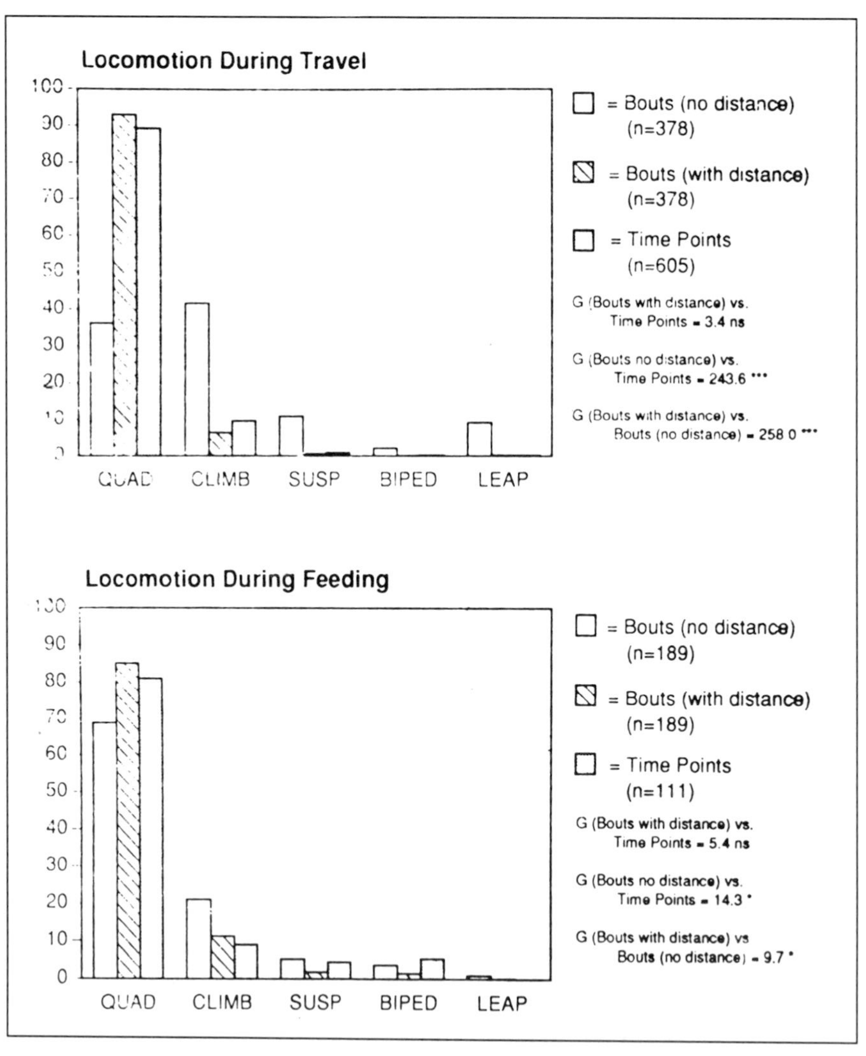

Fig. 4.4. Comparison of three sampling methods on the estimation of frequency of various types of locomotor or behaviour during travel and during feeding by chimpanzees. Different sampling methods yielded significantly different results. Reprinted with permission from Doran DM. Comparison of instantaneous and locomotor bout sampling methods: a case study of adult male chimpanzee behavior and substrate use. Am J Phys Anthropol 1992; 89:85-99.

number of other differences, including size of the enclosure and the enriched environment of the playroom.

In a study on the effects of cocaine on social behavior in Japanese macaques (*Macaca fuscata*), locomotor and positional behaviors were included in an assessment of a variety of behaviors, using a continuous sampling technique including distance.[25] Monkeys were group housed in a corral, and observers made eighteen 15-sec scoring cycles per 15 minute interval, for a total of four hours. Distance travelled was estimated from landmarks in the corral, although vertical and horizontal movements were not scored separately. Effects were found on positional behaviors (sit, lie) and distance travelled. There was also a differential effect of cocaine on vertical position in the corral, depending on whether the animal was socially dominant or submissive. Such analyses revealed effects that would not have been apparent if frequency or duration of locomotion had been the only dependent variable relating to locomotor behavior.

Subjective rating systems have long been part of pharmacological research, being used to assess symptoms of overt toxicity after acute exposure to drugs. In studies of the effects of various dopaminergic drugs on dyskinesia and locomotor behavior in squirrel monkeys rendered Parkinsonian,[26-28] a continuous sampling technique was used in which motor activity was scored from -1 (hypoactivity) to +4 (continuous, severe). In another study on the effects of MAO inhibitors in

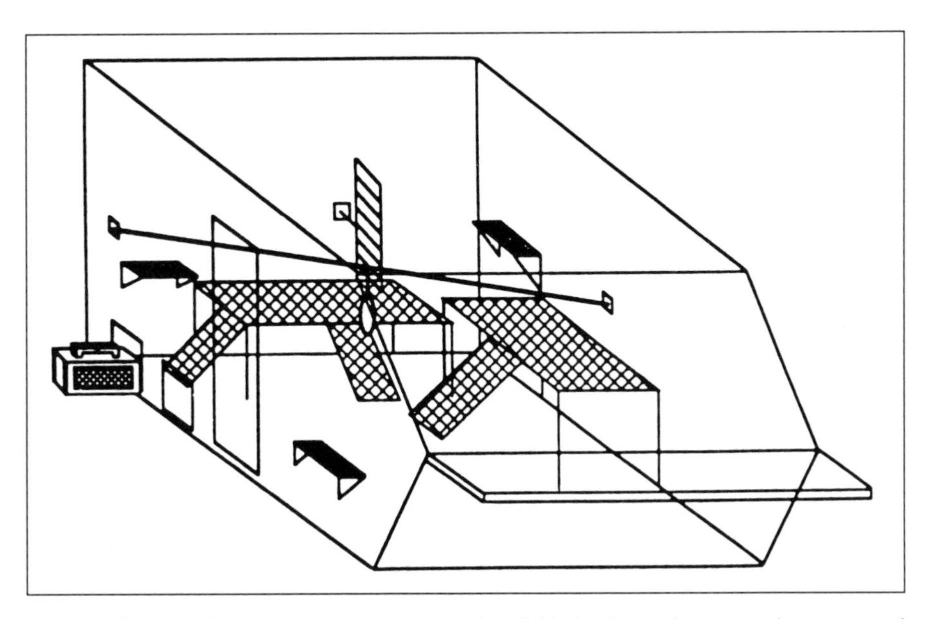

Fig. 4.5. Playroom for assessing locomotor and social behavior in rhesus monkeys exposed developmentally to various neurotoxic agents. Dimensions were 2.0 m x 2.4 m x 2.2 m high. Reprinted with permission from Ferguson SA, Bowman RE. A nonhuman primate version of the open field test for use in behavioral toxicology and teratology. Neurotoxicol Teratol 1990; 12:477-481.

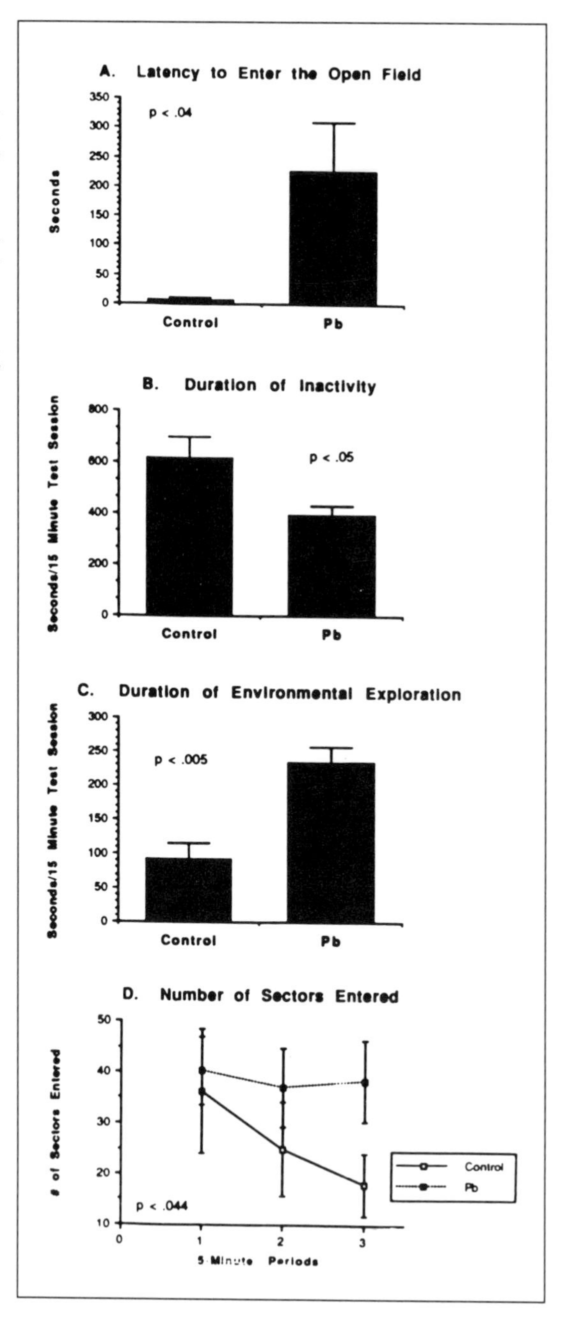

Fig. 4.6. Latency to enter the playroom depicted in Figure 4.5, duration of inactivity, duration of environmental exploration, and number of sectors entered by 1.5-year-old rhesus monkeys exposed to vehicle or lead from birth to one year of age (p values refer to interaction terms). Reprinted with permission from Ferguson SA, Bowman RE. A nonhuman primate version of the open-field test for use in behavioral toxicology and teratology. Neurotoxicol. Teratol. 1990; 12:477-481.

squirrel monkeys,[29] frequency and duration of locomotor behaviors were scored continuously from videotape for 15 min, along with vocalization and head turning. Although the authors mentioned the acts of walking, running, climbing, and jumping, these were either not recorded or not reported separately.

The use of observational scoring systems provides a number of advantages. Different types of locomotor and positional behaviors may be quantified separately, in conjunction with other types of behaviors. Animals may be monitored individually, even in a group setting. The significant disadvantage is the labor-intensive nature of the methodology; the opportunity to collect a relatively small amount of data coupled with choice of sampling technique may result in significant skewing of the data.

ANALYSIS OF GAIT PATTERN

A literature that is largely independent of that discussed in the previous sections is analysis of gait pattern in various primate species. Appearing mostly in the anthropology literature, it includes studies on comparative morphology and muscle physiology between various primate species, including humans. The present section of this chapter is restricted to a discussion of the analysis of observational locomotor patterns in primates. Primates exhibit a wide variety of locomotor patterns. They use a number of substrates, both within and between species, including ground, large and small trees and branches. Some nonhuman primate species use bipedal locomotion under some circumstances, others use a "three-legged" gait, during food-carrying, for example. Even in terms of purely quadrupedal motion, however, primate species and individuals have a larger repertoire of locomotor patterns than nonprimate species.

One of the original studies of gait pattern in primates was an exhaustive analysis by Prost,[30] who studied motion pictures of two individuals from different species of monkey moving at various speeds on the ground. He described a large number of footfall sequences, although clearly a few sequences dominated. Recent literature continues to examine various aspects of footfall sequence. For example, in recent studies by Vilensky and coworkers[31-36] and others[37-40] gaits and gait transitions at different speeds and as a function of a number of variables were examined. Primate locomotion along the ground is different from that of nonprimates quadrupeds in almost every aspect: footfall patterns, variables controlling gait transitions, relative stride length, weight support, and mechanisms of propulsion.

Primate locomotor patterns appear to be more plastic than those of other quadrupeds. For example, horses have three or four gaits, and gait transitions occur at specific energy output levels, related to speed. Individual monkeys, on the other hand, may use any of several footfall patterns at the same speed. Monkeys exhibit both lateral and diagonal footfall patterns, as well as two different gallop patterns (Fig. 4.7). Such behavioral plasticity may be more easily disrupted than the more rigid patterns of other animals. In addition, neural control of locomotion in primates is (at least predominantly) central; unlike other quadrupeds, primates do not exhibit spinal stepping.

Other research has focused on the interrelationship between primate locomotion and environmental variables. For example, in a series of papers, Cant[41-44] has examined the relationship between positional behavior of various species of monkeys and apes and its structural (natural) habitat. He assessed various types of locomotion (leaping, climbing, quadrupedalism, bipedalism, etc.) in relation to various substrates and types of activity (traveling, feeding on plants, foraging for insects). The basic unit of observation was bout of distance moved. A similar analysis has been performed in prosimians.[45] Like the detailed assessment of quadrupedal behavior described above, such careful assessment provides normative data against which locomotor behavior, particularly in captive primates, can be assessed under conditions of various experimental manipulations. For example, locomotor behaviors of free-ranging rhesus monkeys on Cayo Santiago were compared with those of captive monkeys, to determine qualitative similarities and differences (Fig. 4.8).[46] It was observed that free-ranging infant and juvenile monkeys use a much wider range of locomotor behavioral patterns among small tree branches than are observed in captive monkeys. In addition, infants on Cayo Santiago begin to walk using a diagonal-sequence pattern of footfalls, in contrast to literature reports of a lateral-sequence pattern in captive-born infants. The author suggests that these distinctions are impor-

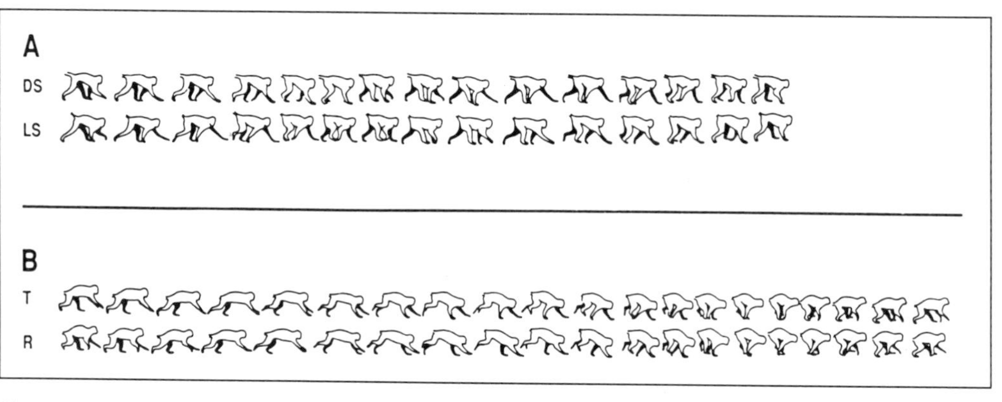

Fig. 4.7. Tracings from a film of a vervet monkey locomoting on a treadmill. (A.) limb movement during diagonal-sequence (DS) and lateral-sequence (LS) symmetrical gaits. Primate quadripedalism is characterized by the relatively frequent use of DS gaits, in contrast to other quadrupeds. (B.) Limb movement during transverse (T) and rotary (R) gallop. Reprinted with permission from Vilensky JA, Larson SG. Primate locomotion: Utilization and control of symmetrical gaits. Annu Rev Anthropol 1989; 18:17-35.

tant for the study of motor development and its neural control, as well as for designing substrates for captive monkeys.

Such analyses provide an apparently untapped source of information on primate locomotion that may be more sensitive to disruption by manipulations of various sorts than simply the fact that the animal moved. This may be especially true in such areas as developmental toxicology or pharmacology, since developmental exposure to neurotoxic agents may interrupt the development of the complex repertoire of locomotor behaviors observed in primates.

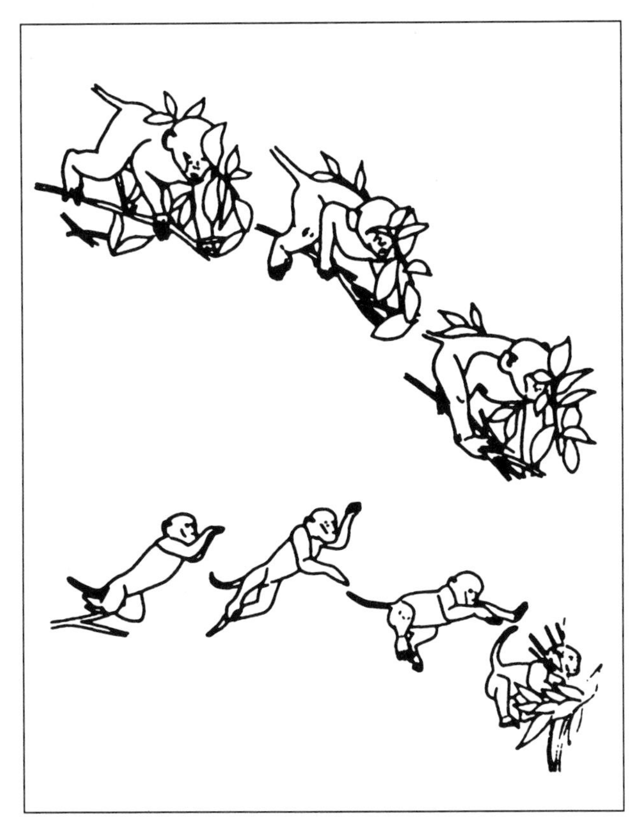

*Fig. 4.8. Analysis of locomotor patterns of juvenile rhesus monkeys observed on Cayo Santiago, but not observed in captive-born monkeys. The upper panel depicts quadrupedal walking on a small branch; the monkey is taking a step with its right hindlimb while the remaining three limbs maintain secure grasps. The lower panel depicts the sequence of leaping between flexible supports in a small-branch setting. Such small-branch settings provide the opportunity for development of strength, balance, and coordination. Reprinted with permission from Dunbar DC. Locomotor behavior of rhesus macaques (*Macaca mulatta*) on Cayo Santiago. Puerto Rico Health Sciences Journal 1989; 8:79-85.*

CONCLUSION

A variety of techniques is currently utilized for assessing locomotor behavior in primates, depending on the experimental question. In fact, there are perhaps more diverse approaches being used to study primate locomotion than are utilized in studying many other species. The three approaches described in this chapter—the use of automated equipment to measure activity, observational scoring systems, and analysis of gait patterns—explore different aspects of locomotor behavior, and are generally used to address different experimental questions. "Counting" activity in some respects supplies the least amount of information concerning locomotor behavior (even when methodology is adequately described), because what the animal(s) is actually doing is unknown. It has the advantage of not being labor intensive, in contrast to the other two methodologies. Data may be collected by computer continuously for long periods of time, and analyzed quickly and easily. This approach may be adequate in situations in which the experimental question is simply "Did the animal move more or less than usual?" Observational scoring systems provide the opportunity to monitor a number of specified behaviors from individuals in either an isolated or group setting, including various classes of locomotor or positional behavior. It has the disadvantage that only a relatively small time sample may be measured, which may result in sampling bias of various forms depending on the sampling method chosen. Analysis of gait pattern per se under various conditions assesses a different set of variables than the scoring of "how often and how long" and provides data that may be used to address a number of experimental questions. For example, the plasticity of locomotor patterns in primates may render them more easily disrupted by physiological or pharmacological manipulation than those of other species, particularly during the developmental period.

REFERENCES

1. Lange KW, Löschmann P-A, Wachtel H et al. Tesuride stimulates locomotor activity at 2 months but not 10 months after 1-methyl-4-phenyl-1, 2, 3, 6-tetrahydropixidine treatment of common marmosets. Euro J Pharmacol 1992; 212:247-252.
2. Löschmann P-A, Smith LA, Lange KW et al. Motor activity following the administration of selective D-1 and D-2 dopaminergic drugs to normal common marmosets. Psychopharmacol 1991; 105:303-309.
3. Wüllner U, Kupsch A, Arnold G et al. The competitive NMDA antagonist CGP40.116 enhances L-Dopa response in MPTP-treated marmosets. Neuropharmacol 1992; 31:713-715.
4. Boyce S, Rupniak NMJ, Tye S et al. Modulatory role for CCK-B antagonists in Parkinson's disease. Clin Neuropharmacol 1990; 13(4):339-347.
5. Bowman RE, Hieronimus MP, Barsotti DA. Locomotor hyperactivity in PCB-exposed Rhesus monkeys. Neurotoxicol 1981; 2:251-258.

6. Bowman RE, Hieronimus MP. Hypoactivity in adolescent monkeys perinatally exposed to PCBs and hyperactive as juveniles. Neurobehav Toxicol Teratol 1981; 3:15-18.
7. Rice DC, Gilbert SG, Willes RF. Neonatal low-level lead exposure in monkeys (*Macaca fascicularis*): Locomotor activity, schedule-controlled behavior, and the effects of amphetamine. Toxicol Appl Pharmacol 1979; 51:503-513.
8. Mistlberger RE, Houpt TA, Moore-Ede MC. The benzodiazepine triazolam phase-shifts circadian activity rhythms in a diurnal primate, the squirrel monkey (*Saimire sciureus*). Neurosci Letts 1991; 124:27-30.
9. Turkkan JS, Allen RP, Hienz RD. Chronic hydrochlorothiazide and verapamil effects on motor activity in hypertensive baboons. Pharmacol Biochem Behav 1992; 41:567-572.
10. Turkkan JS, Hienz RD, Allen RP et al. β-Blocker effects on 24-h activity in normotensive and renovascular hypertensive baboons. Pharmacol Biochem Behav 1992; 42:465-471.
11. Hienz RD, Turkkan JS, Spear DJ et al. General activity in baboons measured with a computerized, lightweight piezoelectric motion sensor: Effects of drugs. Pharmacol Biochem Behav 1992; 42:497-507.
12. Rauth-Widmann B, Thiemann-Jager A, Erkert HG. Significance of nonparametric light effects in entrainment of circadian rhythms in owl monkeys (*Aotus lemurinus Griseimembra*) by light-dark cycles. Chronobiol Internat 1991; 8:251-266.
13. Holtzman SG, Young CW. Motor activity of squirrel monkeys measured with an ultrasonic motion detector. Pharmacol Biochem Behav 1991; 38:633-637.
14. Duteil J, Rambert FA, Pessonnier J et al. Central α_1-adrenergic stimulation in relation to the behavior stimulating effect of modafinil; studies with experimental animals. Eur J Pharmacol 1990; 180:49-58.
15. Hermant J-F, Rambert FA, Duteil J. Awakening properties of modafinil: Effect on nocturnal activity in monkeys (*Macaca mulatta*) after acute and repeated administration. Psychofarmacol 1991; 103:28-32.
16. Lilienthal H, Winneke G, Brockhaus A et al. Pre- and postnatal lead exposure in monkeys: Effects on activity and learning set formation. Neurobehav Toxicol Teratol 1986; 8:265-272.
17. Altmann J. Observational study of behavior: sampling methods. Behaviour 1974; 49:227-267.
18. Fleagle J. Locomotion and posture of the Malayan Siamang and implications for hominid evolution. Folia Primatol 1976; 26:245-269.
19. Doran DM. Comparison of instantaneous and locomotor bout sampling methods: a case study of adult male chimpanzee behavior and substrate use. Am J Phys Anthropol 1992; 89:85-99.
20. Rose MD. Positional behaviour of olive baboons (*Papio anubis*) and its relationship to maintenance of social activities. Primates 1977; 18:59-116.
21. Ferguson SA, Bowman RE. Effects of postnatal lead exposure on open field behavior in monkeys. Neurotoxicol Teratol 1990; 12:91-97.

22. Ferguson SA, Bowman RE. A nonhuman primate version of the open field test for use in behavioral toxicology and teratology. Neurotoxicol Teratol 1990; 12:477-481.
23. Schantz SL, Ferguson SA, Bowman RE. Effects of 2, 3, 7, 8-tetrachlorodibenzo-p-dioxin on behavior of monkeys in peer groups. Neurotoxicol Teratol 1992; 14:433-446.
24. Ferguson SA, Medina RO, Bowman RE. Home cage behavior and lead treatment in rhesus monkeys: A comparison with open-field behavior. Neurotoxicol Teratol 1993; 15:145-149.
25. Crowley TJ, Mikulich SK, Williams EA et al. Cocaine, social behavior, and alcohol-solution drinking in monkeys. Drug Alcohol Depend 1992; 29:205-223.
26. Rupniak NMJ, Boyce S, Steventon M et al. Weak antiparkinsonian activity of the D_1 agonist COAPB (SKF 82958) and lack of synergism with a D_2 agonist in primates. Clin Neuropharmacol 1992; 15:307-309.
27. Rupniak NMJ, Boyce S, Steventon MJ et al. Dystonia induced by combined treatment with L-dopa and MK-801 in parkinsonian monkeys. Ann Neurol 1992; 32:103-105.
28. Boyce S, Rupniak NMJ, Steventon MJ et al. Differential effects of D_1 and D_2 agonists in MPTP-treated primates: functional implications for Parkinson's disease. Neurol 1990; 40:927-933.
29. Newman JD, Winslow JT, Murphy DL. Modulation of vocal and nonvocal behavior in adult squirrel monkeys by selective MAO-A and MAO-B inhibition. Brain Res 1991; 538:24-28.
30. Prost JH. The methodology of gait analysis and gaits of monkeys. Am J Phys Anthropol 1965; 23:215-240.
31. Vilensky JA. Primate quadrupedalism: How and why does it differ from that of typical quadrupeds? Br Behav Eval 1989; 34:357-364.
32. Vilensky JA. Locomotor behavior and control in human and non-human primates: comparisons with cats and dogs. Neurosci Biobehav Rev 1987; 11:263-274.
33. Vilensky JA, Libii JN, Moore AM. Trot-gallop gait transitions in quadrupeds. Physiol Behav 1991; 50:835-842.
34. Vilensky JA, Gankiewicz E, Townsend DW. Effects of size on Vervet (*Cercopithecus aethiops*) gait parameters: a longitudinal approach. Am J Phys Anthropol 1990; 81:429-439.
35. Vilensky JA, Gankiewicz E. Effects of growth and speed on hindlimb joint angular displacement patterns in Vervet monkeys (*Cercopithecus aethiops*). Am J Phys Anthropol 1990; 81:441-449.
36. Vilensky JA, Larson SG. Primate locomotion: Utilization and control of symmetrical gaits. Annu Rev Anthropol 1989; 18:17-35.
37. Kimura T. Hindlimb dominance during primate high-speed locomotion. Primates 1992; 33:465-476.
38. Meldrum DJ. Kinematics of the cercopithecine foot on arboreal and terrestrial substrates with implications for the interpretation of hominid terrestrial adaptations. Am J Phys Antropol 1991; 84:273-289.

39. Reynolds TR. Stride length and its determinants in humans, early hominids, primates, and mammals. Am J Phys Anthropol 1987; 72:101-115.
40. Hurov JR. Monkey locomotion during gait transitions: how do interlimb time intervals, step sequences, and kinematics change? Am J Phys Anthropol 1985; 66:417-427.
41. Cant JGH. Positional behavior and body size of arboreal primates: a theoretical framework for field studies and an illustration of its application. Am J Phys Anthropol 1992; 88:273-283.
42. Cant JGH. Positional behavior of long-tailed macaques (*Macaca fascicularis*) in northern Sumatra. Am J Phys Anthropol 1988; 76:29-37.
43. Cant JGH. Positional behaviour of female Bornean orangutans (*Pongo pygmaeus*). Am J Primatol 1987; 46:1-14.
44. Cant JGH. Effects of sexual dimorphism in body size on feeding postural behavior of Sumatran orangutans (*Pongo pygmaeus*). Am J Phys Anthropol 1987; 74:143-148.
45. Crompton RH, Lieberman SS, Oxnard CE. Morphometrics and niche metrics in prosimian locomotion: an approach to measuring locomotion, habitat, and diet. Am J Phys Anthropol 1987; 73:149-177.
46. Dunbar DC. Locomotor behavior of rhesus macaques (*Macaca mulatta*) on Cayo Santiago. Puerto Rico Health Sciences Journal 1989; 8:79-85.

CHAPTER 5

Measuring Human Individual Differences in General Motor Activity with Actometers

Warren O. Eaton, Nancy A. McKeen and Kimberly J. Saudino

INTRODUCTION

Important insights about motor development in humans have emerged from elegant laboratory studies,[1,2] but the role of the larger context is often overlooked with such focused, small sample approaches. Laboratory performance may inadequately represent behavior that is characteristic in the outside world. Moreover, pre-existing individual differences can influence behavior in the lab. For example, it has been noted[2] that infants of differing activity levels solved the problem of learning to reach in distinctive ways. Hence, it is important to complement laboratory investigations with field studies of in vivo behavior. Measuring such behavior well presents many difficulties, and the present chapter describes one unobtrusive and technically simple approach for assessing individual differences in human motor activity levels.

Methods for the measurement of movement or physical activity, as this volume attests, are many.[3] Some years ago, more than 30 techniques were identified,[4] and they ranged from the highly precise, such as direct calorimetry, for which subjects are required to remain in special chambers that allow measurement of heat production, to the approximate, such as diary techniques, for which respondents estimate their time spent in various activities.[5] In choosing a method, a researcher normally has to trade precision for ecological validity because

Measuring Movement and Locomotion: From Invertebrates to Humans, edited by Klaus-Peter Ossenkopp, Martin Kavaliers and Paul R. Sanberg.

precise techniques do not generally lend themselves for use in daily life. On the other hand, the techniques that are convenient for participants to use in their typical environments are often both imprecise and subjective. In our attempt to avoid techniques that were either precise but unacceptable or acceptable but subjective, we have opted for a middle ground, a measurement technique that is objective, technologically simple, yet easily used by research participants in their daily lives for substantial periods of time. This last attribute is critically important because it allows for the aggregation of information from large samples of behavior that are drawn from many situations. Aggregation, as Epstein[6,7] has convincingly demonstrated, cancels out uncontrollable and incidental factors, and such canceling contributes to the reliability, replicability, and generality of the resultant measurement. Thus, we have made methodological choices that maximize the size of the behavioral sample from which we draw our information in our study of the motor activity levels in infants, children, and adults.

Specifically, we have used instrumented motion recorders more commonly known as actometers. These instruments are modified wristwatches, which, given their size and appearance, can be worn for several days in naturalistic settings with minimal monitoring by the investigator and without disturbing the routines of the participant's daily life. Thus, it is possible to obtain samples of behavior over prolonged time periods from individuals in their typical environments. Over the past decade we have successfully used them with infants as young as five weeks, with preschoolers, with school-aged children, with adolescents, and with adults. We will next describe the basic measurement paradigm that we have used with infants, the subject population with which we have the most experience. However, the basic paradigm can be adapted, with minor variations, for other research populations.

INSTRUMENT

The instrument we have used is the Kaulins and Willis Model 101 Motion Recorder, which is commercially available from Alan Willis, 282 Watertown Road, Middlebury, CT 06762, USA (phone: 203-758-2861, fax: 203-598-3933). This recorder is a modified, woman's mechanical wristwatch (watchcase diameter of 25mm, weight of 10g excluding band). In an unmodified instrument, time-keeping is regulated by a balance wheel that oscillates at a frequency determined by its inertia and the stiffness of a hair spring, which is attached to the balance wheel at one end and the case at the other. A cam on the balance wheel allows a pin on a pallet lever to swing by, one swing of the lever for each swing of the balance wheel. The swing of the pallet lever, in turn, allows an escape wheel to advance one tooth, which, in turn, drives the entire gear train and the watch hands at the far end of the train. In a modified watch (see Fig. 5.1), the balance wheel and the hair spring have been removed, and the watch no longer keeps time. With the addition of a small weight to the pallet lever, it becomes unbalanced, and if the watch is tilted or moved, the pallet lever will swing, causing the escape wheel to advance the hands of the watch. In the modified watch, the apparent passage of time (as read by the hands) is proportional to the number of times the recorder is tilted or oscillated. The actometer is not responsive to intensity of movement, but does provide a frequency or count measure of motor activity.

The Model 101 version of the Kaulins and Willis recorder does not allow for the watch hands to be set, thus rendering it virtually tamper-proof, which is an advantage when using the instruments with young children. Because the actometer cannot be set to "00:00:00" when beginning a data collection session, the calculation of the number of movement registrations that occur is complicated slightly. However, one needs only to calculate the difference in "seconds" between two readings to obtain a total of the number of "seconds," which we refer to as activity units (AUs). Calculation of the difference between two readings is much facilitated by use of a computer program to be described in Appendix A.

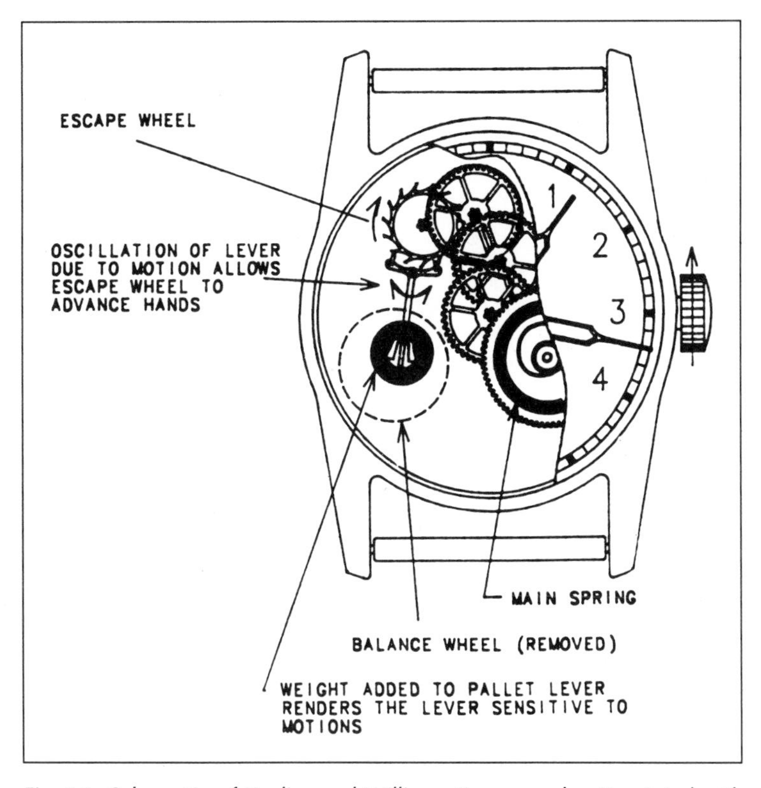

Fig. 5.1. Schematic of Kaulins and Willis motion recorder. Reprinted with permission from A. Willis.

PARADIGM

From the outset, the goal of our research program was to measure individual differences in general motor activity level. We assumed that brief samples of behavior would be much like single items on an aptitude test, subject to substantial error variance and unreliability. Consequently, we tried in various ways to aggregate over as large a sample of behavior as we could manage practically. What evolved was a general protocol that has been used in a number of studies.[8,9,10] Most of these investigations have been carried out with infants, but others have been done, or are being done, with older children, adolescents, and adults.

In a typical infancy study, two visits are made by an examiner to the home of each participating infant. The first visit is to initiate data collection with the motion recorders, and the second is to collect the instruments and to take final readings. During the initial visit, parents are interviewed and other observations are carried out, according to the requirements of the specific study. Then, after demonstrating an actometer to the parent, the examiner straps four instruments to the child, one per limb on either the outside of the wrist or on the outer aspect of the ankle, where they remain, more or less continuously, for 48 hours.

In our infant studies, the actometers are attached to the limbs with homemade bands made of elasticized fabric and Velcro closures. These adjustable bands will fit a wide range of infant wrist and ankle sizes. Before attaching the actometers, we first put a stretchy cotton cuff on the baby's arm or leg. These soft cuffs are cut from the tops of infant socks and prevent skin irritation from the straps and instrument. The actometer is then attached and enfolded in the cuff, which also prevents the accidental opening of the Velcro closures by the infant's brushing an arm or leg against something. An infant so equipped with four motion recorders gives an impression to the casual observer of a baby wearing sports bands and ready for a workout.

For child subjects, attachment is more problematic because it is critical that the actometers not be removed without a recording of the off-time duration. Young children do not appreciate such methodological nuance but, unlike infants, have the curiosity and motor skills to remove the Velcro-attached fabric watchbands. Thus, for preschoolers and elementary school-aged children we have used plastic hospital-style identification bands that, once attached, can only be removed by cutting them off with bandage scissors. Parents are provided with extra bands and bandage scissors for supervised removals and re-attachments, which are necessary for baths, figure skating performances, swimming lessons, and the like.

Unlike younger children, adolescents can appreciate the necessity for recording the durations of instrument removals, so in an ongoing study of adolescents we have not used the difficult-to-remove bands necessary for younger children. Instead, we again employed the elastic and Velcro bands, though in longer sizes and without the enfolding cuffs. Adolescents do not object to wearing the instruments for two days, and they are also willing to maintain a physical activity diary. The leg-attached recorders are not visible under pant legs, and the watch faces of the wrist-worn actometers are covered with tape to forestall the possibility of the subject shaking an arm in order to watch the second hand move. With adults we have, to date, only used wrist-attached actometers and have employed the standard watchbands that come with the instruments.

During the two-day data collection period with infants, the parent records those times when the actometers are removed. To prevent confusion about matching limb to instrument, we color-code the actometers with adhesive labels, which are keyed to a recording sheet maintained by the parent. The matching of instrument to limb, and the color-coding of actometers for that purpose, enables us to track each of our instruments by subject and site of attachment. As a study proceeds and multiple subjects are assessed, we counterbalance actometer assignment over limbs so that a given instrument is worn on the right arm for one subject, on the left arm for a second, on the right leg for the third, etc. Thus, over the entire sample of participants, the instrument is not confounded with a specific site of attachment. This important control protects our results against the possibility of a malfunctioning instrument being linked to a particular site and therefore prevents the introduction of a systematic bias into our results. Also, by tagging each recording to the specific instrument that produced it, we can check our data for any suspicious readings. This is done by sorting all readings from a given instrument by the real times at which readings were made. Because it is impossible for a properly functioning instrument to run backwards, a subsequent reading should always have a larger value than a prior reading.

Figure 5.2 shows a typical data sheet containing sample data in italics. The initial reading, called *BEGIN* on the sample data sheet, is recorded in a specific date-time format that is readable using the widely available *SAS* computer program.[11] When the two-day data collection session is complete, the date and time are recorded again, but as the *END* variable. With such *END* and *BEGIN* values, the actual number of real-time minutes between the attachment and removal of the instruments can be calculated using *SAS* in further data analysis. Because we eventually calculate a rate measure of activity per unit time, the real time during which the motion recorder is worn is required.

One might assume that every subject would wear the instrument for the same length of time, but the exigencies of daily life inevitably mean that instruments are removed for one reason or another, for example, for baths. Thus, it is necessary to adjust the difference between the *END* and *BEGIN* values by subtracting the sum of the minutes a given actometer is off the limb. In the lower part of Figure 5.2, we have reproduced part of a recording sheet, on which the necessary information can be provided by the parent. We total the time the actometer was off of each limb and enter it in our calculations.

The other critical component to those calculations are AUs, the "seconds" that are registered on the actometers during their wearing by the infant. This component requires two readings from the instrument, one at the time of initial attachment, and the second at the time of final removal. These readings are illustrated in Figure 5.2, which includes a start (*STRT*) and stop (*STOP*) reading for each instrument. As before, these readings are recorded in a *SAS* time format

BEGIN (DDMMMYY:hh:mm) *0 6 M A R 9 5 : 1 4 : 1 0*

END (DDMMMYY:hh:mm) *0 8 M A R 9 5 : 1 4 : 1 4*

Limb	Acto #	STRT 0 hours (hh:mm:ss)	STOP +48 hours (hh:mm:ss)	Total mins acto off each limb
Right arm	*27*	*01:43:43*	*02:57:57*	*15*
Left arm	*15*	*04:46:28*	*05:37:29*	*15*
Right leg	*09*	*05:46:32*	*06:34:07*	*26*
Left leg	*36*	*04:18:43*	*05:15:19*	*22*

If you remove a watch, record the times below:

Make a check mark in the column for any watch removed				Time of day in hours and mins		Comments	Sum of mins off
Right Arm	Left Arm	Right Leg	Left Leg	Removed (hh:mm)	Replaced (hh:mm)		
X	*X*	*X*	*X*	*10:05*	*10:20*	*bath*	*15*
		X	*X*	*15:12*	*15:19*	*diaper change*	*7*
		X		*21:38*	*21:42*		*4*

Fig. 5.2. Sample parent recording sheet with specimen data values.

that allows for the subtraction of the *STRT* from the *STOP* value to obtain the number of AUs, or "seconds" (see Appendix A for the program statements that convert data in Figure 5.2 from date-time values into minutes and AUs).

Because of variability in the total time the instruments are worn, we convert the readings to a rate of AUs per 30 minutes real time. Such rate measures are bounded by zero at the low end, and unbounded at the high end, which often results in a positively skewed distribution. Following Tukey,[12] who argues that analytic clarity often results from the re-expression of such skewed distributions, we typically transform the AU rate per 30 minutes variable with a common logarithm. The logged AU score is much more symmetrical and, thus, more psychometrically appropriate in many contexts. The SAS program in Appendix A includes this transformation.

READING AND SCORING CONSIDERATIONS

We have learned that it is not uncommon to misread the minute hand. For example, if the second hand is on the *8* (indicating 40 seconds past the minute), and the minute hand is between the *3* and the *4*, a reading 03:40 would be expected. However, alignment of the minute hand can be such that the minute hand is closer to the *3* than to the *4*, which would not logically occur given the second hand's position at *8*. Should such a reading be treated as *3:40* or *4:40*? A misreading of the minute hand introduces an error of ± 60 AUs (seconds), which could be serious in some contexts. If the total number of AUs registered is large, as it is in our 48-hour sessions, an error of 60 AUs is negligible. However, there could be some low-activity circumstances in which such a misreading could introduce intolerable error variance, and the use of the instruments is inadvisable if an error of 60 AUs would represent a meaningful proportion of the activity score. In any case, reading errors can be minimized by adopting a standard practice. For example, when we remove the actometer from the infant, we take a preliminary reading and then shake the instrument until the second hand reaches *12*. Then, if the minute hand is not pointing directly at a tick mark, we record the closest minute value as the true value. Such a procedure is not convenient or advisable if a parent or adult research subject is taking a daily reading from the actometer while continuing to wear it. In such cases, a possible error of 60 AUs for each recording must be tolerable to the investigator.

Scoring confusion can also arise if the motion recorder hands pass *12:00:00* during the session. For example, if the initial reading was *11:30:00*, and the final reading was *1:15:00*, a negative value would result when the first reading is subtracted from the second by a computer program. We avoid this difficulty by assuming that all initial readings occur during the first 12 hours of a 24-hour clock. If the removal reading is smaller than the attachment reading, as in the preceding example, we record the removal time as occurring during the second 12 hours of a 24-hour clock, e.g., *13:15:00* for the final reading. Another approach to this problem is to add 43,200 (the total number of AUs in a full cycle of the motion recorder hands, i.e. 12 hours x 60 minutes x 60 secs) to the second reading.

The procedures we have just described are premised on the assumption that no subject would accumulate more than 12 hours worth of movement (43,200 AUs) in a recording session. To date, this assumption has been appropriate for the subject populations we have studied. For example, in a sample of 18 university students, no reading exceeded 6,000 AUs over 24 hours. Among a sample of 120 3-year-olds measured over a 48-hour interval, no more than 15,000 AUs were ever registered on the limb of any child over the two days. Thus, there is little danger that the 12-hour AU capacity of the motion recorders will be exceeded in a one- or two-day period by normal individuals. However, an investigator using the instrument with other populations or over longer periods of time, must consider the possibility of a complete revolution of the watch hands during the observation interval. Should such a complete revolution occur, the investigator would not know without other information if the participant had been extremely active or extremely inactive. In our experience, daily reading of the actometer eliminates this potential confusion.

VALIDITY

To assess the validity of the actometers for measuring movement, we have used a chemical shaker bath, which is a commonly available piece of equipment in many laboratories. The shaker bath is designed to agitate racks of test tubes in a bath of liquid maintained at a constant temperature. We omit the liquid, but take advantage of the uniform oscillation of the racks in a constant plane to expose simultaneously a group of actometers to differing amounts of movement by varying the length of the movement session or the rate of rack oscillation. If the actometer readings are valid, they should be sensitive to planned movement variation imposed by the shaker bath.

In a recent validity assessment, we strapped 19 motion recorders face-up to the tops of the shaker bath test tube racks so that the horizontal, to-and-fro movements of the racks passed along the 6-to-12 o'clock axis of the actometer watch faces. Each of the 19 motion recorders traveled the same distance per oscillation (2.5 cm), regardless of its location on the racks. We exposed the actometers to four trials, which varied along two dimensions, time (4- or 8-min sessions) and rate of oscillation (170 or 200 cycles per min). Both the time and rate dimensions varied the total number of movements to which the instruments were exposed. For example, the 8-min session presented 200% as many movements to the actometers as did the 4-min session, and the higher oscillation rate presented 118% more movements than did the lower rate. If the actometers are valid and sensitive in measuring the four trials, which varied in movement amounts, significant effects should emerge for the Minutes (4 vs. 8) and Rate (170 vs 200) factors in an Actometer (19) x Minutes (2) x Rate (2) analysis of variance.

The results, shown in Table 5.1, revealed that the actometers did indeed differentiate among the different movement conditions. The highly significant Minutes effect was due to the 8-min trials mean, 736.2 AUs, being 196% larger than that of the 4-min trials mean, 375.7 AUs. The 200 cycle/min oscillation rate mean, 608.2 AUs, was 121% higher than that of the 170 cycle/min rate, 503.8 AUs, and the Rate effect was also highly significant. Furthermore, the Minutes and Rate effects together accounted for more than 98% of the total variance and did not interact with Actometer, which indicates that the instruments were not differentially responsive to condition differences.

The preceding data unquestionably confirm the actometer's validity for the measurement of moving shaker bath test tube racks. Though encouraging, such validity results do not automatically extend to the more variable limb movements of humans. In an ideal research world, we would conduct validity tests with a model identical to the target situation, but, to date we have been notably unsuccessful in designing a mechanical infant. However, reliability information about the actometers, in conjunction with the preceding validity data, convince us that the actometers provide valid, though imperfect, information about activity level differences among infants, and it is to that reliability information that we now turn.

RELIABILITY

The validity assessment described above also includes information about the reliability of the actometers. Two features of Table 5.1 imply that the actometers are reliable or interchangeable in measuring the movement of the shaker bath. First, as noted earlier there was no

Table 5.1. Shaker bath validity study analysis of variance results

Source of variation	df	*F*-ratio	Percentage total variance
Actometer	18	0.46	0.0
Minutes (4- vs 8-)	1	2480.39**	90.7
Rate (170- vs 200/min)	1	208.00**	7.4
Actometer x Minutes	18	1.78	0.5
Actometer x Rate	18	1.07	0.0
Minutes x Rate	1	6.06*	0.4
Residual (A x M x R, error)	18		1.4

* $p < .05$, ** $p < .0001$

interaction between actometers and the other factors. Second, there was almost no variance associated with between-actometer differences. The reliability implied by both of these facts can be estimated by calculating an intraclass correlation coefficient,[13] which estimates the degree of concordance among the readings of the 19 actometers. That intraclass correlation is .98 for the shaker bath study, and shows a very high level of agreement among the instruments in assessing a common movement criterion. But how reliable are actometers in measuring individual differences in the activity of living humans?

Because our work with actometers was directed towards the measurement of individual differences, our initial strategy was to average over the four limb scores to obtain a single activity measure for each infant. From this perspective, we viewed the four actometers worn on the four limbs as different measures of the same construct, namely the infant's overall level of motor activity. Do these four measurements intercorrelate well for a sample of individuals? If infants differ in general activity levels, we would expect that they do and that an infant with a highly active right arm would have a similarly active left arm, or right leg, or left leg. If so, individual actometer limb readings are alternative and justifiable indices of a common construct, the individual's general activity level. Table 5.2 presents such correlations from a sample of 175 infants, approximately half of whom were 6-weeks-old, and half, 6-months old. For both age groups the interlimb correlations were significantly positive. Such correlations imply that the different limb scores are, to some extent, interchangeable and provide converging information about the overall activity of the infant. Consequently, we aggregated the four measurements to obtain a single, more reliable composite measure of general activity level.

As our work continued we realized that our aggregation procedure, though psychometrically sound, might also mask systematic differences between, say, arms and legs. For example, we have found that infant arm activity is greater than leg activity in the first year of life, a pattern of results consistent with the principle of cephalocaudal de-

Table 5.2. Activity interlimb correlations by age group

	Right arm	Left arm	Right leg	Left leg
Right arm	—	**.60**	*.37*	.39
Left arm	**.72**	—	.49	*.41*
Right leg	*.40*	.43	—	**.60**
Left leg	.36	*.47*	**.62**	—

Within-cephalocaudal axis correlations are bolded; within-lateral axis correlations are italicized. Six-month-olds are above the diagonal; six-week-olds are below. All correlations are significant, $p < .001$.

velopment. From such a perspective, activity differences between arms and legs are not random and should not be considered part of error variance when considering individual differences. To assess reliability in a way that acknowledges such systematic sources of activity variance, we can partition total activity variance into various components and then estimate reliability. We will illustrate this approach using data from two studies.

In the first study of 175 infants, our actometer data fit an Infant (175) by Cephalocaudal Axis (arms vs. legs), by Lateral Axis (right vs. left) design and a corresponding ANOVA. The ANOVA results are shown in Table 5.3A, where it can be seen that there were significant differences among infants as well as between levels of both the cephalocaudal and lateral axes. Between-infant differences were significant and accounted for more than 50% of the total variance. As an illustration that actometers can be used with older participants, we present in Table 5.3B some results from a second unpublished study of 18 university undergraduates who wore two actometers, one on each wrist, for two days (with separate readings for each day). We had hypothesized that the dominant arm would be more active than the nondominant, which turned out not to be the case. Nevertheless, we found, as with infants, that individual differences generalize across other fac-

Table 5.3. Components of variance from actometer scores in two studies

Source of variation	df	*F*-ratio	Percentage total variance
A. Infant study			
Infant (I)	174	21.48****	50.7
Cephalocaudal axis (C)	1	835.41****	25.9
Lateral axis (L)	1	7.31**	0.0
I x C	174	3.07****	11.4
I x L	174	1.03	0.1
C x L	1	12.83***	7.5
Residual (I x C x L, error)	699		11.1
B. Adult study			
Student (S)	17	28.66****	37.1
Day (D)	1	0.16	0.0
Lateral axis (L)	1	6.28*	0.0
S x D	16	9.34****	34.2
S x L	17	5.21**	18.8
D x L	1	2.13	0.6
Residual (S x D x L, error)	16		9.2

* $p < .05$, ** $p < .01$, *** $p < .001$, ****$p < .0001$

ets of measurement interest; between-student differences accounted for more than a 37% of the total variance, somewhat less than in the infancy study. In both studies the main order effect for persons was significant, which is an important condition for arguing that the actometers are reliable in identifying individual differences,[14] because if there are no individual differences to detect, agreement between actometers would not be meaningful.

It is important to note that in both of the above studies individual differences interacted with other facets of measurement. For example, in the infant study the cephalocaudal axis difference between arm and leg activity was not constant across all infants and produced the significant I x C interaction. Similarly, student-to-student differences interacted with day of observation to produce the significant S x D interaction. Such interactions reduce reliability because they mean that the rank ordering of individuals on activity will vary from one condition to another. This complexity and others can be accommodated by using a generalizability approach to reliability issues,[15,16] and we follow this approach to estimate the generalizability (or reliability) for a single actometer score, as well as for composite scores. These estimates are presented in Table 5.4 for both of the preceding studies, and they well illustrate the point that reliability increases with aggregation.

A single actometer reading is clearly not as reliable as a score based on aggregated readings. Moreover, aggregation over some facets of observation is more productive than aggregation over others. For example, in the infancy study, choosing to attach the actometer to an arm or a

Table 5.4. Estimated reliability coefficients for actometer scores from two studies

Pattern of actometer aggregation	Reliability[a]
Infant study (48-hr recording intervals)	
Single limb reading	.69
A left and a right limb combined	.75
An arm and a leg combined	.82
Four limbs combined	.86
Adult study (24-hr recording intervals)	
One arm, one day	.37
Both arms, one day	.43
Both days, one arm	.48
Both arms, both days	.56

[a] More strictly, a generalizability coefficient, which is analogous to a reliability coefficient.[16]

leg, while ignoring whether it was on the right or left side, would have more impact on reliability than choosing a right-side limb or a left-side limb, while ignoring whether it was an arm or leg. Consequently, averaging over arm and leg readings has a greater beneficial effect on the reliability of the composite score than averaging over right-side and left-side readings. Averaging over all limbs produces the most reliable score, as one would expect given the strong positive correlations among limbs (see Table 5.2). The power of aggregation can be seen in other ways. Indeed, it is likely that the lower reliability in the adult sample reflects, at least in part, the 24-hour observation interval (as opposed to a 48-hour interval) in the infant study.

In comparing the level of agreement among actometers for measuring shaker bath movements (.98, as estimated earlier) to their level of agreement for measuring infants (.86) and university students (.56), we see that the vagaries of the real world have manifested themselves in the latter cases. Reliability can not be divorced from the measurement context, and the latter, lower reliabilities are better estimates of the functional reliability of actometers in measuring human limb movements than is the reliability based on shaker bath data. Furthermore, the length of the behavioral sample is quite important. For example, if we had used a 15-min recording period rather than 24- or 48-hour ones, the functional reliability of our scores undoubtedly would have been far lower because of momentary or unrepresentative influences that are canceled out during a longer assessment. Whether or not the real-world reliabilities reported here are adequate for other investigations depends upon the specifics of the research situation and can not be answered in an absolute way.

CONCLUSIONS

Motion recorders attached to the limbs of human infants and adults in their normal, daily environments have repeatedly revealed reliable individual differences. The actometers that have uncovered those differences are relatively inexpensive and technically simple. Despite these modest attributes, they have the great advantage of being unobtrusive and non-intrusive for their wearers. This advantage, in turn, enables the investigator to measure motor activity over relatively long time periods and large samples of behavior in the natural environment. For many research purposes, such seemingly mundane advantages can have important scientific uses.

ACKNOWLEDGMENTS

The research program upon which this is based has been supported by research grants from the Social Sciences and Humanities Research Council of Canada and from the Medical Research Council of Canada to W. Eaton. We thank Alan Willis for providing schematic and mechanical details on the motion recorder.

References

1. Gesell A, Halverson HM. The daily maturation of infant behavior: A cinema study of postures, movements, and laterality. J Gen Psychol, 1942; 61:3-32.
2. Thelen E, Corbetta D, Kamm K et al. The transition to reaching: mapping intention and intrinsic dynamics. Child Dev, 1993; 64:1058-1098.
3. Tryon WW. Activity measurement in psychology and medicine. New York: Plenum, 1991.
4. LaPorte RE, Montoye HJ, Caspersen CJ. Assessment of physical activity in epidemiologic research: problems and prospects. Public Health Rep, 1985; 100:131-146.
5. Blair SN. How to assess exercise habits and physical fitness. In: Matarazzo JD, Weiss SM, Herd JA, eds. Behavioral health: A handbook of health enhancement and disease prevention. New York: Wiley Interscience, 1984: 424-447.
6. Epstein S. The stability of behavior: II. Implications for psychological research. Am Psychol, 1980; 35:790-806.
7. Epstein S. The stability of behavior across time and situations. In: Zucker R, Aronoff J, Rabin AI, eds. Personality and the prediction of behavior. San Diego: Academic Press, 1984: 209-268.
8. Miller AR, Barr RG, Eaton WO. Crying and motor behavior of six-week-old infants and post-partum maternal mood. Pediatrics, 1993; 92:551-558.
9. Saudino KJ, Eaton WO. Continuity and change in objectively assessed temperament: A longitudinal twin study of activity level. Br J Dev Psychol 1995; 13:81-95.
10. Saudino KJ, Eaton WO. Infant temperament and genetics: An objective twin study of motor activity level. Child Dev, 1991; 62:1167-1174.
11. SAS Institute. SAS Language Guide for Personal Computers (Release 6.03 ed.). Cary NC: Author, 1988.
12. Tukey JW. Exploratory data analysis. Reading, MA: Addison-Wesley, 1977.
13. Shrout PE, Fleiss JL. Intraclass correlations: Uses in assessing rater reliability. Psychol Bull, 1979; 86:420-428.
14. Lahey MA, Downey RG, Saal FE. Intraclass correlations: There's more there than meets the eye. Psychol Bull, 1983; 93:586-595.
15. Cronbach LJ, Gleser GC, Nanda H et al. The dependability of behavioral measurements: theory of generalizability of scores and profiles. New York: Wiley, 1972.
16. Shavelson RJ, Webb NM, Rowley GL. Generalizability theory. Am Psychol, 1989; 44:922-932.

PART II

Measuring Other Types of Movement

CHAPTER 6

Developmental Aspects of Movement Sequences in Mammals

J.C. Fentress and V.J. Bolivar

INTRODUCTION

Mammalian movement patterns begin their construction in embryogenesis and continue to develop through the early phases of postnatal life.[1-4] A major challenge for behavioral neuroscience is to trace early changes in motor expression, including the contexts within which specific movement patterns occur.[5,6] In this chapter we emphasize issues of pattern formation as expressed across various levels of organization. To achieve a satisfactory picture of changing patterns in movement it is equally important to isolate individual action properties, to determine how these properties are combined in space and time, and to evaluate how movements allow the developing organism to adapt to changes in external circumstances. The problem of pattern formation in behavior is intimately linked to our ability to recognize patterns across multiple criteria.[7,8]

There are numerous ways that movement can be described, classified and analyzed. As illustration, ethologists have traditionally made the distinction between categorizations of behavior based upon functional consequences and form.[9] Thus movement patterns of similar form can serve different goals, just as common goals may be achieved through potentially variable forms of action (cf.[10] on "motor equivalence"). In each case it is apparent that movement occurs through constellations of actions, restricting the potential degrees of freedom in expression and providing an economy for nervous system control.[11] Adaptive behavior represents a balance between constraint and flexibility;

Measuring Movement and Locomotion: From Invertebrates to Humans, edited by Klaus-Peter Ossenkopp, Martin Kavaliers and Paul R. Sanberg.

the ontogenetic expression of these constraints and flexibilities as observed in specific contexts offers an especially fertile field for future investigation.

Prior to the analysis of mechanism, it is essential to provide objective taxonomic criteria for the particular aspects of movement that are of primary interest. Depending upon the purpose of the analysis, there are numerous potential criteria that might be emphasized. For example, movement elements can be abstracted, and their sequential and hierarchical patterning may clarify levels of neurological as well as ontogenetic control.[1,12-14] Specific phases of a movement sequence can be evaluated developmentally and as an assay for dynamic rules of movement control.[15-17] A variety of movement notation systems can be used to separate individual movement properties, their combinations, and their changes in time.[18-20] More recently, video and computer technology has become available that allows precise quantification of such variables as velocity, trajectory, limb coupling and rhythmicity.[1]

In this chapter we review the potential and limitations of these techniques as they apply to mammalian motor development. Our emphasis is upon the dynamic systems properties of movement, and development. Thus, while static abstractions of movement types, developmental stages, or even individual mechanisms can provide a useful heuristic for initial categorizations, it is important to recognize that these abstractions are limited in their ability to reveal more fluid and fine-grained movement variables. Conversely, sole emphasis upon individual fine details of movement can preclude our perceptions of higher-order pattern properties and their adaptive functions. We have found that it is often valuable to isolate individual properties without losing sight of the broader contexts within which these properties are expressed.

SEQUENTIAL HIERARCHIES

Many mammalian movement patterns can be divided into perceptual sub-elements that are in turn connected in a rule-governed manner. For example, rodent grooming actions can be divided into body regions addressed, such as face, belly and back. These body regions are normally articulated in a face to belly to back sequence.[12] Within these categories, e.g. facial grooming, a number of stroke types can be discerned on the basis of refined geometrical contacts, timing, limb coupling, and so on.[14] While such categories are obviously abstractions that may be based upon multiple criteria,[13,19] they can be useful in highlighting not only sequential but also hierarchical rules of organization. As illustration, in rodent grooming facial strokes form clusters of actions that are in themselves sequentially ordered. Importantly, individual stroke types may participate in more than one cluster, thus indicating the existence of higher-order rules of sequential organization. Interestingly, depending upon circumstances of expression, constraints in movement (invariants) may be more pronounced at any one of these levels. In this sense, it is not necessarily the case that movement profiles become more simple to describe as one descends levels of organization.

The dissection of distinctive layers in movement organization leads to a number of analytical questions. For example, do animals master "notes" of movement before "melodies," or do certain CNS regions have particular influence on one versus other levels of organization? With respect to the former question, data from several laboratories including ours suggest a series of developmental rules. One rule is that grooming of anterior body regions tends to occur developmentally prior to grooming of more posterior body regions, analogous to the sequence observed in full adult sequences.[13,17,21] A second more subtle aspect of grooming development is that movements are both refined (differentiated) and combined into progressively higher clusters (integrated) rather than either alone.[2] As analogy one can think of improved pronunciation of individual words by children as they are also mastering more complex linguistic units. Clearly, then, the analysis of movement across complementary levels of organization is essential to a full developmental evaluation.[5,13] A third property of juvenile rodent movements is that they often occur in more isolated packets than observed in adult animals. Thus, adult rodents often blend ("co-articulate") movement properties as actions are imbedded in variable sequences. Young rodents may also show considerable variability in individual stroke "types," but this variation appears to be more "internal" to the individual strokes and less systematically affected by sequentially neighboring strokes. Fourthly, juvenile movements for a given trajectory and paw to face contact are often temporally slowed in comparison to adults. There are two components to this: first, the movements themselves can be slower; and second, pauses are often inserted between individual movements that in adults appear as uninterrupted cycles.[17]

A challenge for future research is to establish more satisfactory ways to combine sequential and temporal information. Analyses of sequences alone do not necessarily reveal the temporal properties of these sequences (contrast sequences of letters to melodic patterns). Sequential properties may cross-correlate with changes in movement timing, but to date we are unaware of any unified analysis that combines sequential and temporal information in a satisfactory manner. A second limitation of "element plus sequence" analyses can be seen when the form of individually abstracted elements changes ontogenetically. Under these cases the taxonomic decision to label an element as an immature form of the same labeled element in adults, or to provide different labels at different stages is potentially arbitrary and may reflect investigator biases. A third caution is necessary if there is an inconsistent emphasis upon movement function and form across ontogeny. Thus, the term "grooming" implies consequences of certain movement sequences (e.g. cleaning the fur), and does not in itself say anything about movement form. Young rodents may show movements similar in form to those seen in adult grooming, but these movements do not necessarily result in effective care of the body surface. For example, Golani and Fentress[20] found that many early facial "grooming" movements in mice occurred either without any contact between forepaws and face or with contacts with excessive pressure that one or both forelimbs became stuck (immobilized) on one part of the face (thus eliminating contact pathways across the face). As Golani[19] correctly points out in a recent review, the inconsistent use of descriptive criteria in movement studies, including studies of movement ontogeny, can lead to taxonomies that are arbitrary and inadequate.

A final comment about the above mentioned hierarchical ordering of rodent grooming is in order. If one begins with the idea of movement types, it is then possible to isolate underlying ("lower order") variables from which these types are composed (e.g. timing, amplitude). This seems entirely logical, and suggests a clear hierarchical ordering. However, as Berridge et al[22] have noted, characteristics such as movement timing can signal certain types of movement phase properties, and indeed the same timing characteristics may be found across adjacent and qualitatively distinct actions such as forepaw licking and small forepaw to snout contact pathways. It seems to us that in a strictly logical sense one could thus view timing as the "higher order" variable, and the subtypes of movement form the "lower order" variable. Each of these considerations emphasizes the importance of more refined analyses of movement phase structure as well as individual properties of movement form and function.

MOVEMENT NOTATION ANALYSIS

Golani[18,19] has pioneered the application of movement choreography to animals, including their motor development, using the Eshkol-Wachmann movement notation system.[23] This system provides a systematic polar coordinate framework for examining posture, individual limb segment kinematics, and various constellations of movement across limb segments in time. Polar coordinate systems have the advantage of allowing one to visualize each limb segment as anchored within the center of a sphere. The free end of the limb can thus be viewed as tracing one or more curved pathways across the surface of the sphere. There are three logical types of movement possible: (1) planar movements which occur at 90° to the axis of rotation; (2) rotational movements that are parallel to the axis of movement; (3) conical movements which occur between 90° and 0°. Constraints for individual limb segments depend upon mechanical properties of the joint.

Movements of a full limb result from combinations of movement for each participating limb segment. The full limb movement can thus be reconstructed by assembling the polar coordinate transitions for each segment. Five insights become apparent immediately. The first is that static posture involves the relative positioning of limb segments with each other and with respect to the environment; and that movement is thus resolved as dynamic changes in posture. Postural and movement properties can thus be addressed within a single framework. The second insight which follows is that movements can be described from several complementary frames of reference. For example, a movement may be described differently based upon body-wise relations than when based upon environmental reference. Environmental references can vary, such as with respect to fixed objects or relative changes (movements) of these objects (as in a moving social partner). Thirdly, whether or not a given limb segment is viewed to move at all can depend upon whether the body or external environment is used as the frame of reference. Thus active movements of the shoulder only result in movements of the forearm if the sphere at the elbow is held fixed with respect to a fixed point in the external environment, but no movement is recorded in the forearm if the elbow sphere rotates as a result of active movements of the shoulder. Fourthly, measured consequences of movement of a given limb segment can depend upon circumstances as well as reference frame. Thus if flexion occurs at the wrist suspended in space there may be no consequences for leg position referenced externally (wrist movement defined as "light"), whereas the same movement at the wrist will cause the legs to swing if one holds onto a chinning bar (wrist movement defined as "heavy"). This reminds us that in active movement the organism must recalibrate consequences under different circumstances. Note also that when described from a body-wise as opposed to an external referent the changing position of the hand with respect to the legs is identical for each of the two cases described. As Golani[19] has emphasized recently, clarification of an organism's "base of support" (part of body in contact with substrate) is fundamental to understanding the basics of movement. Finally, systematic employment of limb segment polar coordinate descriptions can clarify the important constraints (invariants) in multisegmental movement. One can thus attain invariant passage of a tooth brush across the teeth through highly variable combinations of forelimb and head movements. The former description for combined forelimb and head movements thus becomes more "simple" than descriptions of either the head or forelimb alone. These relative invariants in movement can in turn provide insights into the important control variables in movement (which of course can change during ontogeny, as well as under different momentary circumstances of movement production). Consistencies and changes in numerous properties of movement organization can be compared within a single comprehensive framework, whatever the details of the movement, either in form or functional consequence.

Golani and Fentress[20] took advantage of the complementary perspectives of movement description provided by the Eshkol-Wachmann notation system to separate properties of individual limb segment kinematics, forelimb trajectories in space, and paw to face contacts in mouse grooming ontogeny. Although early precursors to grooming, such as isolated face swipes, appear prenatally in rodents,[4,24] loss of intrauterine support at birth presents the young organism with a number of new gravitational and postural problems that can block grooming expression. These problems can be overridden by providing the young animal with external support. Thus Golani and Fentress[20] designed a "filming chair" that held the newborn mice in a sitting posture similar to that used by adult mice when they groom. When placed within a particular posture, young mammals will often be "trapped" into performing movements relevant to that posture ("motor traps"[25]). Further, moderate activation, such as the result of lightly pinching the tail, can "feed into" the posturally facilitated movement, which in turn increases the efficiency of examining a number of different motor patterns. This type of activation works for adult animals only if their higher CNS functions are compromised.

The filming chair was constructed of mirrors to permit three dimensional images of movement. Before filming, the shoulder, elbow, and wrist joints of the infants were marked to assist precise evaluation of segmental movements. A high speed Locam camera with strobe lighting was used to trace the behavior at 100 fps daily from birth through postnatal day 14 (a time at which relatively mature unsupported grooming sequences are observed). Films were notated frame by frame with the Eshkol-Wachmann system. Movement of the forelimbs was represented as the sum of movements of separate segments, while positions and movements of the neck and head, and of upper arms, were described in relation to the chest. Movements of the forearms were described in relation to the upper arms and those of the forepaws were described in relation to the forearms, etc. From these descriptions individual limb segment motions could be related systematically to forelimb trajectories as well as contact pathways between the forepaws and face.

In two-week old mice facial grooming involves preparatory postural adjustments which become joined by movements of the head and the neck, the upper and lower arms, and the paws. For each grooming stroke the forepaws are raised along the face, then lowered. During the raising phase the forepaws do not make contact with the face, although they do pass through the mystacial vibrissae. Paw-to-face contact is attained during the lowering phase, and these contacts are statistically ordered into progressively larger movements (although with a substructuring within this overall order). Simultaneous and successive spherical movements of the upper arms, forearms, and paws are transformed into curved paths traced by the paws in the air. These movements are joined by spherical movements of the head and neck, which results in contact on the face by the forepaws. This rich pattern is in turn constructed by a collection of rotational, planar and conical movements defined for individual participating segments. The overall pattern of forepaw to face contacts can be maintained through alternative trajectories of the forelimbs (e.g. through compensatory movements of the neck and head), and individual trajectories can be established through different combinations of movement of the body, shoulders, elbows and wrist.

Thus the richness of even a relatively "simple" form of mammalian movement becomes highlighted by the Eshkol-Wachmann system, and this movement can be reconstructed through variable combinations of its subcomponents. The notation system also highlights the fact that movement is not linearly ordered, but consists of "movement chords" in which simultaneous and partially overlapping processes are assembled together in parallel. In very young mice (0-100 hours), grooming consists of isolated strokes, or bouts of strokes, which vary in amplitude and symmetry. Later (100-200 hours), the bouts of strokes disappear, asymmetry is eliminated, and contact pathways are restricted but reliable. Subsequently (200-300 hours), bouts reappear with increasingly rich combinations of participating movement properties.

Golani has applied the Eshkol-Wachmann notation system in a number of insightful studies of movement ontogeny (cf.[19]). By extracting basic geometrical measures he has succeeded in clarifying developmental principles that are general in nature but not readily apparent by more traditional descriptive and analytical methods. For example, relatively independent of a particular movement class, movements tend to progress in a cephalocaudal direction, and progressively incorporate transitions along horizontal, forward and vertical domains. He and his colleagues have also shown that when young animals are placed within a novel environment, they commonly repeat movement patterns observed earlier in ontogeny prior to expressing their full capacities of the moment ("warm up"). An important lesson from these studies is that it is easy for the investigator to bring pre-existing perceptual and conceptual biases into studies of movement and its ontogeny, and these biases can blind one to organizational principles that cross traditional categories.[13] The value of the Eskhol-Wachmann system is that it provides an objective and unifying approach that can be applied to many classes of movement including their ontogeny.

PHASE STRUCTURE IN MOVEMENT

Given the richness of movement, as illustrated by the Eskhol-Wachmann method, it is sometimes valuable to extract rules of sequencing ("action syntax"[22]). These sequencing rules can then be used to highlight both the perfection of individual movement elements and the means by which these elements are combined. This can be valuable for developmental analyses in that one can document both the refinement of individual actions ("differentiation") and the establishment of higher-order patterns ("integration").[17,26]

Berridge et al[22] articulated a number of additional rules for rodent facial grooming. These included overall stochastic profiles, a tendency for animals to oscillate between actions ("perseverant alternation") while also going through linear sequences, and the existence of sub-phases in grooming where the same individual actions could be embedded either in highly variable or strictly stereotyped sequences.[12] This phase structure turns out to provide an important window for the analysis of mechanism. Thus, as predicted on theoretical grounds,[12,27] movements that are rapid and occur within stereotyped sequences are less sensitive to peripheral perturbations than are slower movements within more flexible sequences. There is also a consistent positive correlation between movement speed and sequential stereotypy. As illustration, deafferentation of the face by sectioning the sensory branches of the trigeminal nerve had much less pronounced consequences upon movements within the stereotyped sequence phase of grooming than upon the variable phase of grooming (even when these two phases were analyzed for otherwise identical individual actions).[28,29] Interestingly, even when movement form was somewhat affected by the trigeminal deafferentation procedures, the basic rules of sequencing among actions in the stereotyped grooming phase were not.

Finally, the extent to which grooming form and sequencing were affected depended upon the (motivational) context within which grooming actions were observed. Thus, deformations were found in rhythmic tongue protrusions when emitted in ingestive but not in grooming contexts. Conversely, alterations in forelimb action were not found during ingestive contexts, but could occur during postprandial grooming (especially during the flexible sequence phase). A general implication of such findings is that central as opposed to peripheral processes in integrated action are dynamically organized. These rules of dynamical organization can also help clarify relative contributions of central mechanisms. Thus Berridge and Fentress[29] found that kainic acid lesions of the striatum have their primary effect upon the sequential integrity ("syntax") of stereotyped action phases, with little effect upon the form of individual movements. Conversely, cerebellar lesions are more likely to disrupt movement form while leaving action sequencing relatively intact.[30]

Berridge and his students[17] have examined grooming in both altricial (rats) and precocial (guinea pigs) rodents. As expected, grooming undergoes more substantial postnatal developmental changes in the altricial (developmentally immature) animals. In rats there is no evidence for syntactic chaining before postnatal day 7. Elliptical strokes first appear on day 7 or 8, and at first almost always occur singly. Syntactic chains develop over days 9 to 15 through the addition of successive grooming phases. In the early syntactic chains the individual phases are less distinct than they are later, and the full sequence of phases is not typically observed until day 14. Both phase sequence completion and perfection of individual strokes occur together over the first two weeks of life. Such observations indicate that movement development can occur simultaneously across several levels of organization. This in turn offers rich opportunities to relate data at the level of brain maturation with data on overt movement expression.

MOVEMENT SYSTEM EPIGENESIS

As with all developmental events, the emergence of movement patterns during ontogeny results from a still poorly understood interplay between genetic variables, experience, and opportunities for expression.[2-4,16] Both central and peripheral processes work together in movement production, as do specific regions of the brain. It is often impossible to disentangle these interlocking contributions entirely, but individual contributions can be evaluated and then synthesized together. The comparative approach to movement allows one to examine genetic distinctions between similarly reared animals, and also to trace changes in movement phenotypes under different conditions across time. Recent advances in studies of genetically altered brain structure and function offer the opportunity to relate developmental time tables in cellular, circuit and behavioral terms.

Attempts to relate issues of movement ontogeny to brain function represent an important area that has still received remarkably little attention. Neurological mutant mice provide one way to investigate these issues. Many mutant mice have single gene recessive mutations that affect specific cell types in particular brain regions, the developmental history of which has now been documented in detail.[31] One such mouse is weaver (wv/wv), a single gene mutation that in the homozygous state results in deficiencies in cerebellar Purkinje, granule, and Bergmann glia cells,[32-36] as well as dopaminergic deficits including loss of midbrain dopamine neurons and reduced dopamine uptake and levels in the striatum.[37-42] As some of these deficits appear very early in postnatal development it is important to explore the emergence of related movement abnormalities during the same time period. Over the past few years we have developed a battery of movement tests that permit the early detection and separation of these CNS degenerative disorders.

The two motor patterns examined in our recent research are grooming and swimming. As indicated previously, grooming has been examined extensively in rodents. Swimming has also been examined in mice and rats and is frequently used as an assay of CNS function and dysfunction.[12,43,44] One value of swimming for ontogenetic studies is that buoyancy provided by water allows newborn animals to exhibit cyclical movements of the four limbs without the impediment of full gravitational force. Grooming was measured both before and after swimming, thus swimming also serves as a source of grooming activation during the post-swim period. In the first phase each individual mouse was placed into a warmed circular glass container for 150 seconds and allowed to groom at will. During the next phase, the mouse was placed into a partitioned aquarium maintained at 38 ± 2°C and allowed to swim for a maximum of 30 seconds. While swimming, the mouse was supported by a rubber band around its midsection to keep the head above water while at the same time not restricting limb movement. It also allowed us to hold the mouse in a fixed position with respect to the video camera used to collect data (shutter speed 1/2000 second and film speed of 30 fps). The supported swimming technique also enabled us to study the swimming behavior of very young mice (postnatal day 3) making our procedure useful for the entire preweaning period.

Video frames were digitized with Peak Performance Technologies software, which subdivides each frame into two component pictures (resulting in 60 pictures per second). For each picture a manual digitization of the points of interest on the animal's body was necessary, which in our case included limb joints (i.e., shoulder, hip, knee) and the end points of limbs (i.e., paw). The digital picture was displayed along with a cross-hair cursor which was controlled by a computer mouse. Using the mouse, the points were selected and stored as "X-Y" coordinates in a data file. The data were scaled and then filtered using a fourth order, zero-lag Butterworth digital filter. A cutoff value of 21 was used for the filtering process due to the high frequency of the limb movements. Software was used to calculate displacements, velocities, accelerations, angular velocities and angular accelerations. Data were then displayed as stick figures (Figs. 6.1 and 6.2), trajectories of particular points (Fig. 6.3), or as parameter graphs (Fig. 6.4). Figures 6.1-6.4 illustrate typical examples of swimming and grooming movements from weaver control and mutant (wv/wv) mice.

Stick figure reconstructions of swimming in an 11-day old control (Panel A) and a same-age mutant (wv/wv) mouse (Panel B) are illustrated in Figure 6.1. Stick figure representations of grooming postures are shown in Figure 6.2 for a 15-day-old control (Panel A) and a same-age mutant (wv/wv) mouse (Panel B). These stick figures are obtained by overlapping several frames, and help the observer visualize the characteristically more jagged and less regularly coordinated movements in the mutant animals.

Swimming trajectory reconstructions for the left forepaw and hindpaws of an 11-day-old control and a same-age (wv/wv) mouse indicate the relatively "jagged" or "irregular" nature of paw movements in the mutant animal as compared with the control. The larger ellipses of the mutant's paws also suggest a less efficient swimming style for this animal. In Figure 6.4 resultant displacement and velocity, plotted against time, of the movement of the left forepaw and left hindpaw

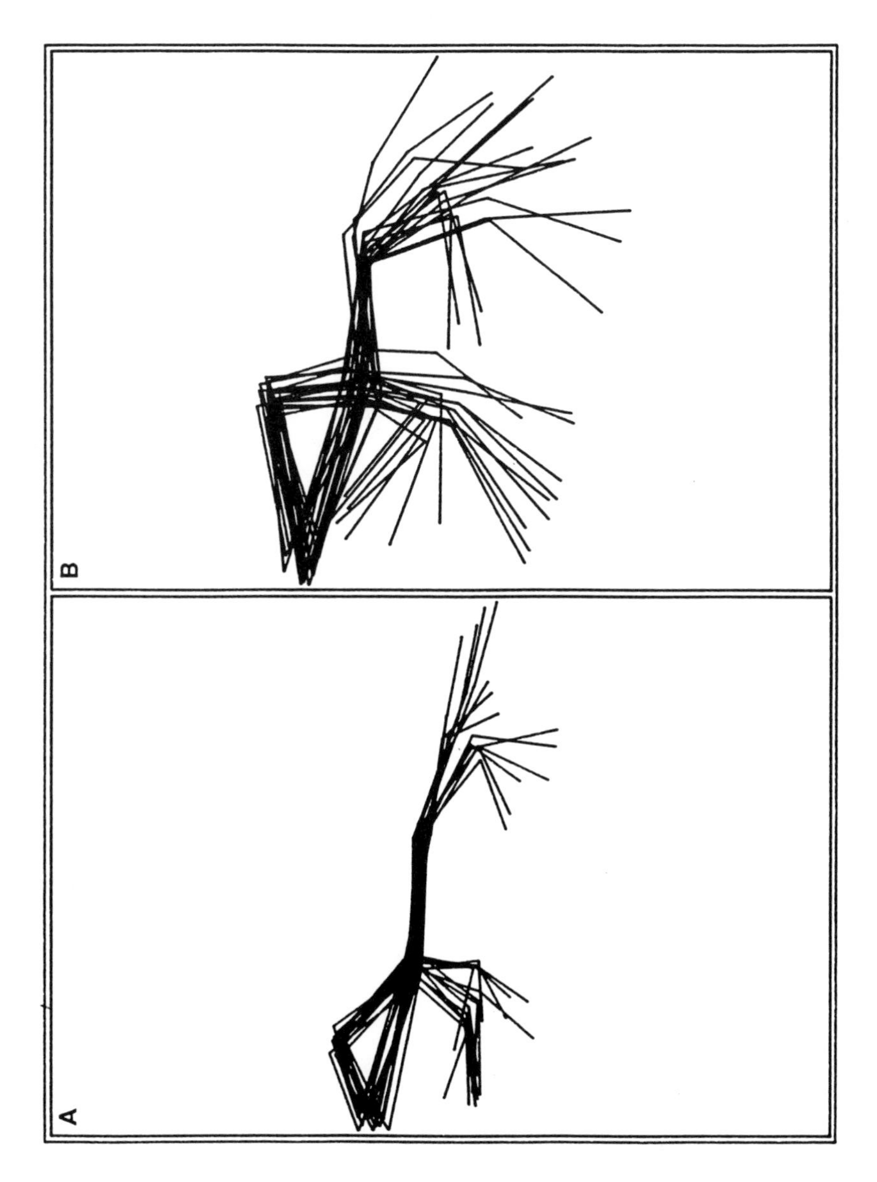

Fig. 6.1. Stick figure representations of swimming 11-day-old control (Panel A) and wv/wv (Panel B) mice.

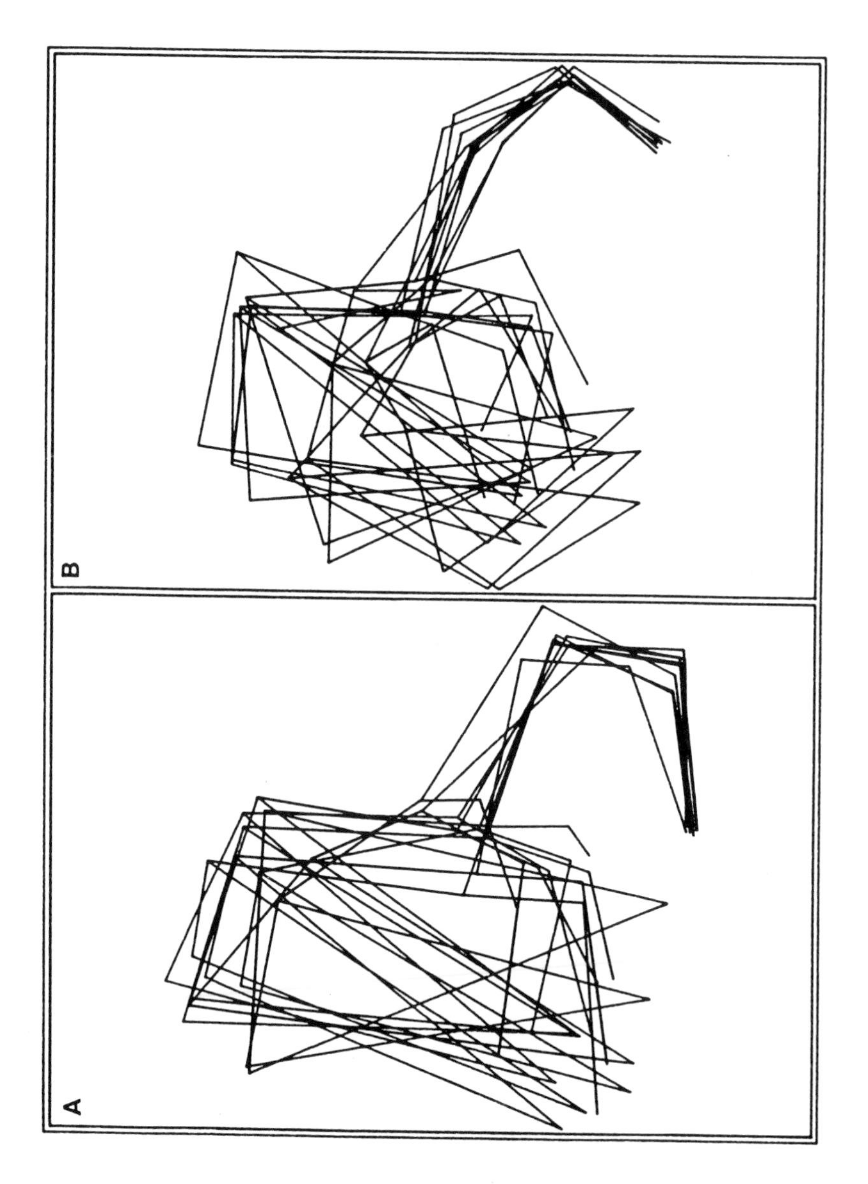

Fig. 6.2. Stick figure representations of grooming in 15-day-old control (Panel A) and wv/wv (Panel B) mice.

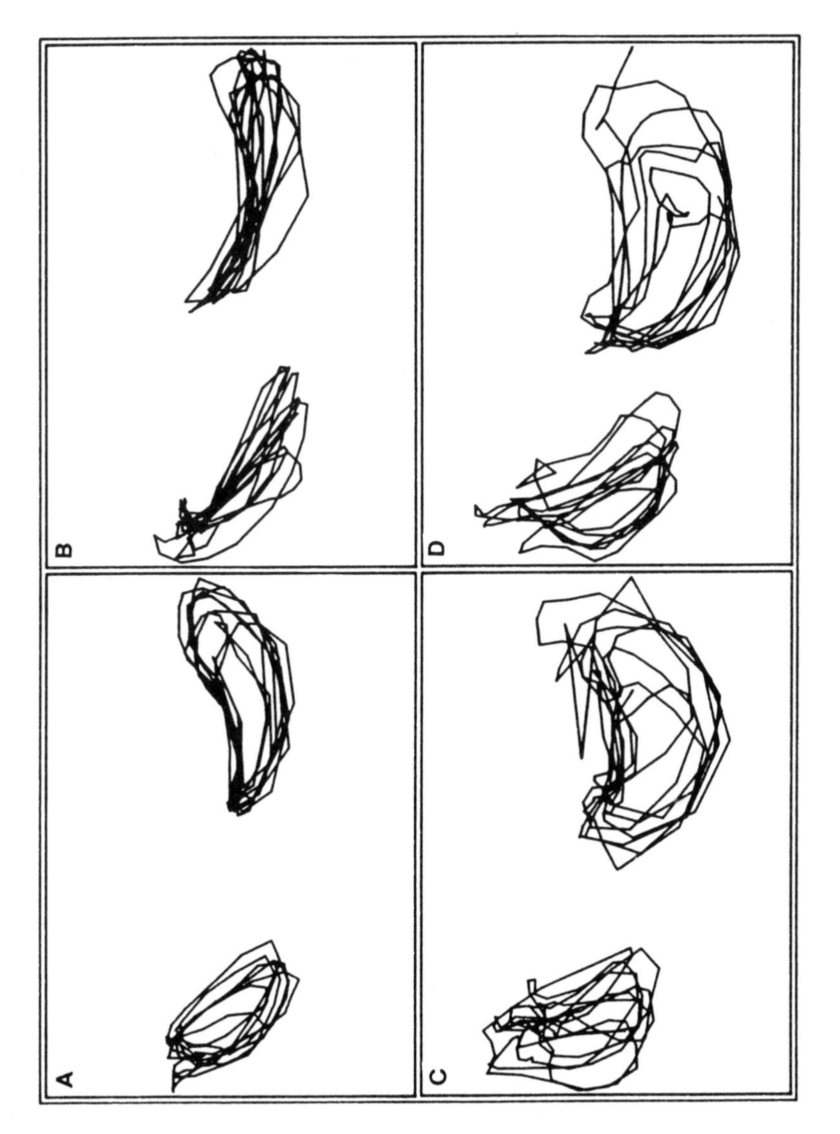

Fig. 6.3. Left forepaw and hindpaw trajectories of swimming movements in 11-day-old control (Panels A and B) and wv/wv (Panels C and D) mice.

for both animals is depicted. For both mutant and control, the relationship between stroke cycle and velocity at this age can be summarized as follows: (i) maximum velocities are attained shortly after the beginning of the stroke cycle; (ii) secondary velocity peaks occur close to the end of stroke cycles; and (iii) minimum velocities are attained at the transition between stroke cycles and at the midpoint of stroke cycles.

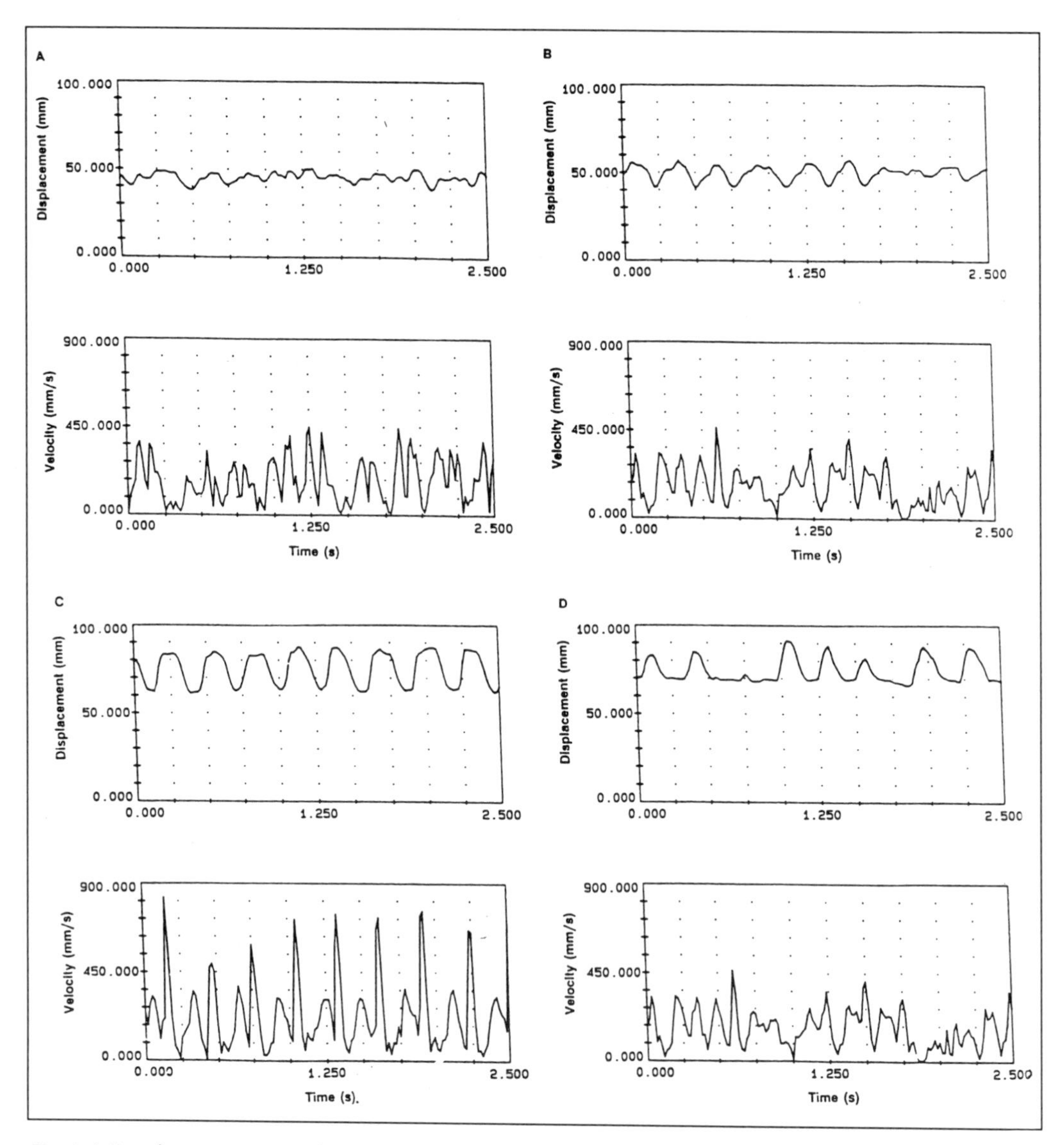

Fig. 6.4. Resultant position and velocity, plotted against time during swimming for the left forepaw (Panel A) and left hindpaw (Panel C) of an 11-day-old control mouse and for the left forepaw (Panel B) and left hindpaw (Panel D) of an 11-day-old wv/wv mouse.

Note that the mutant animal's forepaw moves more and displays more consistent velocity cycles during swimming than the control. The control mouse of the same age uses its frontlimbs only occasionally, whereas its hindlimbs provide the major propulsive thrust for swimming. This illustrates a developmental lag on the part of the mutant. In both mice[12] and rats[44] use of the forepaws in swimming precedes regular use of the hindpaws, at which time forepaw use becomes irregular and then disappears altogether. This developmental sequence is useful in reminding us that ontogeny consists not just of new actions being added, but also of early forms of behavior being replaced.[2,4,16] The data also suggest that in addition to various facets of motor coordination, the weaver mutation can affect the time course of development.

Interestingly, in spite of early signs of CNS degeneration in cerebellum (granule and Purkinje cells) and striatum (dopamine deficiency), early behavioral studies on the weaver mouse have suggested that abnormalities are not detectable until 10-14 days after birth.[45] Part of this conclusion may derive from lack of sufficiently sensitive measures. In a detailed study of the ontogeny of swimming behavior, Bolivar et al[8] examined weaver mice from postnatal day 3 to 19. Mutant mice displayed a developmental lag in terms of swimming style in comparison to controls, and also displayed a generalized slowness in limb movements during swimming. This slowness correlated with the developmental onset of use of a particular limb during the swim. Distinctions between control and wv/wv mice could be traced from as early as postnatal day 3 for stroke cycle duration and stroke latency of limbs. Thus careful dissection of both individual limb movement parameters and comparisons across limbs allowed a much earlier detection of mutant gene effects than had previously been possible.[8]

Coscia and Fentress[46] demonstrated that multiple measures of grooming, such as bout number versus bout duration, can clarify early distinctions between control and wv/wv mice after a swimming task. They also showed that mutant mice would often support themselves during grooming, and continue to increase both the number and duration of grooming bouts after other signs of motor ataxia became apparent. This indicates that different classes of motor action, such as grooming versus locomotion, can differentially reflect degenerative disorders of the nervous system.

Distinctions between mutant and control animals during grooming behavior proved to be measurement, age, and context specific.[6] For time spent grooming, mutants can reach the grooming levels of control mice pre-swim after day 13 even though overall wv/wv mice spent less time grooming than did controls. The mutant animals also showed an increase in the number of grooming bouts post-swim relative to pre-swim from day 15—a fact that illustrates movement deficits can result from activational deficits; i.e. impoverished movement does not necessarily reflect an animal's maximum ability. By examining grooming sequences for their stroke types, it was also found that wv/wv mice frequently failed to display strokes used in later sequence phases by control mice. Both the activational effects and loss of sequential integrity of grooming correspond to experimentally produced striatal deficits,[15,30] and contrast with deficits in fine motor control more commonly associated with cerebellar disorders.[47,48] Thus, careful dissection of movement during development may in principle be used to distinguish the contribution of mutant genes to more than one brain structure.

There are numerous opportunities for future experimentation to elaborate upon these descriptive findings. For example, chimera mice can be constructed that are composed of variable mixtures of mutant and normal cell populations.[49,50] Selective CNS lesions and pharmacological treatments[17] can be applied to litter-mate control animals in an attempt to mimic specific consequences of the mutant gene, and it may prove possible to provide selective methods for "rescuing" genetically compromised CNS function as has been done experimentally in conjunction with the application of teratological agents.[51]

CONCLUSIONS

In this chapter we have surveyed several types of movement analysis that can be applied within a developmental context. In doing so, we have tried to argue that no one movement recording system is necessarily "best" for all purposes. We have also tried to argue that development provides a method of natural dissection in movement, including its spatial, temporal and sequential properties. New techniques, such as those involving mutant mice, offer considerable potential for linking epigenetic substrates to normal and abnormal movement control. These mutant animals also permit one to examine brain and behavior in an animal that, through degeneration, is becoming progressively "disassembled." Independent experimental manipulations of both the mutant and control individuals can help bridge developmental analyses with many other branches of the movement system literature. This promise will only be fulfilled, however, if care is taken to describe and classify movement at its various levels and across its various contexts of expression.

Obviously the value of mutant mice or any other single model depends upon the specific issues one wishes to address. At the same time we have tried to show that there are also more general issues in movement and its ontogeny that transcend any particular model system. One issue is how to deal with both separable and combined properties of movement as these change over different temporal dimensions including ontogeny. Clarification of these diverse dynamic principles may clarify how underlying movement and developmental systems achieve their adaptive balance between intrinsic organization and sensitivity to contextual influences.

ACKNOWLEDGMENTS

The authors thank Peter Ossenkopp for giving us the opportunity to contribute to this book. We also thank Wanda Danilchuk for her invaluable help in preparing the final version and Kevin Manley for his technical assistance with the "Peak" system and for producing the "Peak" figures. This research has been supported by grants to J.C.F. from the Medical Research Council of Canada and the Natural Sciences and Engineering Research Council of Canada.

REFERENCES

1. Fentress JC. Emergence of pattern in the development of mammalian movement sequences. J Neurobiol 1992; 23(10):1529-1556.
2. Fentress JC, McLeod PJ. Motor patterns in development. In: Blass EM, ed. Handbook of behavioral neurobiology. Vol 8. Developmental processes in psychobiology and neurobiology. New York: Plenum Press, 1986:35-97.
3. Fentress JC, McLeod PJ. Pattern construction in behavior. In: Smotherman WP, Robinson SR, eds. Behavior of the fetus. Caldwell, NJ: Telford Press, 1988: 63-76.
4. Smotherman WP, Robinson SR. The development of behavior before birth. Dev Psychol, in press.
5. Fentress JC. The role of timing in motor development. In: Fagard J, Wolff PH, eds. The development of timing control and temporal organization in coordinated action. Elsevier Science Publishers B.V. (North-Holland), 1991:341-366.
6. Bolivar VJ, Danilchuk W, Fentress JC. Separation of activation and pattern in grooming development of weaver mice. Behav Brain Res (in press).
7. Alkon DL, Blackwell KT, Barbour GS et al. Pattern-recognition by an artificial network derived from biologic neuronal systems. Biol Cybern 1990; 62:363-76.
8. Bolivar VJ, Manley K, Fentress JC. The development of swimming behavior in the neurological mutant weaver mouse. Dev Psychobiol (in press).
9. Hinde RA. Animal behavior: A synthesis of ethology and comparative psychology. 2nd ed. New York: McGraw-Hill, 1970.
10. Lashley KS. The problem of serial order in behavior. In: Jeffries LA, ed. Cerebral mechanisms in behavior. New York: John Wiley & Sons, 1951:112-136.
11. Bernstein N. The co-ordination and regulation of movements. New York: Pergamon Press, 1967.
12. Fentress JC. Development and patterning of movement sequences in inbred mice. In: Kiger J, ed. The biology of behavior. Corvallis: Oregon State University Press, 1972:83-131.
13. Fentress JC. Organizational patterns in action: Local and global issues in action pattern formation. In: Edelman GM, Gall WE, Cowan WM, eds. Signal and sense: local and global order in perceptual maps. New York: Wiley-Liss, 1990:357-382.

14. Fentress JC, Stilwell FP. Grammar of a movement sequence in inbred mice. Nature 1973; 244:52-53.
15. Berridge KC, Fentress JC. Disruption of natural grooming chains after striatopallidal lesions. Psychobiol 1987; 15(4):336-342.
16. Smith LB, Thelen E, eds. A dynamic systems approach to development. Cambridge, MA: The MIT Press, 1993.
17. Berridge KC. The development of action patterns. In: Hogan JA, Bolhuis JJ, eds. Causal mechanisms of behavioural development. New York: Cambridge University Press, 1994:147-80.
18. Golani I. Homeostatic motor processes in mammalian interactions: a choreography of display. In: Bateson PPG, Klopfer PH, eds. Perspectives in ethology. Vol. 2. New York: Plenum Press, 1976:69-134.
19. Golani I. A mobility gradient in the organization of vertebrate movement: The perception of movement through symbolic language. Behav Brain Sci 1992; 15:249-308.
20. Golani I, Fentress JC. Early ontogeny of face grooming in mice. Dev Psychobiol 1985; 18:529-544.
21. Richmond G, Sachs BD. Grooming in Norway rats: the development and adult expression of a complex motor pattern. Behav 1980; 75:82-96.
22. Berridge KC, Fentress JC, Parr H. Natural syntax rules control action sequence of rats. Behav Brain Res 1987; 23:59-68.
23. Eshkol N, Wachmann A. Movement notation. London: Weidenfeld & Nicholson, 1958.
24. Smotherman WP, Robinson SR. The prenatal origins of behavioral organization. Psychol Sci 1990; 1:97-106.
25. Fentress JC. The development of coordination. J Motor Behav 1984; 16:99-134.
26. Fentress JC. Expressive contexts, fine structure, and central mediation of rodent grooming. Ann NY Acad Sci 1988; 525:18-26.
27. Fentress JC. Specific and non-specific factors in the causation of behavior. In: Bateson PPG, Klopfer P, eds. Perspectives in ethology. New York: Plenum Press, 1973:155-255.
28. Berridge KC, Fentress JC. Contextual control of trigeminal sensorimotor function. J Neurosci 1986; 6:325-330.
29. Berridge KC, Fentress JC. Deafferentation does not disrupt natural rules of action syntax. Behav Brain Res 1987; 23:69-76.
30. Berridge KC, Whishaw IQ. Cortex, striatum and cerebellum: control of serial order in a grooming sequence. Exp Brain Res 1992; 90:275-90.
31. Lyon MF, Searle AG. Genetic variants and strains of the laboratory mouse. Oxford: Oxford University Press, 1989.
32. Blatt GJ, Eisenman LM. A qualitative and quantitative light microscopic study of the inferior olivary complex of normal, reeler, and weaver mutant mice. J Comp Neurol 1985; 232:117-128.
33. Hirano A, Dembitzer HM. Cerebellar alterations in the weaver mouse. J Cell Biol 1973; 56:478-486.

34. Rakic P, Sidman RL. Sequence of developmental abnormalities leading to granule cell deficit in cerebellar cortex of weaver mutant mice. J Comp Neurol 1973; 152:103-132.
35. Rakic P, Sidman RL. Weaver mutant mouse cerebellum: defective neuronal migration secondary to abnormality of Bergmann glia. Proc Natl Acad Sci 1973; 70:240-244.
36. Smeyne RJ, Goldowitz D. Development and death of external granular layer cells in the weaver mutant cerebellum: a quantitative study. J Neurosci 1989; 9:1608-1620.
37. Simon JR, Ghetti B. Topographic distribution of dopamine uptake, choline uptake, choline acetyltransferase, and GABA uptake in the striata of weaver mutant mice. Neurochem Res 1992; 17:431-436.
38. Richter JA, Stotz EH, Ghetti B et al. Comparison of alterations in tyrosine hydroxylase, dopamine levels, and dopamine uptake in the striatum of the weaver mutant mouse. Neurochem Res 1992; 17:437-441.
39. Schmidt MJ, Sawyer BD, Perry KW et al. Dopamine deficiency in the weaver mutant mouse. J Neurosci 1982; 2:376-380.
40. Roffler-Tarlov S, Graybiel AM. Weaver mutation has differential effects on the dopamine-containing innervation of the limbic and nonlimbic striatum. Nature 1984; 307:62-66.
41. Roffler-Tarlov S, Graybiel AM. Expression of the weaver gene in dopamine-containing neural systems is dose-dependent and affects both striatal and nonstriatal regions. J Neurosci 1986; 6:3319-3330.
42. Triarhou LC, Norton J, Ghetti B. Mesencephalic dopamine cell deficit involves areas A8, A9 and A10 in weaver mutant mice. Exp Brain Res 1988; 70:256-265.
43. Schapiro S, Salas M, Vukovich K. Hormonal effects on ontogeny of swimming ability in the rat: assessment of central nervous system development. Sci 1970; 168:147-151.
44. Bekoff A, Trainer W. The development of interlimb coordination during swimming in postnatal rats. J Exp Biol 1979; 83:1-11.
45. Simon JR, Richter JA, Ghetti B. Age-dependent alterations in dopamine content, tyrosine hydroxylase activity, and dopamine uptake in the striatum of the weaver mutant mouse. J Neurochem 1994; 62:543-548.
46. Coscia EM & Fentress JC. Neurological dysfunction expressed in the grooming behavior of developing weaver mutant mice. Behav Gen 1993; 23(6):533-541.
47. Weiner WJ, Lang AE. Movement disorders: a comprehensive survey. New York: Futura Publishing Company, 1989.
48. Thach WT, Goodkin HP, Keating JG. The cerebellum and the adaptive coordination of movement. Ann Rev Neurosci 1992; 15:403-442.
49. Goldowitz D, Eisenman LM. Genetic mutations affecting murine cerebellar structure and function. In: Driscoll P, ed. Genetically defined animal models of neurobehavioral dysfunctions. Boston: Birkhauser, 1992:66-88.

50. Goldowitz D, Moran TH, Wetts R. Mouse chimeras in the study of genetic and structural determinants of behavior. In: Goldowitz D, Wahlsten D, Wimer RE, eds. Techniques for the genetic analysis of brain and behavior. Amsterdam: Elsevier Science Publishers, 1992:271-290.
51. Tatton WG, Greenwood CE. Rescue of dying neurons: A new action for deprenyl in MPTP Parkinsonism. J Neuroscience Res 1991; 30:666-672.

CHAPTER 7

Righting and the Modular Organization of Motor Programs

Sergio M. Pellis

INTRODUCTION

Righting is a postural support behavior that is fundamental to the performance of other motor behaviors such as standing and locomotion.[1] Under normal circumstances, our ability to gain or maintain an upright posture is automatic, and we take it for granted. The importance of this seemingly simple, reflexive activity only becomes evident when this behavior is impaired by disease.[2] For example, as some Parkinsonian patients have a specific loss of normal righting behavior, getting out of bed becomes a major chore.[3] Given the importance of righting, surprisingly little is known about the neural systems that regulate this behavior, although the ability to regain an upright posture is thought to involve a midbrain center that is responsive to information about the position of the head and perhaps also to information concerning the center of gravity of the whole body. This requires "the integration of afferent signals from a variety of sensors located in different parts of the body" (Ito, ref. 4, p. 516). In this chapter, I will show that the kinds of neural circuits to be looked for are influenced by the physiological models we develop from our descriptions of the behavior. For instance, by referring to righting as a reflex, as is often done,[4-6] one makes particular assumptions about the underlying neural organization. Firstly, it assumes that it is a unitary response which can be triggered by multiple sensory inputs; and secondly, it assumes there is a particular relationship between the stimuli and the response. This review will illustrate that righting is composed of a cluster of relatively independent sen-

Measuring Movement and Locomotion: From Invertebrates to Humans, edited by Klaus-Peter Ossenkopp, Martin Kavaliers and Paul R. Sanberg.

sorimotor patterns. Furthermore, righting will be shown to be more like a motor program, where multiple motor elements are combined in slightly different ways so as to produce a flexible, adaptive response.

THE CLASSICAL MODEL

Righting involves turning the head and body from a recumbent position to prone. The classic work of Magnus,[5] Rademaker[7] and others has shown that righting can be triggered independently by several different sensory modalities. The terminology adopted by these researchers is still widely used and descriptively incorporates both the sensory input that triggers the righting and the part of the body that rights.[6,8,9]

Two forms of tactile righting were identified by Magnus and his coworkers; both involved asymmetrical tactile input on the body. One triggers the righting of the body, usually the hindquarters, and is termed body-on-body righting. The other triggers righting of the head and is termed body-on-head righting.[10] The third known form of tactile righting was demonstrated more recently by Troiani et al.[11] This involves contact on the face (i.e., trigeminal nerve) which triggers rotation of the head and neck towards prone, and is referred to as trigeminal-on-head righting, or more simply, trigeminal righting. Body-on-body and body-on-head righting systems have been widely documented in a variety of mammalian species including cats, dogs, primates, guinea pigs[5,7] and rats.[12,13] Trigeminal righting was originally documented for guinea pigs,[11] and was subsequently observed in adult and infant rats,[12,13] and in the marsupial cat, *Dasyurus hallucatus*.[14]

Vestibular righting involves righting the head to the normal prone position from some abnormal orientation.[10] However, this vestibular-on-head righting system may involve distinct systems, depending on the initial orientation of the head. If the subject is held supine, the vestibular apparatus on each side of the head receives equal stimulation, and so the resulting head righting is referred to as symmetrical vestibular righting.[6] An animal held by the pelvis laterally in the air will also right the head to prone. In this case, however, the vestibular apparatus on the side facing the ground receives different stimulation to that on the side facing skyward; this is referred to as asymmetrical vestibular righting.[6] In altricial mammals, these both mature early postnatally; for example, in humans, these mature in the first 6 months of postnatal life.[15] We found that in rats, a response to asymmetrical stimulation was earlier and of a stronger intensity than the response to symmetrical stimulation.[13] In the more immature young of *Dasyurus*, asymmetrical righting matures up to 10 days earlier than the symmetrical.[14] This developmental dissociation suggests that vestibular righting from an abnormal stationary position may be composed of two independent systems—symmetrical and asymmetrical.

Righting can also be triggered visually in some species.[5,10] That is, visual stimuli can trigger the righting of the head when inverted. However, such righting only appears to occur in species with well-developed visual cortical systems, such as cats and monkeys.[5] Rats cannot use vision to trigger righting[16] but can, as do cats,[17-19] modulate the onset and speed of vestibularly triggered air-righting.[20] This modulating function is controlled subcortically, involving the superior colliculus.[21]

During air-righting, vestibular (or visual) righting occurs in the absence of tactile righting systems, and thus provides a simpler basis for a descriptive model of how righting occurs. "The typical course of falling in air in a normal cat, as determined from pictures which Magnus himself has taken and reproduced, involves a series of stages including the following: First, the animal falls for a short distance through the air back down. The head then begins to turn while the rest of the body remains undisturbed. When the head has turned through 90° the thorax begins to turn, the hind portion of the body still remaining immobile. Soon, however, this rear portion begins to turn, and finally the body is completely re-oriented, so that the animal lands on all four legs." (Carmichael, ref. 22, p. 455). Basically, the model established by Magnus involves the concept of a chain-reflex,[23] where the action of one reflex creates the appropriate stimuli for triggering the next. In this case, the vestibular reflex triggers cervical righting, which in turn triggers rotation of the rest of the body.[24] This model is summarized in Figure 7.1. It shows that there is a common set of body movements that can be triggered independently by diverse sensory modalities. The only one that differs is body-on-body which has the reverse direction in the sequencing of body movements. Nonethe-

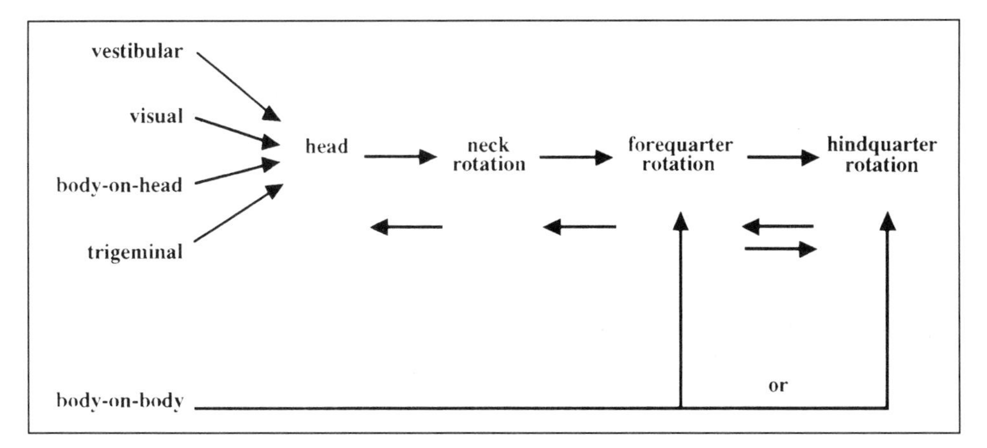

Fig. 7.1. The traditional model for righting is summarized schematically. That is, all sensory modalities (except body-on-body) trigger cephalocaudal rotation. Body-on-body is an exception in that the body is triggered to right first, which then results in the recruitment of the head and neck. Some species' differences should also be noted. In cats[5] and rats,[12] body-on-body commences with righting by the hindquarters, whereas in monkeys[6] and some ungulates,[9] it commences with the forequarters. Also, only mammals with a well-developed visual cortex, such as cats and monkeys, can trigger righting visually.[5]

less, this model suggests that righting is a reflex that can be triggered by multiple sensory inputs.

Such a model makes certain predictions about how the nervous system works and directs the search for neural mechanisms in particular ways. I shall now present evidence that suggests righting is not a reflex and does not involve motor responses of equal access to all sensory modalities.

IS RIGHTING A REFLEX OR A PROGRAM?

Adult rats, unlike adult cats, do not rotate the head and neck independently of the shoulders during righting.[25-27] Therefore, in rats, vestibularly- or body tactually-triggered righting does not require the action of the neck-righting reflex to trigger shoulder rotation—thus bypassing one link in the chain of this chain-reflex. However, Magnus[5] did provide experimental evidence for such a mechanism. That is, if the head and neck of a cat held by the pelvis is rotated by the experimenter, then the shoulders are recruited, and also rotate. That this is true for a bilabyrinthectomized and blind-folded cat shows that the shoulder recruitment is via the cervical righting reflex. Clearly, neck rotation is sufficient to recruit shoulder rotation. In the adult rat, however, such cervical righting is not necessary to recruit the shoulders during unrestrained righting. One possibility is that in cats, the mechanism is as described by Magnus, whereas in rats it is different, with the mid-brain righting mechanisms having direct connections to the shoulders, rather than indirectly via the neck.

An alternative possibility is suggested by a developmental study of the rat by Laouris et al.[28] They analyzed the development of air righting in rats tested with a harness that prevented independent head, neck and shoulder rotation, and compared them with rats which were unrestrained. If the shoulder rotation during air righting in infant rats were actually caused by the preceding head and neck rotation, one would expect that in a harness that prevents independent head and neck rotation, independent shoulder rotation should clearly be delayed. However, in the unrestrained rats, head and neck rotation occurred as early as about 5 days; and shoulder rotation, following head and neck rotation, occurred by about day 7. In the harnessed infants, shoulder rotation also commenced at day 7, suggesting that the developmental onset of shoulder rotation may not depend upon the cervical righting reflex. Therefore, for the rat, there is no independent evidence for shoulder rotation being recruited via the cervical righting reflex when falling supine in the air. Cervical rotation occurs during trigeminal righting throughout this early developmental period,[13] and into adulthood.[12] In order to verify that in such instances (on the ground) neck rotation is necessary for the recruitment of shoulder rotation, a harness that blocks independent head, neck and shoulder rotation, as used by Laouris et al[28] would be necessary. The same reasoning applies to the supposed recruitment of the shoulders by neck rotation that is found in cats.

Even if cats use the cervical righting reflex to recruit shoulder rotation during air-righting, the movements of the head, neck and shoulders during righting suggest that there is a physiological mechanism not accounted for by the classical model. The traditional description by Magnus[5] of righting while falling involves a spiral movement around the longitudinal axis starting with the head and neck, followed by the shoulders, and finally the pelvis. A detailed modern description of the ontogeny of air-righting by rabbits confirms this view[29]—the head and neck rotate, followed by the shoulders catching up with the head. In Figure 7.2, using a simplified version of the Eshkol-Wachman movement notation system (EWMNS),[30] the incompleteness of this description is revealed. In brief, EWMNS is designed to express the relations and changes in the relation between the parts of the body. The body is treated as a system of articulated axes (i.e., body and limb segments). A limb is any part of the body which either lies between two joints or has a joint and a free extremity. These are imagined as straight lines (axes) of constant length which move with one end fixed to the center of a sphere (see ref. 31, and references therein).

In Figure 7.2A, the head and neck rotate 90° (or 2 units in EWMNS); this is then followed by a forequarter rotation, in the same direction, for 180°. However, if the head does nothing, it will be passively carried further around by the motion of the shoulders. That is, even after ceasing its own movement, the head travels another 180° due to the rotation of the shoulders. Thus, if the head continues to rotate, albeit slowly, or ceases to rotate on its own, it is impossible for the shoulders to catch up, since their movement will always be added to that of the head. Since the shoulders do 'catch up' with the head, the necessary revision is illustrated in Figure 7.2B. After making its 90° rotation to the right, the head has to rotate actively in the opposite direction to counteract the equal and opposite movement by the shoulders. Thus only by actively rotating to the left will the head remain in the same place, which will enable the shoulders to catch-up. Then as the shoulders continue to rotate, both they and the head will achieve the fully righted position. This second neck rotation does not stimulate the cervical righting reflex, for if it did so, the shoulders would flip from right to left and back again. In order to maintain the chain reflex model, an inhibitory control over the cervical righting reflex is needed for this second neck movement. An analysis of the pelvic rotation that follows and catches up to the shoulders reveals a similar problem (i.e., a hitherto undescribed counter rotation by the shoulders), and thus the need for a similar solution.

The above analyses reveal that righting can involve the bypassing of steps (i.e. direct shoulder-led rotation), and must include oscillatory, rather than unidirectional movements by the head-neck and shoulders. Such modifications weaken the explanatory simplicity of the chain-reflex model. In my view, the behavior of the tail during air-righting completely invalidates this model. The movements of the tail became apparent to me when we made high speed films (500 and 1000 frame/s) of air-righting by rats.[27] These films showed that as the rat's shoulders began to rotate to one side, the tail began to rotate to the opposite side. If the chain-reflex model were correct, such tail movement should not occur until pelvic rotation has commenced. The biomechanical utility of this tail movement further illustrates the inadequacy of the

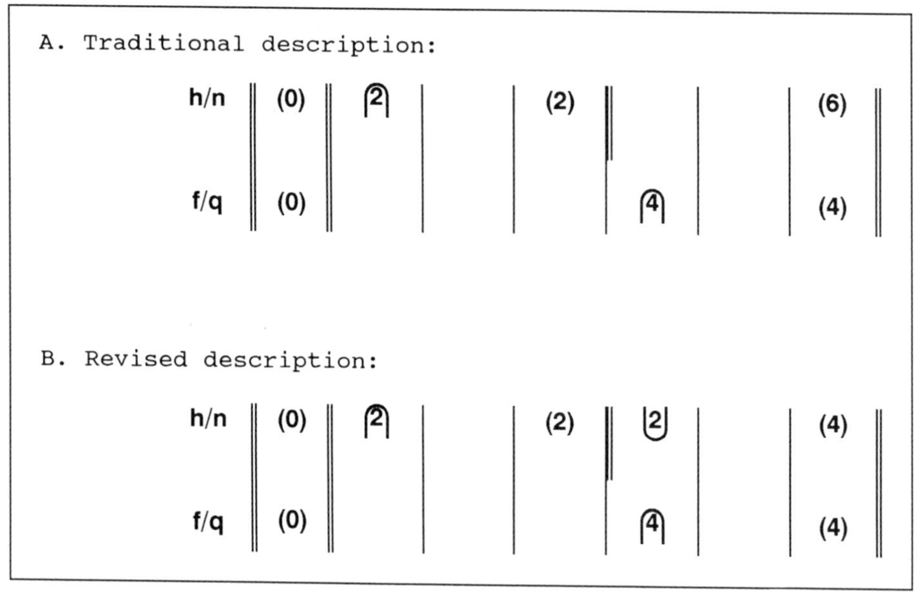

Fig. 7.2. The kinematic pattern of righting movements between the head, neck and shoulders during air-righting is illustrated using the Eshkol-Wachman movement notation. The head and neck (h/n) are shown as a unit, as are the forequarters (f/q). The numbers in parentheses represent the position of the respective body parts. Imagine that the top of head is labelled 4, the ventral surface labelled 0, the right surface 2 and the left surface 6. These numbers represent points about 90° apart from one another, so that intermediate points would be labelled 1, 3, 5 and 7. In this way, each unit of movement is approximated to the nearest 45°, and this is shown by the numbers inside the signs for this type of movement. Rotation around the longitudinal axis is represented by ∪ for negative movements, and by ∩ for positive movements. The viewpoint for seeing changes in the rotation of the body parts is directly from above. Thus if this top view sees a change from facing the ventrum to the right side, then this is shown as that body part going from (0) to (2). Furthermore, a positive movement is so designated if the numbers increase (i.e. 0 to 1 to 2); if the numbers decrease (0 to 7 to 6 to 5 to ... 2) then it is a negative movement. The columns represent units of time (e.g. video frames), the two sets of double bar lines encompassing the first column represents the position of the body parts prior to any movement. The double bar lines in other columns represent the end of movement. In A, the traditional description is translated into notated form, and in B, the revised description represented. Note that in A, the head turns further around than the shoulders, whereas in B, a counterrotation of the head and neck is introduced to re-align the head and forequarters, matching the actual behavior observed. See text.

chain-reflex model. The most common explanation takes into account the moments of inertia of the body parts that interact when an angular action is initiated. Thus, for the forequarters to rotate to the right, the hindquarters must rotate to the left. Of course, differences in the relative mass of the body parts influence the degree of counterrotation needed.[32] In rats, the heavy tail probably provides a considerable counterrotatory force for the forequarters to act upon. Therefore, the act of air-righting appears more like a programmed act than a chain-reflex, with different body parts simultaneously activated, not sequentially recruited.

MULTIPLE ACCESS PROGRAM OR MULTIPLE MODULES?

Even if the organization of righting is better described as a motor program rather than as a reflex, the classical model would not be rejected in its entirety. Different sensory modalities could still trigger the onset of the same response. That is, righting could still be one behavior pattern, albeit variable, that is activated by any one of several sensory inputs (Fig. 7.1). Several lines of evidence, however, suggest that righting is not one behavior pattern, but several distinct righting programs.

Movement Patterns

Righting triggered by different sensory modalities involves qualitative differences in the pattern of the movements used. Symmetrical vestibular righting, as noted above, involves cephalocaudal axial rotation, which in infancy begins with the head and neck and ends with the pelvis. In species such as cats, vestibular righting continues to be led by the head and neck into adulthood.[5,19] In rats[13,27,28] and many other small mammals (Pellis and Pellis, unpublished observations), vestibular righting begins with the axial rotation of the shoulders and then the pelvis. The head and neck are thus passively carried to prone by shoulder rotation.[27] Asymmetrical vestibular righting involves rotation of the head and neck to prone.[6] In addition, during development, infant rats appear to undergo a transitional phase in which the head is raised skyward.[13] At first, the head raises vertically and remains there. Later, the head rotates to prone after first lifting skyward. Finally, the head, neck and shoulders directly rotate to prone without the initial skyward movement.[14] Trigeminal righting also involves a cephalocaudal axial rotation which begins with head and neck rotation. For both rats[12,13] and guinea pigs,[11] the anterior portion of the head and face maintains contact with the ground throughout the act of trigeminal righting (see Figure 2 in ref. 14). Such continuous contact with the ground makes trigeminal righting behaviorally distinguishable from vestibular righting.

Body-on-head and body-on-body righting have three distinguishable patterns of righting. The first pattern involves the animal's limb that is closest to the ground being flexed and placed onto the ground. The limb is then extended; this flips either the shoulders or the pelvis over to prone. Simultaneously, with the flexion of one limb, the homologous limb extends. This tends to overbalance the pelvis or the shoulders, and so moves the center of gravity over the paw which has been placed on the ground. A diagnostic feature of this pattern of righting which distinguishes it from the crossed-extensor reflex[9] is that the paw is placed onto the ground and is rotated inward, with the digits facing the ventrum. Failure to maintain a grip on the ground leads the limb to extend upward and across the ventrum. The homologous paw does not rotate when extended (see Figures 4 and 9 in ref. 13). The second pattern of righting involves the flexing and placing of the paw closest to the ground onto the ground, but instead of pushing to flip the shoulders or the pelvis over to prone, active axial rotation completes the movement to prone. The third pattern involves direct rotation of either the shoulders or pelvis to prone with the limbs closest to the ground flexing to accommodate the rotation, and only placing when the body axis reaches the prone position. In *Dasyurus,* body-on-head righting matures before vestibular righting, and it is apparent that in its earliest onset, body-on-head involves head and neck rotation to prone. Only later is this replaced by a direct shoulder-led rotation.[14] That such direct shoulder-led rotation is triggered by the body-on-head righting system is demonstrated in its occurrence when righting on the ground by bilabyrinthectomized rats.[12,33]

In adult animals, body-on-body righting does not normally occur when the head is free to move; instead, vestibular, trigeminal and body-on-head righting take place.[6,10,12,26] However, body-on-body righting can be triggered if the animal's head is restrained.[10] Although in early infancy, body-on-body righting can occur in combination with the various head righting systems,[13,14,34,35] it can be studied in isolation by restraining the head. During both recovery from lateral hypothalamic damage and normal development, this righting system progresses from pushing with the limb to axial rotation triggered by placing the paw onto the ground, and finally, to independent axial rotation, which is the form typically seen in adults.[12,13] This suggests that for body-on-body, pushing with the limb is the most immature pattern of righting. For body-on-head righting, it appears that head and neck rotation precede the onset of forelimb righting movements.[14] Therefore, righting triggered by different sensory modalities does not involve a common set of body movements. Instead, the righting triggered by each sensory modality involves characteristic motor elements, or combinations of motor elements.

Context of Righting

As pointed out above, in air-righting, vestibular triggering of righting (where visual righting is not present) occurs in the absence of tactile righting systems. Air-righting, therefore, can be viewed as vestibular righting in pure form, and so can be understood as a simplified model for the study of vestibular righting. This assumption, however, underestimates the modular organization of righting behavior.

Upon recovery from anesthesia, rats with large electrolytic lesions of the lateral hypothalamus are somnolent,[36] and when gently laid onto their backs may not right themselves. When dropped supine in the air however, such rats will execute the normal righting response.[33] This may be interpreted as showing that in their somnolent state, the rats require a stronger vestibular stimulus to trigger the righting response. The development of righting on the ground and in the air suggests an alternative explanation. In ontogeny, righting on the ground develops before righting in the air.[13,14] This is not simply due to tactile righting systems having an earlier onset than vestibular righting systems but is due to there being an important difference in the types of vestibular righting involved. When placed supine on the ground, both vestibular and tactile forms of righting are triggered. To test for the presence of vestibular righting in the absence of tactile righting, the subject can be placed in a tub of warm water.[13,14,37] In the water, the subject slowly sinks to the bottom, and so does not experience the acceleratory fall when falling supine in the air. Therefore, supine placement in water provides a test for symmetrical vestibular righting, where only the labyrinths provide information about the abnormal position of the head. In rats, while some neonates show the vestibular righting response, albeit incomplete, on the day of birth, all will do so in the first 5 days.[13] In contrast, in rats, the air-righting version of vestibular righting does not begin to appear until after 5-6 days,[28] and it is only by about 14 days that they succeed in landing fully prone.[38] In *Dasyurus,* the difference in the age of onset between positional and acceleratory vestibular righting is around 15 days.[14] This developmental dissociation suggests that these two contexts for vestibular righting reflect a major difference in the underlying neural organization.

A simpler possibility is that the young rats do not have the skeletomuscular necessary means to right themselves when falling in the air. To test for this possibility, the ontogeny of air-righting in rats was compared to their righting when falling backwards from a bipedally standing position (for an illustration see Figures 11 and 12 in ref. 26). From this posture, the rats had not only proprioceptive-tactile, in addition to vestibular, information about their orientation, but also a base of support from which to gain leverage. As the age for the onset of righting from bipedal falling is about 6 days, it was more like air-righting than contact-righting.[39] The marginally earlier onset of righting or falling bipedally compared to air-righting may reflect a developmental dissociation between proprioceptive-tactile and vestibular righting from falling. Indeed, vestibular and proprioceptive-tactile righting from the bipedal position have been dissociated pharmacologically.[26] Adult rats made cataleptic with high doses of haloperidol exhibit righting from the bipedal posture whether bilabyrinthectomized or intact. When treated with morphine in addition to haloperidol, only rats with intact labyrinths can right themselves when falling from the bipedal position. Therefore, righting during falling from the bipedal position can be triggered and guided by the proprioceptive-tactile system alone or the vestibular system alone.

The difference between righting from a stationary versus a falling context is not due to differences in the sensory modalities themselves, but is due to differences in the central organization dealing with these different contexts. That is, there is a neural system that deals with righting when in an inverted stationary position, and there is another neural system that deals with righting when in an inverted falling position.

Chronology of Maturation of Righting Systems

Righting triggered by different sensory modalities has distinct chronological onsets. The general mammalian pattern appears to involve tactile systems coming on-line sooner than vestibular; these, in turn, are available sooner than visual systems. In each case, the use of these sensory modalities in static contexts emerges earlier than their use in dynamic contexts (Fig. 7.3). At this stage, inclusion of the visual systems is partly inferential. Nonetheless, it does appear that visually triggered righting in cats develops after the completion of vestibularly triggered air-righting, and visual modulation appears to mature prior to visual righting.[19] Also, a visual triggering of righting in cats has been reported in both stationary and falling contexts. In rats, the visual modulation of air-righting is not matured until early adulthood,[40] well after all other righting systems are fully developed.[13]

This order in the onset of righting systems reflects a true dissociation of these systems; it is not simply the following of the same order as the maturation of these sensory systems.[41] In *Dasyurus*, the trigeminal is functional at birth, and probably serves an important role in guiding the embryo towards the mother's pouch.[42] However, we could find no evidence of trigeminal righting until 40 days after birth, when the young were still attached to the teats.[14] Similarly, the vestibular apparatus is partly in place by birth,[43] and the rest is structurally complete by 21 days.[44] This is 25-50 days earlier than the onset of the vestibular righting systems.[14] Therefore, the sequence of onset is not merely due to the sequence of maturation of the sensory systems, but also reflects the sequential central organization of these righting systems. In *Dasyurus*, this is strikingly illustrated by the body-on-body and body-on-head righting systems. Like all marsupials, the embryonic neonate has to physically navigate, unaided, from the mother's cloaca to her pouch. In order to do this, the neonate has well developed forelimbs, with the tips of its digits possessing long, curved claws. In contrast, the hindlimbs are still undifferentiated buds.[45] During development, the forelimbs continue to lead in their ontogenetic maturation. Therefore, by the time body-on-body and body-on-head systems appear (about 42-46 days), the forelimbs are better developed; yet body-on-body appears first, and involves hindlimb righting movements. If the rate of overall maturation dictates the onset of righting systems, the body-on-head system should appear first, as the forelimbs are more mature.

Furthermore, these body-tactile righting systems progress through the same stages during recovery following lateral hypothalamic damage.[12] The limbs at first push the body to prone, then limb placement on the ground triggers axial rotation, and finally direct axial rotation occurs. Importantly, as the body-on-body system reaches its terminal phase of axial rotation, the body-on-head emerges involving a more primitive phase, that of limb pushing. Therefore, even though the animal has axial rotation as part of its movement repertoire, it cannot be accessed via body-on-head at this time. Therefore, it appears that each righting system only has access to righting movements via some central organization unique to that system. This strongly suggests that these righting systems have a modular organization. That is, every righting

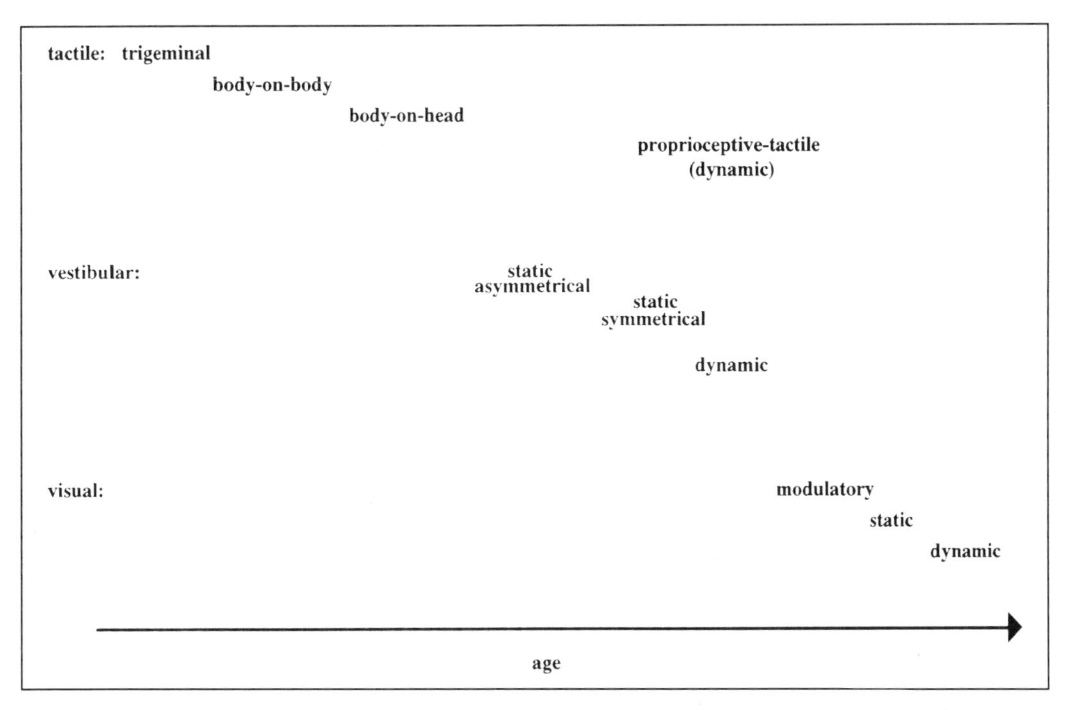

Fig. 7.3. The age of onset of all righting programs are schematically juxtaposed. All tactile, vestibular and visual programs are shown. In all cases, the dynamic programs triggered by each sensory modality are the last to appear. The independence of such programs, even when triggered by the same sensory modality, is markedly illustrated by the tactile systems. The first to appear is trigeminal, which is cephalocaudal, followed by body-on-body which is caudocephalic, and then by body-on-head, which is cephalocaudal. Much later, a dynamic cephalocaudal program emerges.

system is a distinct module, each having its own access networks to motor acts typical of that system.

REVISED MODEL

When the constituent motor elements in the recovery following brain damage and in normal development are analyzed, the organization of righting behavior appears to differ markedly from the classical model. Firstly, the motor elements are not linked together in a chain-reflex-like manner. Rather, motor elements are packaged together in a manner that reflects context-specific adaptability. Secondly, each sensory modality capable of activating a righting response does not simply appear to gain access to a common set of motor elements. Instead, each sensory modality seems to have its own motor program at its disposal, with some motor elements being unique to specific righting programs. For example, all vestibular righting programs involve axial rotation, whereas body-tactile righting programs have both axial rotation and limb pushing motor elements. Therefore, a revised model of righting involves a set of righting programs organized in a modular manner, with each righting program being classified by the activating sensory modality. To complete the classification, another dimension is needed, that of context. Recall that righting from a static (or positional) context is dissociable from righting from a dynamic (or acceleratory) context, irrespective of the sensory modality involved (Table 7.1). Here, the model envisaged is a nested hierarchy of modules. The two main submodules of righting are static versus dynamic. Each of these submodules are themselves composed of further submodules, which are characterized by the activating sensory modality. In turn, righting is a submodule of a module which includes other postural support responses.[2,5]

IMPLICATIONS

When a rat is dropped supine in the air, the righting program that is activated is easily discernible: dynamic vestibular righting. The

Table 7.1. The classification of righting programs along two dimensions

		Sensorimotor systems		
Context	**static**	trigeminal body-on-body body-on-head	vestibular asymmetrical vestibular symmetrical	visual
	dynamic	proprioceptive-tactile	vestibular	visual

situation is more complex when a rat rights on the ground where multiple activating sensory modalities are involved. Here, systems are either all coactivated, or a dominance relationship exists among them. The evidence would seem to favor the latter case. Firstly, body-on-body righting (identified by pelvis-led righting) does not occur; instead, one of the head righting systems occurs. Furthermore, an intact adult rat rarely uses trigeminal righting (diagnosed by head-led rotation), but uses a shoulder-led rotation characteristic of both vestibular and body-on-head righting. Secondly, in the recovery from lateral hypothalamic damage, righting which is shoulder-led appears earlier (2-3 days) when they have intact labyrinths than when they are bilabyrinthectomized (up to 3 weeks).[33] This suggests that vestibular righting recovers sooner than body-on-head righting. Righting programs, then, are not equally likely to be activated; instead, on the ground, vestibular righting is probably the dominant program, with body-on-body being the lowest in the hierarchy. This arrangement would predict that one of the roles of the neural control systems involved in righting is to select among the available righting programs. During infantile development, righting programs co-occur, so that body-on-body righting occurs simultaneously with body-on-head, vestibular and trigeminal; this leads to bizarre patterns of movement which appear counterproductive to righting.[13] However, as the young mature, shoulder-led righting becomes the predominant form of righting. This suggests that one aspect of development involves the maturation of this 'selecting circuit.' That such a circuit exists is further supported by a lesion study. Electrolytic lesions of the red nucleus have a disorganizing effect on righting behavior. When righting on the ground, such rats exhibit a mixture of righting programs reminiscent of early infancy (see Figure 7 in ref. 46). A comparison with neurotoxic lesions of the red nucleus suggests that this disruption is not caused by damage to the red nucleus itself, but to fibers of passage coursing through and around the red nucleus.[46] Since there is also a loss of righting after lesions to the lateral hypothalamus, which is then followed by its gradual re-integration,[12,33] part of this circuit is likely to involve the basal ganglia and pontine-cerebellar systems.

Once a righting program, or combination of programs, is selected, then presumably there are other neural circuits specific to those programs that act to organize the appropriate elements into suitable responses. This suitable response would be appropriate given the stimulus conditions under which righting is to occur. Finally, the motor elements must have their neural control circuits as well. At least some of these are likely to be in the lower parts of the brain. Indeed, I have observed decapitated adult rats performing hindleg righting movements; this suggests that at least some of the motor elements of body-on-body righting are organized in the spinal cord. My suspicion is that the mid-brain system that organizes righting[4] involves the systems needed for selecting between righting programs, and some other systems are responsible for coordinating the motor elements of the selected righting program. The program-selecting mechanism must integrate the general stimulus context, and then select the program based on some hierarchical arrangement. In contrast, the mechanism responsible for the selected program itself must use the specific features of the stimulus context in order to adaptively alter the arrangement of the motor elements to be used. Therefore, we should be searching for multiple neural control systems over righting, not a single system.

Another implication of this modular organization of righting is in the interpretation of pathology. Some Parkinsonian patients have been shown to have difficulty initiating righting movements when recumbent.[3] Such patients cannot use axial rotation, but instead use the limbs to push or pull the body over. Lakke[3] argues that because axial rotation can occur in these patients under appropriate sensory stimulation (i.e., when falling backwards or sidewards), this disability reflects the inability to 'call up' appropriate motor programs; he therefore calls this deficit 'axial apraxia.' Unlike other parkinsonian motor disabilities, this axial apraxia is not ameliorated by L-dopa therapy.[47] Several animal models of Parkinson's disease, in which the ascending nigrostriatal dopaminergic system is disrupted,[48] do not mimic this deficit, but rather, such rats appear to show the normal shoulder-led axial rotation form of righting.[25,26] Electrolytic damage to the lateral hypothalamus, which includes systems beyond the nigrostriatal bundle, does disrupt righting, producing axial apraxia-like deficits.[12,33] Therefore, although nigrostriatal dopamine depletion constitutes a major component of Parkinson's disease,[49] additional degeneration of other non-dopaminergic neural systems must be involved, especially in the later phases of the disease.[2] The search for the relevant neural systems is in part guided by the behavioral description which is the basis for the physiological model proposed. In Lakke's conception, the inability for these patients to right themselves results from axial apraxia. The modular model of righting suggests an alternative interpretation.

That righting occurs on falling, but not when stationary,[50] suggests that the dynamic module is intact, while the static is not. Lakke[3] also provides examples of Parkinsonian patients using different motor strategies to right themselves in the absence of axial rotation. For example, one patient first uses his legs and then his arms to pull and push himself to prone, and another patient, who was unable to right on the ground, reaches over with her arm and touches the experimenter's hand, which triggers axial rotation of the shoulders. In the first example, the patient may be using the most primitive motor elements of the body-on-body and/or body-on-head righting programs. In the second example, the patient seems to be using the intermediate form of the body-on-head righting program. Vestibular dysfunction is also present in some Parkinsonian patients.[51] This possibly limits the righting on the ground to the tactile systems. From this perspective, the righting strategies of different patients may not be idiosyncratic techniques to overcome axial apraxia, but instead may be seen to reflect stages of functional deterioration; that is, as the disease progresses, more of the righting programs become unavailable. Given the evidence from studies of recovery from brain damage[12] and from normal ontogeny[13,14] (which should be opposite to the progressive degeneration of Parkinson's disease), the first patient described should be in a more advanced stage of the disease than the second patient.

That striatal mechanisms are important for integrating tactile-motor systems,[52] may account for the regression to more primitive forms of tactile-righting in cases of advanced Parkinsonism as described above. Recently, my colleagues and I have found that the body-on-body righting of unilaterally 6-OHDA lesioned rats is of the most primitive form, that is, hind leg pushing. Recall, that body-on-body righting is triggered by asymmetrical body-on-ground contact and can be observed in isolation from the head-initiated patterns of righting by restraining the head. On the side contralateral to the lesion about 78% of all righting involves pushing with the hind leg. For intact controls, only about 5% of such righting does so (Pellis, Martens and Whishaw, work in progress). These findings suggest that at least some of the regression in righting systems by Parkinson patients may be due to disruption of the dopaminergic input to the basal ganglia, but only for those righting systems involving body contact with the ground.

Righting is also frequently used as a means of assessing pathologies induced by various environmental toxins,[53,54] as well as other experimental manipulations of the nervous system.[55,56] Typically, unitary measures, such as the latency to right, are used to evaluate effects on righting.[57] The modular model of righting suggests that the use of such unitary measures is inadequate. An experimental manipulation may affect one righting system but leave the others intact, or it may interfere with the righting selection mechanism, or it may alter the availability of motor elements to different righting programs. Any or all these changes may or may not be revealed by measures such as the latency to right. Therefore, the modular righting model suggests that in order to adequately evaluate the neurological effects of various treatments, each righting program needs to be tested separately, as well as when interacting with other righting programs.[12-14]

CONCLUSION

The modular organization of righting behaviors shows there is a level of organization of intermediate complexity between motor elements and the highest levels of motor control. These movement subsystems of intermediate complexity[58,59] may be viewed as a hierarchy of nested modules, with the rules of organization making each module more like a motor program than a simple reflex. This is similar to the ethological conception of behavior systems,[60] where sensory, motor and integrative mechanisms are connected so as to form a hierarchically structured, functional system.[61] A neglected area of research in motor behavior is on the organization of these intermediate sensorimotor systems.[62] There are rules for module organization and inter-module interaction that need to be understood. This is true not only for righting, but for other postural and movement modules as well.

Acknowledgments

I wish to thank my various colleagues without whom this sketch of righting would not have been possible. I especially wish to thank Philip Teitelbaum and Vivien Pellis for their unceasing participation in solving the puzzle. Also I would like to thank Vivien Pellis for her helpful comments on earlier drafts, and Adria Allen for typing the manuscript. In part, this chapter was financed by a grant from the University of Lethbridge to the author.

References

1. Langworthy DR. The Sensory Control of Posture and Movement. A Review of the Studies of Derek Denny-Brown. Baltimore, MA: The Williams and Williams Company, 1970.
2. Martin JP. The Basal Ganglia and Posture. London, UK: Pitman Medical Publishing, 1967.
3. Lakke JPWF. Axial apraxia in Parkinson's disease. J Neurol Sci 1985; 69:37-46.
4. Ito M. Neural systems controlling movement. Trends NeuroSci 1986; 9:515-18.
5. Magnus R. Körperstellung. Berlin: Springer, 1924. (A 1987 English translation of Body Posture is available from the U. S. Department of Commerce.)
6. Monnier M. Functions of the Nervous System: Volume II, Motor and Sensorimotor Functions. Amsterdam: Elsevier, 1970.
7. Rademaker GGJ. The Physiology of Standing. Minneapolis, MN: University of Minnesota Press, 1980. (Original work published 1931)
8. O'Connell AL, Gardner EB. Understanding the Scientific Bases of Human Movement. Baltimore, MD: Williams and Williams, 1972.
9. Roberts TDM. Neurophysiology of Postural Mechanisms. (2nd ed.). London: Butterworths, 1978.
10. Magnus R. On the co-operation and interference of reflexes from other sense organs with those of the labyrinths. Laryngoscope 1926; 36:701-12.
11. Troiani O, Petrosini L, Passani F. Trigeminal contribution to the head righting reflex. Physiol Behav 1981; 27:157-60.
12. Pellis SM, Pellis VC, Chen YC et al. Recovery from axial apraxia in the lateral hypothalamic labyrinthectomized rat reveals three elements of contact righting: Cephalocaudal dominance, axial rotation and distal limb action. Behav Brain Res 1989; 35:241-51.

13. Pellis VC, Pellis SM, Teitelbaum P. A descriptive analysis of the post-natal development of contact-righting in rats (*Rattus norvegicus*). Dev Psychobiol 1991; 24:237-63.
14. Pellis SM, Pellis VC, Nelson JE. The development of righting reflexes in the pouch young of the marsupial *Dasyurus hallucatus*. Dev Psychobiol 1992; 25:105-25.
15. Peiper A. Cerebral Function in Infancy and Childhood. New York: Consultants Bureau, 1963.
16. Chen YC, Pellis SM, Sirkin DW et al. Bandage backfall: Labyrinthine and non-labyrinthine components. Physiol Behav 1986; 37:805-14.
17. Cremieux J, Veraart C, Wanet MC. Development of the air righting reflex in cats visually deprived since birth. Exp Brain Res 1984; 54:564-66.
18. Muller HR, Weed LH. Notes on the falling reflex of cats. Am J Physiol 1916; 40:373-79.
19. Warkentin J, Carmichael L. A study of the development of the air-righting reflex in cats and rabbits. J Genet Psychol 1939; 55:67-80.
20. Pellis SM, Pellis VC, Morrissey TK et al. Visual modulation of vestibularly-triggered air-righting in the rat. Behav Brain Res 1989; 35:23-26.
21. Pellis SM, Whishaw IQ, Pellis VC. Visual modulation of vestibularly-triggered air-righting in rats involves the superior colliculus. Behav Brain Res 1991; 46:151-56.
22. Carmichael L. The genetic development of the kitten's capacity to right itself in the air when falling. J Genet, Psychol 1934; 44:453-58.
23. Sherrington CS. The Integrative Action of the Nervous System. New York: Scribner's, 1906.
24. Fukuda T. Statokinetic Refexes in Equilibrium and Movement. Tokyo: University of Tokyo Press, 1984.
25. De Ryck M, Schallert T, Teitelbaum P. Morphine versus haloperidol catalepsy in the rat: A behavioral analysis of postural mechanisms. Brain Res 1980; 201:143-72.
26. Pellis SM, De La Cruz F, Pellis VC et al. Morphine subtracts subcomponents of haloperidol-isolated postural support reflexes to reveal gradients of their integration. Behav Neurosci 1986;100:631-46.
27. Pellis SM, Pellis VC, Teitelbaum P. Air righting without the cervical righting reflex in adult rats. Behav Brain Res 1991; 45:185-88.
28. Laouris Y, Kalli-Laouri J, Schwartze P. The postnatal development of the air-righting reaction in albino rats. Quantitative analysis of normal development and the effect of preventing neck-torso and torso-pelvis rotations. Behav Brain Res 1990; 37:37-44.
29. Schoenfelder J The development of air-righting reflex in postnatal growing rabbits. Behav Brain Res 1984; 11:213-21.
30. Eshkol N, Wachmann A. Movement Notation. London: Weidenfeld and Nicholson, 1958.
31. Whishaw IQ, Pellis SM. The structure of skilled forelimb reaching in the rat: A proximally driven movement with a single distal rotatory component. Behav Brain Res 1990; 41:49-59.

32. Hay JG. The Biomechanics of Sports Techniques. Englewood Cliffs, NJ: Prentice-Hall, Inc., 1973.
33. Pellis SM, Pellis VC, Teitelbaum P. 'Axial apraxia' in labyrinthectomized lateral hypothalamic-damaged rats. Neurosci. Lett 1987; 82:217-20.
34. Fox MW. Reflex development and behavioral organization. In: Himwich MA, ed. Developmental Neurobiology. Springfield, IL: Charles C. Thomas, 1970: 553-81.
35. Villablanca JR, Olmstead CB. Neurological development of kittens. Dev Psychobiol 1979; 12:101-27.
36. Levitt D, Teitelbaum P. Somnolence, akinesia and sensory activation of motivated behavior in the lateral hypothalamic syndrome. Proc Natl Acad Sci USA 1975; 72:2819-23.
37. Windle WF, Fish MW. The development of the vestibular righting reflex in the cat. J Comp Neurol 1932; 54:85-96.
38. Hård E, Larsson K. Development of air righting in rats. Brain Behav Evol 1975; 11:53-9.
39. Pellis SM, Pellis VC. The development of righting when falling from a bipedal standing posture: Evidence for the dissociation of dynamic and static righting reflexes in rats. Physiol Behav 1994; 56:659-663.
40. Pellis SM, Pellis VC, Whishaw IQ. Visual modulation of air righting by rats involves calculation of time-to-impact, but does not involve the detection of the looming stimulus of the approaching ground. Behav Brain Res 1995; in press.
41. Gottlieb G. Ontogenesis of sensory function in birds and mammals. In: Tobach E, Aronson LR, Shaw E, eds. The Biopsychology of Development. New York: Academic Press, 1971:67-128.
42. Nelson JE. Growth of the brain. In: Tyndale-Biscoe, CH, Janssens PA, eds. The Developing Marsupial. Models for Biomedical Research. Berlin: Springer-Verlag, 1988:86-100.
43. Gemmell RT, Nelson J. The vestibular system of the newborn marsupial cat, *Dasyurus hallucatus*. Anat Rec 1989; 225:203-8.
44. Gemmell RT, Nelson J. Development of the vestibular and auditory system of the Northern native cat, *Dasyurus hallucatus*. Anat Rec 1989; 234:136-43.
45. Sharman GB. Adaptations of marsupial pouch young for extra-uterine existence. In: Austin, CR, ed. The Mammalian Fetus in Vitro. London: Chapman and Hall, 1973:67-90.
46. Whishaw IQ, Pellis SM, Pellis VC. A behavioral study of the contribution of cells and fibres of passage in the red nucleus of the rat to postural righting, skilled movements, and learning. Behav Brain Res 1992; 52:29-44.
47. Lakke JPWF, DeJong PJ, Koppejan EH et al. Observations on Postural Behavior—Axial Rotation in Recumbent Position in Parkinson Patients after L-dopa Treatment. In: Rinne VK, Klinger M, Stamm G. eds. Parkinson's Disease—Current Progress, Problems and Management. Amsterdam: Elsevier, 1980:187-96.

48. Schultz W. Depletion of dopamine in the striatum as an experimental model of parkinsonism: Direct effects and adaptive mechanisms. Progress Neurobiol 1982; 18:121-66.
49. Bernheimer H, Birkmayer W, Hornykiewicz O et al. Brain dopamine and the syndromes of Parkinson and Huntington: clinical, morphological and neurochemical correlates. J Neuro Sci 1973; 20:415-55.
50. Lakke JPWF, van den Burg W, Wiegman J Abnormalities in postural reflexes and voluntarily induced automatic movements in Parkinson patients. Clin Neurol Neurosurg 1982; 84:227-35.
51. Reichert WH, Doolittle J, McDowell FH. Vestibular dysfunction in Parkinson disease. Neurology 1982; 32:1133-38.
52. Lidksy TI, Manetto C, Schneider JS. Consideration of the sensory factors involved in motor functions of the basal ganglia. Brain Res Rev 1985; 9:133-146.
53. Frieder B, Epstein S, Grimm VE. The effects of exposure to diazepam during various stages of gestation or during lactation on the development of behavior of rat pups. Psychopharmacol 1984; 83:51-55.
54. Henderson MG, McMillen BA. Effects of prenatal exposure to cocaine or related drugs on rat developmental and neurological indices. Brain Res Bull 1990; 24:207-12.
55. Almli RC, Fisher RS. Infant rats: Sensorimotor ontogeny and effects of substantia nigra destruction. Brain Res Bull 1977; 2:425-39.
56. Bignall KE. Ontogeny of levels of neural organization: The righting reflex as a model. Exp Neurol 1974; 42:566-73.
57. Markus EJ, Petit TL. Neocortical synaptogenesis, aging and behavior: Lifespan development in the motor-sensory system of the rat. Exp Neurol 1987; 96:262-79.
58. Teitelbaum P. Disconnection and antagonistic interaction of movement subsystems in motivated behavior. In: Morrison, AR, Strick, P, eds. Changing Concepts of the Nervous System: Proceedings of the First Institute of Neurological Sciences Symposium in Neurobiology and Learning. New York: Academic Press, 1982:127-43.
59. Teitelbaum P, Schallert T, DeRyck M et al. Motor subsystems in motivated behavior. In: Thompson RF, Hicks LH, Shvyrkov VB, eds. Neural Mechanisms of Goal-Directed Behavior and Learning. New York: Academic Press, 1980:127-43.
60. Hogan JA. Cause and function in the development of behavior systems. In: Blass EM, ed. Handbook of Behavioral Neurobiology. Vol. 9. Developmental Psychobiology and Behavioral Ecology. New York: Plenum Press, 1988:63-106.
61. Baerends GP. The functional organization of behaviour. Anim Behav 1976; 24:726-738.
62. Teitelbaum P, Pellis SM. Toward a synthetic physiological psychology. Psychol. Sci 1992; 3:4-20.

CHAPTER 8

A Rat's Reach Should Exceed Its Grasp: Analysis of Independent Limb and Digit Use in the Laboratory Rat

Ian Q. Whishaw and Elena I. Miklyaeva

The rodents are a mighty group
Of many shapes and sizes.
They reach for food with little paws
And eat it with incisors.
—iqw

INTRODUCTION

We define skilled movements of the limbs as those made by an animal when it uses its limbs, paws and digits for catching, manipulating, and holding objects. These movements are special. They can be compromised by brain damage that seemingly spares the coordinated limb movements that are used for walking, climbing, swimming, and grooming.[1] This review features the rat and describes observational, end point, and kinematic methods used to study the limb, paw, and digit movements that it uses to catch prey, to handle food, and to reach for objects.

In demonstrating some of the features of these movements, we will argue that the rat can be used as a convenient and inexpensive

Measuring Movement and Locomotion: From Invertebrates to Humans, edited by Klaus-Peter Ossenkopp, Martin Kavaliers and Paul R. Sanberg.

analog for studying a variety of applied neuroscience problems related to skilled movements, including those associated with loss, recovery, and restoration of function. It can also be used for the study of basic neuroscience problems including those related to the organization of the motor system, the ability of the motor system to undergo changes that permit learning and remembering skilled movements, and the neurochemical connections that allow its many components to interact in the production of skilled movement.

WHY RATS?

The rat has been overlooked as a good subject for studying skilled movements. It has been believed that its neocortex is too simple to produce the skilled movements characteristic of primates,[2] that primate movements are characteristic of only that phylogenetic lineage,[3,4] and that it lacks the anatomical connections between the central motor system and spinal motor neurons thought to be prerequisite for skilled movement.[5]

None of these ideas has received much experimental support. The rat has a well-developed motor system in that its motor cortex as a percentage of total cortex is among the largest of mammals while primates are only average.[6] The portion of motor cortex representing the forelimbs is disproportionately large.[7,8] It displays good forelimb use, as the many papers dedicated to this topic testify. Finally, it does have direct connections between corticospinal projections and motor neurons.[9,10] Although we do not wish to deny obvious differences between primates and rodents, we are of the view that the rat, and rodents more generally, has a well developed motor system and so provides a good resource for studying the function and organization of the motor systems.[11,12] In fact, Wise and Donoghue[12] have argued that comparative anatomical and behavioral studies of the many kinds of rodents could provide a rich resource for arriving at an understanding of the motor systems.

Ironically, even though Karl Lashley[13] promoted the idea that functions could not be localized in the neocortex, his graduate student Peterson demonstrated a close relation between limb preference and the motor cortex. Peterson[14] first showed that rats could use a single limb for prehension. Then in a series of experiments, beginning with studies demonstrating that rats have an individual limb preference, but not a population preference, Peterson showed that limb preference could be both biased and changed by lesions to motor cortex but not by lesions to other areas of the neocortex.[14-18]

Since Peterson's studies, there has been a growing list of papers in which the success of limb movement has been used as a measure of nervous system function. In these studies, rats have reached into slots, down tubes, onto conveyor belts, off shelves, and through bars to get food. Also, they have performed allied tasks of manipulating puzzle latches, pushing force transducers, and pushing bars.[19-22] Rats have also been observed as they spontaneously pick up food,[23,24] and other rodents have been observed as they spontaneously manipulate food to eat it.[25,26] In addition to revealing the ingenuity with which the rat can perform motor tasks, these studies have shown that a variety of brain structures, in addition to motor cortex, such as the pyramidal tract, basal ganglia, nigrostriatal dopaminergic system, cerebellum, red nucleus, and various structures within the medulla are in some way involved in limb use.[11,19,27,28]

HOW DO YOU STUDY RAT MOVEMENTS?

The answer to this question is, "watch them." One wag we know has stated that his criteria when searching for graduate students is to find those who will watch an animal for three hours without a coffee break. Furthermore, while watching, it is helpful to say periodically, "now what is it doing?" One of us once observed a coworker watching a film of a sleeping rat and mumbling from time to time, "now what is it doing?" It was surprising to see how many people gathered around, each trying to formulate an answer to this enigmatic question.

Although rats are small and their movements take place quickly, they can be videotaped with a video camera that has a fast shutter speed option (about 2,000 of a second is optimal). Films made with a fast shutter speed produce an image that is clear. Although such filming requires a good deal of light, we find that with very little habituation, rats will work well in bright light provided by a cold light source. Light levels can be reduced if a camera that is sensitive at low light levels is used. Many small hand-held video cameras provide both variable shutter speed and low light level recording options at low cost. Video recording can be combined with other measures of movement.[29,30]

BUT THE MOVEMENTS ARE JUST AS FAST ON VIDEOTAPE!

Video film can be replayed by video cassette recorder (VCR) that has a frame-by-frame option and that can hold a jitter-free image on the screen, and many commercial VCRs do this. Conventional video tapes are replayed at 30 frames per second, which allows behavior to be analyzed at 1/30th of a second. For many behaviors this is adequate. Each video frame, however, is composed of two fields. A frame grabber attached to a computer can be used to grab individual fields so that behavior can be viewed at 1/60th of a second. For some problems, still faster filming is required, and this requires a special video camera. Cameras that record up to 1,000 frames per second are available, but we have found that for most limb movements a conventional camera is adequate and one that gives 60 frames per second (120 fields) can solve most special problems. Video cameras that film at 60 frames a second are gradually becoming affordable.[31] Video images can be printed on a video printer and they can be grabbed using a frame grabber and computer, edited or combined with a graphics program and then printed in color or black and white. These manipulations produce sequences of "before" and "after" movements that can be assembled for direct comparison. To perform these functions we use a hand-held Hi-8 camera, a high-8 VCR, a frame grabber attached to a Macintosh computer, a graphics program, and a video printer.

THE ELEMENTS OF REACHING

Although it is not necessary to have a theory before observing behavior, it is helpful to know that there are some recognized features of primate reaching (including our own reaching) that are shared by rats and possibly by most animals that grasp objects.[32] The object has to be detected, the body needs to be oriented so that the limb can be appropriately positioned, the limb needs to be advanced toward the target, grasping must take place, and the object must be retrieved and released.[33]

Rats Locate and Identify Objects by Sniffing and Touching

We and other primates use vision to detect objects. Before reaching, we orient our head to the object and look at it to estimate its distance, size and texture, and so identify it to decide how it should be grasped. Rats have a well-developed visual system and can see objects at a distance that have a size of about one degree of visual angle. They may not use vision to detect objects that are very close to them, however.[34] We trained rats to reach for different sized white food pellets that were placed on a black shelf in front of one of 21 slots. The rats' ability to detect the objects was inferred by their latency to reach for the object and their accuracy. Once animals were well trained their vision was blocked by placing patches on their eyes. This had no effect on reaching performance. The rats still "scanned" the slots to look for food and they reached only into slots that contained food. When olfaction was disrupted by removing the olfactory bulbs, the rats behaved as if they were "blind." They reached well, but they reached into every slot sequentially until they found the one that contained the food. Since rats generally sniff objects before they pick them up, it seems likely that olfaction is used for detecting objects under most circumstances. Interestingly, many animals, including cats and dogs, sniff objects before picking them up, suggesting that olfaction is quite widely used for "grasping detection" by mammals.

As rats contact objects with their snout and pick them up by mouth, they probably use tactile information to make judgments about the size, shape, and weight. Rats make decisions about whether to eat food on site or carry it to a refuge to eat on the basis of the time that will be required to eat the food. This time judgment is based on food size and type as judged by tactile information from receptors located around the mouth.[35] As we will see below, tactile information also plays a role in instructing the paws in how to grasp.

Even though rodents and primates use different sensory systems for object identification, their orienting movements are similar. For example, we humans point our nose at, and lean toward, objects that we are identifying visually for grasping in just the same way that rats point their nose at, and lean toward, objects that they are identifying. How different sensory systems might guide movement is as yet an almost unexplored question. Goodale et al[36] have suggested that humans have a visual system for "hand guidance" and so it is possible to imagine that rats have olfactory and tactile systems for "paw guidance."

Reaching Requires Making Two Movements at Once

Animals have to maintain their posture when they move. When humans lift an arm to reach or when rats lift a paw, they risk falling over unless they make compensatory postural adjustments. When humans move their arm forward, they also move the upper part of their body backward to maintain a constant center of gravity. Dogs shift their weight to other limbs when they lift a forelimb, usually to the contralateral forelimb and the ipsilateral hindlimb.[37] When rats lift a paw to reach, they shift their weight onto the contralateral forelimb and ipsilateral hindlimb. This diagonal couplet both supports the rat's weight and adjusts the rat's posture as it reaches. The hindlimb contralateral to the reaching forelimb may also move as the forelimb moves. The movements of reaching and postural adjustment are not sequential but concurrent. Thus, a reaching movement really involves two quite different concurrent movements: the limb movement of reaching and the simultaneous postural adjustment necessary to balance the body against displacement. Thus, one can only talk quite loosely of reaching being the act of a single limb; in reality, it is an action in which the whole body participates.

The notion that a voluntary movement requires two quite different movements to occur almost simultaneously has profound implications for the study of movement control. First, it is likely that these coordinated actions need to be learned. Most of the learning-to-move, at which infants spend such a long time, likely involves learning to coordinate skilled movements and their concurrent postural adjustments. Similarly, learning a motor skill, such as skiing, is almost entirely a matter of learning to maintain a center of gravity while at the same time moving the feet to control speed and direction. Second, it is possible that different components of the nervous system are involved in postural adjustments and voluntary movements[38,39] and so these systems must learn to cooperate. For example, the loss of brain dopamine in human Parkinson's disease, reduces the person to a condition in which they can either defend body posture or make a voluntary movement, but not both.[40] Rats depleted either bilaterally or unilaterally of dopamine appear to suffer a similar impairment. Rather than reaching and adjusting body posture at the same time, they engage in a series of actions that involve first adjusting posture, and then moving, and so on.[41,42] Third, since limb movement requires a compensatory body movement, it must be that the neural representation of function can never really be reduced to body parts but must nearly always involve the body as a whole.[43,44] The implication of this notion is that almost any damage to motor systems could potentially change skilled movements.

Limb Transport and Withdrawal

Transport is the term given to the movement of using the limb to carry a hand or paw toward an object that is to be grasped and *withdrawal* is the term for moving it back again.[45] Transport and withdrawal are produced mainly by the musculature of the upper arm and shoulder and so they are sometimes also called *proximal movements.* They may be controlled by specialized neural systems. Lawrence and Kuypers[46] have suggested that the ventromedial pathways of the spinal cord control axial (trunk and shoulder) movements, the dorsolateral rubrospinal tracts and corticospinal tracts control limb and hand movements; and the lateral corticospinal tracts also control digit movements. Thus, the ventromedial pathways as well as the lateral corticospinal and rubrospinal pathways are likely involved in transport and withdrawal of the limb.

Hand and Digit Movements

There are a variety of hand and digit movements that can occur during grasping, and these are sometimes referred to as *distal movements.* When the hand is moved toward an object it is usually held in an aiming position with perpendicular posture, palm facing inward. *Pronation* is the term given to the movement that it makes when it is turned palm down to grasp an object. *Supination* is the term used to describe the movement of turning the palm back to the perpendicular position or to turning it so that it faces upward. As the hand is moved toward an object the digits are usually *semiclosed*, or *semiflexed.* To grasp they are usually *opened* or *extended* and then *closed* or *flexed.* When the digits are extended they are usually also opened (*abducted*) and when they are flexed they are usually also closed (*adducted*).

Primates have a variety of grasping postures, depending upon the species of animal and the purpose for which they use their paws. For brevity, we will define only the three main grasping patterns of humans. Human grasping actually begins before the object is touched. As the hand is transported toward the target the fingers are shaped to the size of the target. Then an object may be grasped using most or all of the digits, called a *whole hand grasp*, or it may be grasped by the tips of the first digit (thumb) and second digit, called a *pincer grasp*. It might also be grasped between the sides of the thumb and the first digit, as a screw driver is grasped, called a *power grasp*. Whole hand grasping is thought to be different from the other grasping patterns since the digits are moved together in a coordinated pattern while for the other movements they are moved *relatively independently*. Digits can also be used almost singly, such as in the action of removing an object from a small hole. In primates it is thought that the ability of an animal to make the pincer grasp and independent digit movements in removing objects from a hole depends upon direct connections of the crossed corticospinal tract onto motor neurons.[46]

The two main contemporary theories of limb movement are somewhat confusing in that they use different terms for movements but in their broad outlines the theories are similar. They both postulate that at least two different subcomponents of the motor system control limb movements. One theory emphasizes limb parts. According to this theory, proximal movements are controlled largely by brain stem to spinal cord pathways while distal movements are controlled mainly by cortex to spinal cord pathways. Some of these corticospinal projections make direct connections with motor neurons in the spinal cord, and these are thought to control very skilled or independent movements, particularly movements of the digits.[46] The second theory emphasizes movements. It proposes that the transport and grasping components of reaching can be disassociated with respect to their neural control. Corticospinal pathways control grasping while other pathways control limb transport and withdrawal component.[45]

SKELETAL, MUSCLE AND SENSORY BASIS OF MOVEMENT

The skeletal and musculature structure of the rat forelimb is described and illustrated by Green.[47] The rat is able to generate approximately the same range of movements with a forelimb as do primates, although there are some differences in the way the movements are produced (Fig. 8.1). The extent of movement of the scapula is difficult to describe since there is no fixed reference point. Relative to the humerus, it can make about 10° ventral and dorsal movements and 45° anterior and posterior movements. It can also move together with the humerus and clavicle, which together form the shoulder joint as in primates, giving it an additional range of movement. The main tether of the shoulder is by muscles and they also are the main restriction on its movement. The humerus can rotate about 10° to 20° in its socket with the scapula, move from 20° at flexion to 180° (almost straight) in the anterior-posterior plane, and move over a 145° range (75° medially to 75° laterally) in the medial-lateral plane. The ulna and radius can make almost no rotation in their elbow joint with the humerus. At this joint they can move about 10° in the medial to lateral direction in the horizontal plane. They can flex to an angle of 10° and extend to an angle of 160° (almost straight) in the anterior posterior plane. The paw, in relation to the ulna and radius, can rotate by about 20°, flex and extend by about 90° in each direction, and move laterally about 45° in each direction. In comparison to humans, rats have more parasagittal movement and less horizontal movement at the scapula, less rotation but otherwise similar movement at the shoulder, and more limited backward but otherwise similar movement at the elbow. Humans pronate and supinate the hand by rotating the radius over the ulna, but these bones are fused in the rat preventing this movement. In compensation, whereas humans can not rotate the wrist, the rat wrist is much more flexible and so can contribute to the rotatory movements of the paw.

The digits can flex and extend in the way that the digits of humans flex and extend but whereas humans both flex and adduct the thumb, the rat seems only able to flex the thumb (digit 1). Although

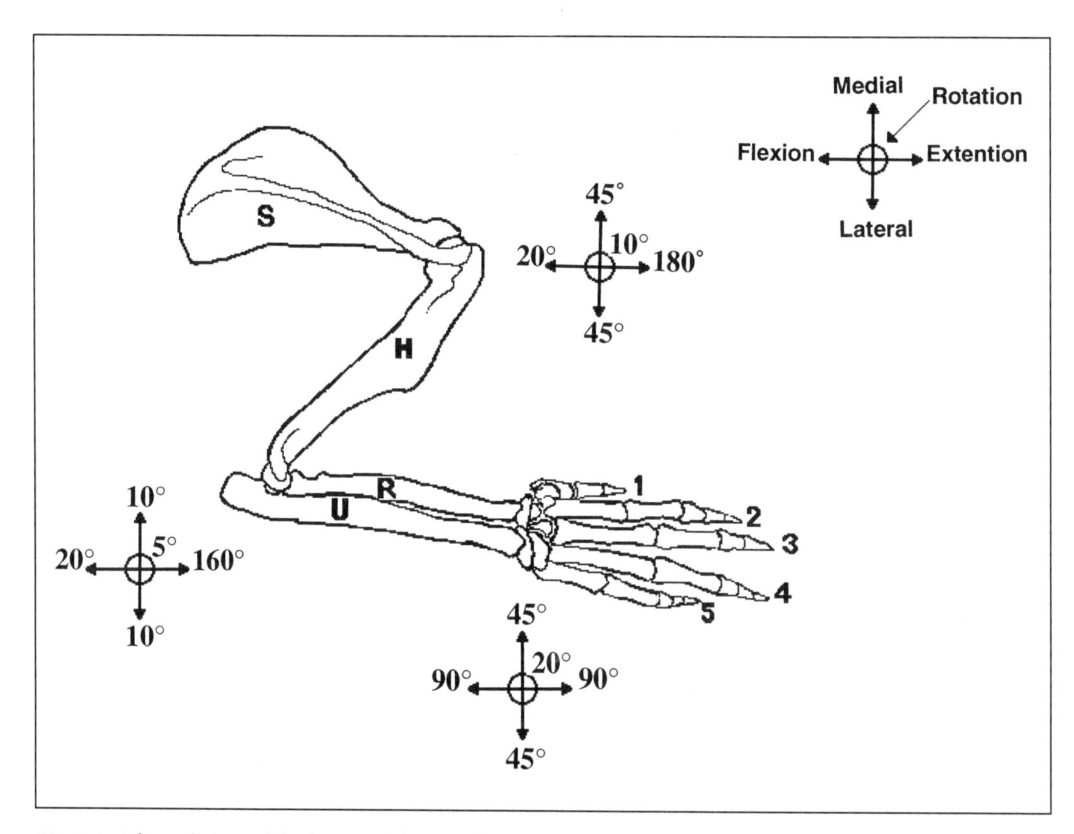

Fig. 8.1. A lateral view of the bones of the arm illustrating the approximate limits of movement at each joint. The inset indicates the direction of movement. The digits are number 1 to 5, medial to lateral. S, scapula; H, humerus; R, radius; U, ulna. See text for an account of the difficulty in specifying movement of the scapula.

the thumb is small, it is not vestigial. Curiously, whereas all of the other digits have claws, the thumb has a nail, which suggests it may be used for skilled manipulation. Digit 5 also appears to adduct to some extent, which makes it more versatile than the human small finger. Very little study has been made of forelimb muscle activity during movement: however, Hyland and Reynolds[48] have described the activity of some muscles during movements of reaching for food.

We are not aware of studies on the sensory receptors on the digits and paws of rats but the animals do have pads on which there is a rich array of sensory receptors. Additionally, they have large hairs on their wrists, which are like those on the vibrissae, that may be related to guiding limb movements. We have used kinematic measures to evaluate their function and find that if they are removed, there are subtle changes in the trajectory of reaches.

SPONTANEOUS AND LEARNED LIMB MOVEMENTS

Limb movements have not been examined in all situations in which rats use them. Movements that we have studied include those used in predation, such as catching and handling crickets, those used in the spontaneous handling of food, and those used in grasping food in test boxes, in what is euphemistically called skilled reaching. These three kinds of limb movements provide a rich repertoire of acts for drawing conclusions about a variety of topics of interest including the evolution of movements, species differences, laterality of function, and neural control.

PREDATION

Rats will hunt crickets as will many small nocturnal animals (Whishaw, Ivanco and Pellis, unpublished). We have studied cricket catching and manipulation in the laboratory rat and contrasted the rats' behavior with *Monodelphis domestica*, a small marsupial opossum whose main food source are insects.

The strategy that *Monodelphis* uses for catching crickets is simple. Once it locates a cricket it lifts a forepaw and smashes it down on the cricket and then grasps the cricket in the paw and stuffs it into the side of its mouth for chomping. In lifting, smashing, and grasping the cricket, there is very little pronation or supination of the paw. If the cricket is large or is not well placed in the mouth, the animal will use both forepaws to reposition the cricket. To do so the forepaws are turned palm inward. The decision about which paw to use in the attack seems to be based entirely on the location of the cricket with respect to the midline of the snout. If the cricket is located to the left, the left paw is used, if it is located to the right, the right paw is used.

When experienced rats catch crickets, the movements that they make are similar to those of *Monodelphis*. Once the cricket is grasped, however, the rat is much more skilled in its handling of the cricket than is *Monodelphis*. The rat sits back with the cricket and brings the other paw up to aid in holding. The cricket is then manipulated so that its head points upward. Then the head, wings, and the limbs of the cricket are removed, and the cricket is positioned so that its ventrum faces the rat, which the rat then eats. While this series of actions is occurring, the rat is continually manipulating the cricket to the appropriate position for biting and shredding. These limb and paw movements must be both delicate and precise, as the crickets have sharp spines on their legs which the rats do not like to touch.

Since rats and opossums share the ability to use a single limb in prey catching, it must be that this is an evolutionary old movement, dating to at least 60 million years ago when these families are thought to have diverged.[49] Since the rat makes skilled movements that are not shared by the opossum, it is likely that the rat has developed neural structures that the opossum does not have. Indeed, Kuypers[5] reports that corticospinal projections in the opossum do not connect with the pools of interneurons and motor neurons as they do in the rat. Thus, these connections may be necessary for the skilled movements of the rat.

Since the forelimb that the animals use to grasp the cricket is that which can most easily reach the prey, it is likely that there are constraints against the development of limb preferences, and in favor of ambidexterity, in both species. This leads us to suppose that the absence of a population limb bias in the rat[50] and only weak limb preferences in individual rats[51] may have its origins in a need to conserve symmetry for effective predatory behavior.

Picking Up Food

The movements that rats use in picking up food are initially different from those used for predation in that food is first grasped in the mouth and only later do the paws reach for the food and take it from the mouth.[23]

A single movement sequence takes place in the following way (Fig. 8.2): When the rat encounters food, it first sniffs the food while at the same time probably also palpating it with its vibrissae and perioral receptors. It then grasps the food in its mouth and sits back to transfer the food to its paws, from which it eventually eats it. In taking the sitting posture, it first lifts the forelimb that is least involved in supporting the weight of the forequarters and then secondarily, as its weight is completely transferred onto the hindquarters, it lifts the other forelimb. The forelimbs are lifted so that the elbows are brought toward the midline of the body and the palms of the paws are rotated so that they face medially. The paw that is lifted first does not immediately contact the food but is held in a "waiting" position until the second forelimb is lifted. Positioning of the limb to the waiting position is done mainly by the upper arm. Then by adduction of the upper arm, both paws are moved medially to grasp the food. As the paws are brought toward the food by upper arm movements, the digits are adjusted so that their aperture is appropriate to the size of the piece of food that is being grasped. If the food is small, the digits are closed. If the food is of an intermediate size, the aperture of the digits may not change. If the food is large, then the digits open as they approach the food. In all cases the food is grasped with the tips of the digits and thereafter it is largely manipulated with the digit tips for eating. Photographs illustrating the anticipatory changes in digit aperture for food pellets of different sizes are shown in Figure 8.3.

During limb transport, humans position the digits to a size for grasping that is appropriate for the object. Thus the anticipatory change in digit size prior to grasping in the rat is similar to that which has been described for humans. Humans, however, use vision to guide digit aperture, whereas rats must use tactile information from the perioral area to instruct the digit movements. That rats do change the aperture of their digits in anticipation of grasping suggests that the theories derived from primate and human studies, which suggest that proximal vs. distal or transport vs. manipulative movements are neurally dissociable, can be applied to rats.

Food Handling

Rats are opportunistic foragers and will consume a wide range of foodstuffs including grasses, nuts, leaves, roots and almost any type of food discarded by humans. We have filmed rats eating a wide range of objects (pasta, grapes, peanuts, rice, etc.) and have found that the paw postures and digit movements that they make are appropriate for the food that they are eating.[24] Thus, the variations in digit postures and the range of grips that they use seem almost as versatile as those used by primates. For example, they may hold food items between digit 1 and 2 in to what appears to be a pincer grip (thumb and fore

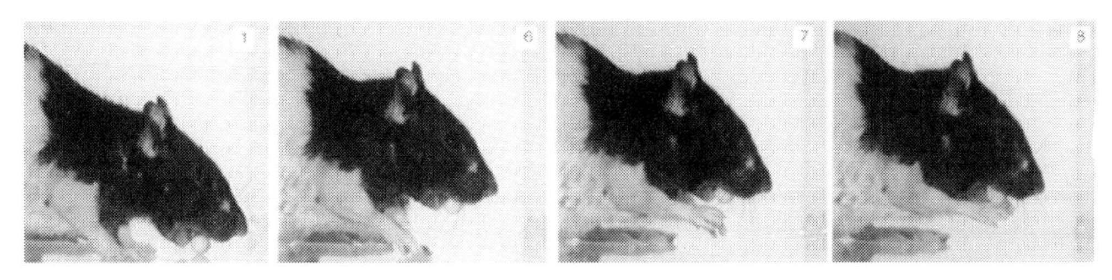

Fig. 8.2. Spontaneous food pickup. After sniffing the food, the rat grasps it in its mouth and sits back on its haunches. It then lifts its paws and positions them to grasp the food. The first paw lifted is generally that which is least involved in weight support. Movement of the limbs is accomplished mainly with upper arm movement, as is the movement to grasp the food. Prior to grasping the digits are adjusted to the size of the object to be grasped.

finger in humans) and they may hold items in a scissor grip between the other digits. Additionally, they may use one limb to support a food item and the other limb to manipulate it to the mouth. Thus, they are capable of bimanual coordination when eating.

Skilled Reaching

Test boxes

Although there are many different kinds of test boxes used for studying reaching, we will only describe the two boxes that we use (Fig. 8.4). In Figure 8.4A, the rat reaches through bars to grasp food

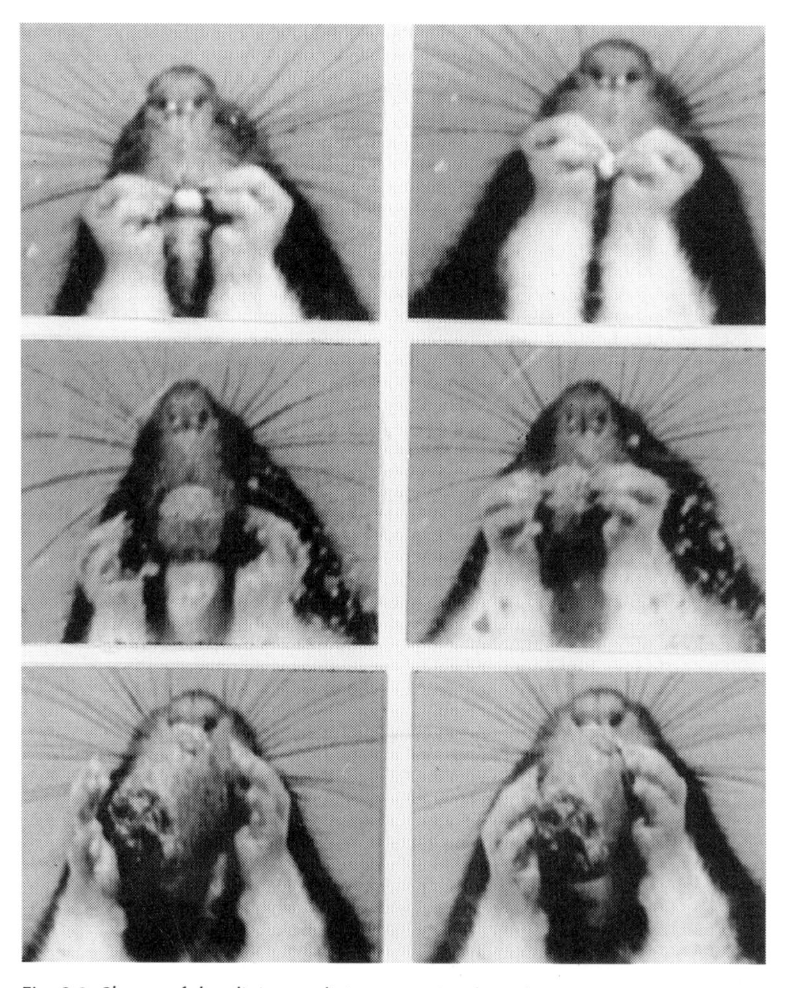

Fig. 8.3. Shape of the digits, or digit aperture, when the paws were positioned to grasp food from the mouth (left) and when they grasped the food (right). Note that the digit aperture is adjusted relative to the size of the food before the food is grasped. Food: top, rice; middle, 500 mg food pellet; bottom, lab chow.

that is piled up on a tray. We use chick feed obtained from a local feed mill since it is inexpensive and we use training sessions lasting up to an hour so the animals eat a lot. In Figure 8.4B, the rat reaches through a slot for a single round commercial food pellet that is located on a shelf. The second test can be thought of as more complex or demanding in that the rat must place its paw correctly to obtain the food. In the second test, the size of the food can also be changed to challenge the rat to alter its movements. The second box is constructed of clear Plexiglas to allow filming from different angles, including ventrally through an inclined mirror.

Bracelets

There are situations in which the experimenter might wish to specify the limb that the rat should use. Humans, who have motor system damage, are asked to sit on the good limb in order to force use of the bad limb. With monkeys, the good limb is simply tied up. A small

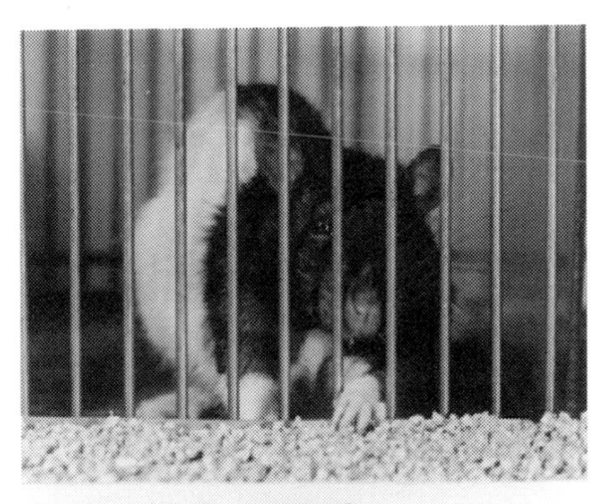

A. Food Tray Task

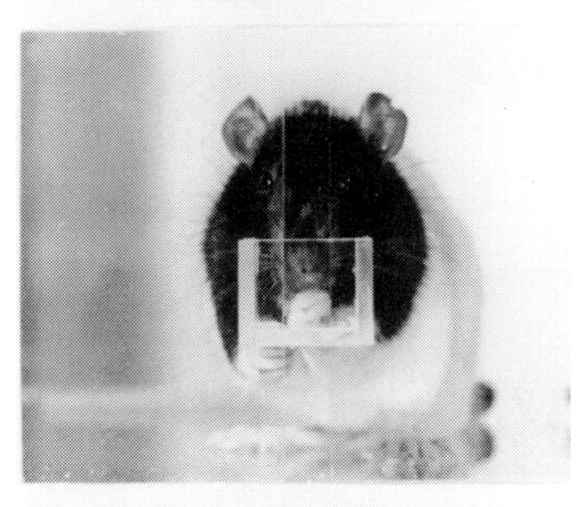

B. Single Food Pellet Task

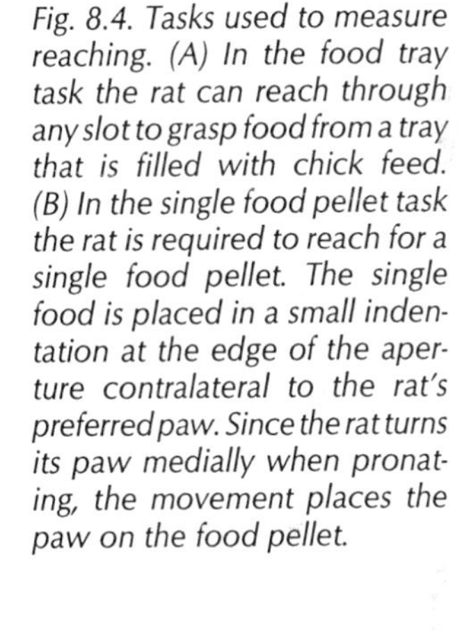

Fig. 8.4. Tasks used to measure reaching. (A) In the food tray task the rat can reach through any slot to grasp food from a tray that is filled with chick feed. (B) In the single food pellet task the rat is required to reach for a single food pellet. The single food is placed in a small indentation at the edge of the aperture contralateral to the rat's preferred paw. Since the rat turns its paw medially when pronating, the movement places the paw on the food pellet.

bracelet can be placed around the wrist of a rat to make it difficult for the animal to reach through the bars or apertures of the test boxes (Fig. 8.5). Elastoplast is an excellent material because the rat cannot shred it with its teeth. After worrying the bracelet for a few minutes they learn to ignore it. If the material is cut and folded as is illustrated in Figure 8.5, it is easy to place on the wrist and remove. The bracelet does not denude the hair on the wrist, impede walking, postural adjustments, or the movements of the paw for holding and manipulating food.

We use these tasks and procedures for a number of reasons. (1) They keep a rat in a relatively fixed position to facilitate filming and kinematic analysis. (2) They allow for the same movement to occur repeatedly in a relatively short period of time. (3) They provide a good sample of the movements used in spontaneous reaching (above), including proximal and distal movements and grasping and releasing food. (4) The reaching movements have a number of unique features suggesting that they are not simply a modification of some other movement such as digging, walking or climbing, as has been suggested.[52] Rather the characteristics of the movement suggest that it is a biologically useful action in its own right (Whishaw and Pellis, 1990). (5) They provide a reasonable approximation to the movements made by primates and humans when they reach, including the component movements that are used, their sequencing, and their execution.[32] This strengthens the argument that rats can be used to model diseases of the motor systems that occur in humans. (6) Finally, whatever move-

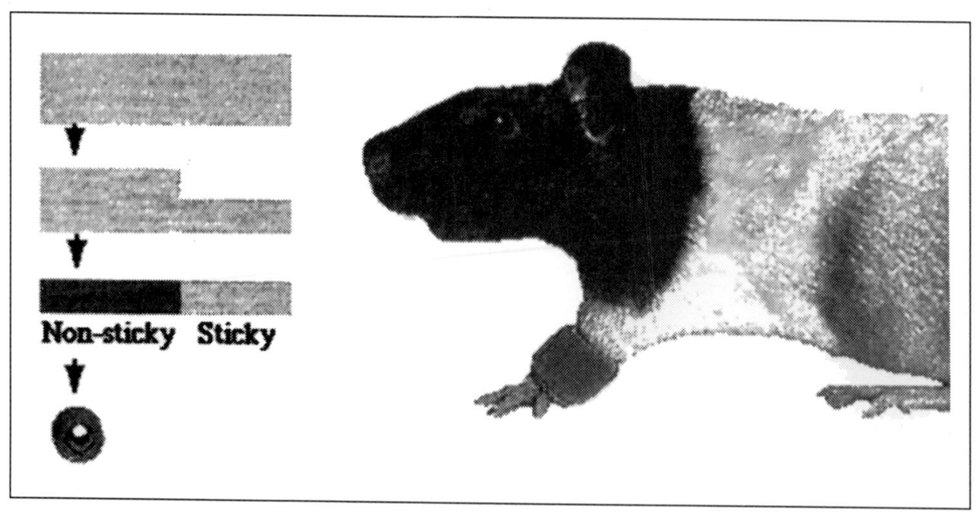

Fig. 8.5. A bracelet placed on the rat's wrist impedes movement through a slot to grasp food and forces the rat to use the other limb. The bracelet is made from elastoplast which is cut and folded so that when it is rolled the adhesive (sticky) surface can be fixed to the nonadhesive surface. When wrapped onto a rat's wrist it does not impede movement or posture.

ments and neural mechanisms that control this form of reaching, they are likely to be the same ones that contribute to spontaneous independent limb use.

MEASURING AND REACHING

ASYMMETRIES

Most animals show asymmetries in the selection of limb use at the individual level and some show asymmetries at the population level. We use *limb preference* as a term to describe a preference of an individual animal for a particular limb in a task and *limb dominance* for the similar expression of a preference in a population of animals. As noted above, the ecology of the rat may have actively selected against limb dominance. Nevertheless, limb preference is a pervasive feature of the animal's behavior in laboratory tests. As such, it is a very useful first measure of real or possible central nervous system damage. Even so, an animal may display different limb preferences in different test situations.[51]

Beginning with the exhaustive study of Peterson,[14] there have been a large number of studies directed toward attempts to understand limb preferences.[28,50,51,53-57] These studies show that rats have limb preferences, but no statistically significant limb dominance. About 13% of rats are ambidextrous and the remainder are almost equally left and right limbed. Ambidexterity itself may not be so much an absence of limb preference as an indication of a lack of motor skill.[50] There are no sex differences (but see Collins[58]). Limb preferences are displayed as soon as a rat begins to use a limb and they remain stable thereafter. Even a single session of 10 reaches will accurately identify a limb preference displayed on a more exhaustive test given as long as 4 months later.

Limb preference can be specified or changed by brain damage. Peterson and his coworkers demonstrated that small lesions in motor cortex will result in the selection of the ipsilateral limb when rats are first trained,[15] and will result in a change in limb preference away from the affected limb in rats that have been trained prior to surgery.[16] Damage to other cortical areas is less effective in influencing limb preference.[18,59,60] Limb preference can be similarly influenced by damage to the caudate-putamen and nigrostriatal dopamine projection[28] but not by damage to the red nucleus.[61] What is surprising in the studies of limb preference is how resilient preferences are to central damage. Animals only seem to change use of limbs when central damage almost completely incapacitates the use of a preferred limb.[62] A demonstration of this resilience is illustrated by observing the use of a limb after either peripheral restriction or central blockade of neurons with tetrodotoxin.[54] Whereas both treatments incapacitated limb use, peripheral blockade is much more effective in changing limb preference than central blockade. These results suggest that once established, limb preferences are dependent upon very distributed neural networks.

End Point Measures

The characteristic feature of much of the research on rat skilled movements is that it consists of *end-point* measures. That is, the *success* or *failure* of a motor act is recorded and that measure in turn is used to make inferences about nervous system status. Most people divide the number of successful reaches by the total number of reaches to obtain a *hit percent* score. Figure 8.6 gives an example of an end point measure of reaching performance in the food tray task in rats that received unilateral motor cortex damage. The rats were trained to reach with either paw by moving a bracelet back and forth between their two forelimbs on daily preoperative tests. With a few days training, the rats quickly changed limb use on "command." After the rats were trained, hit percent was measured in 10 min daily tests. The rats then received a unilateral motor cortex lesion and daily tests of the performance of each limb was measured over the next 15 days, beginning on the day after surgery. Note that performance with the *good limb*, the limb ipsilateral to the lesion, is not impaired by the lesion but that performance with the *bad limb,* the limb contralateral to the lesion, is initially severely impaired but then shows gradual recovery over the postoperative test period. The rats never quite recover postoperative performance levels with the bad limb. Sparing of function in the good limb and initial loss with incomplete recovery in the bad limb are typical characteristics of end point measures of motor cortex damage.[22,28] Although end point measures say a lot about the status of motor behavior, they can leave a good deal out. For example, rats with pyramidal tract lesions have good success in reaching immediately after lesions in that they do not display the loss and recovery observed after motor cortex lesions. Visual observation indicates that their behavior is impaired in much the same way as is the behavior of

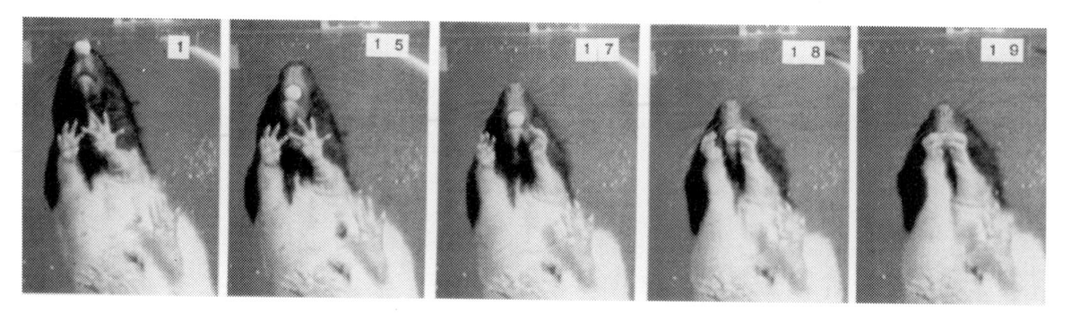

Fig. 8.6. End point measures of reaching success (successful reaches/total reaches) in rats prior to surgery (single dot) and after unilateral motor cortex lesions. Using the bracelet technique, the performance of the good paw (ipsilateral to lesion) and bad paw (contralateral to lesion) was evaluated each day for 15 days in 10 min reaching tests in the food tray task. Note that the lesions produce loss followed by incomplete recovery in the bad paw. The change in performance in the good paw may have been related to changes in reaching strategy involved in learning how to use the bad paw.

motor cortex damaged rats, however.[63] End point measures are not sensitive to this or the following kinds of differences: (1) Animals with different kinds of brain damage may perform equally badly on a task, but do so for quite different reasons. (2) Animals may do very well and yet still be impaired. (3) Animals may do very badly but not have a brain lesion. (4) Animals may seemingly show relatively equal recovery after a brain lesion, but the process of recovery may be different. In pointing out weakness, we are not dismissing the usefulness of end point measurement. They provide an admirable assay of motor status and, if used in different ways, they may even redress some of their own weaknesses.

Kinematics

Kinematics is the art of describing movements using measures such as velocity, trajectory, duration, etc. Figure 8.7A (top) illustrates the situation in which a rat is filmed making a single reach for a food pellet and shows the trajectory of the forelimb. Figure 8.7B gives the vertical, horizontal, and resultant velocities for this movement. The limb is extended above and beyond the target (the reach exceeds the grasp). When the limb is lifted the movement is rapid and then gradually slows to the point that the food pellet is grasped. The limb may sometimes come to a stop in the aiming position before being advanced again.

To perform kinematic analysis of movement from videotape, the simplest procedure is to place a transparent sheet of plastic on the screen of the television set and draw points of a body part or joint from successive video frames (i.e., digitize). Such images provide both trajectory and velocity profiles of the movements. Commercial computer systems can also be used to catch and digitize movements and to provide coordinates and graphic representations. To make these measurements, we use a Peak Performance Technologies system. This is a VHS format system, but videotape copied from other formats to VHS provides accurate copy.

Kinematic measures give wonderful representations of individual reaches but much of their richness is lost in trying to use them to make comparisons between individuals and especially groups. The mathematical difficulties of comparing the many points of these curves are horrendous. In the end one is usually reduced to the rather sad condition of comparing mean durations and velocities.

Notating behavior

The richest, most rewarding, and perhaps least used, measure of behavior is description. Description is little used because it is seen as unreliable, but there are methods that can be used to make it both accurate and replicable. The descriptive technique we use is called Eshkol-Wachman movement notation system or EWMNS.[64]

The EWMNS has been adapted from human dance for the study of animal motor behavior.[65] It is designed to express relation and changes of relation between the parts of the body. The body is treated as a system of articulated axes (i.e., body and limb segments). A limb is any part of the body which either lies between two joints or has a joint and a free extremity. These are imagined as straight lines (axes) of constant length, which move with one end fixed to the center of a sphere. The body is represented on a horizontally ruled page. Each horizontal space represents a part of the body; e.g., left limb, right limb, head, trunk, etc. Vertical lines divide the manuscript page into columns which denote units of time (e.g., frames of a video film). Thus, movements of body parts can be read sequentially against time.

An important feature of EWMNS is that the same movements can be notated in several polar coordinate systems. The coordinates of each system are determined with reference to the environment, to the animal's body midline axis, and to the next proximal or distal limb or body segment. By transforming the description of the same behavior from one coordinate system to the next, invariances in that behavior may emerge in some coordinate systems but not in others. Thus, the behavior may be invariant in relation to some or all of the following: the animal's

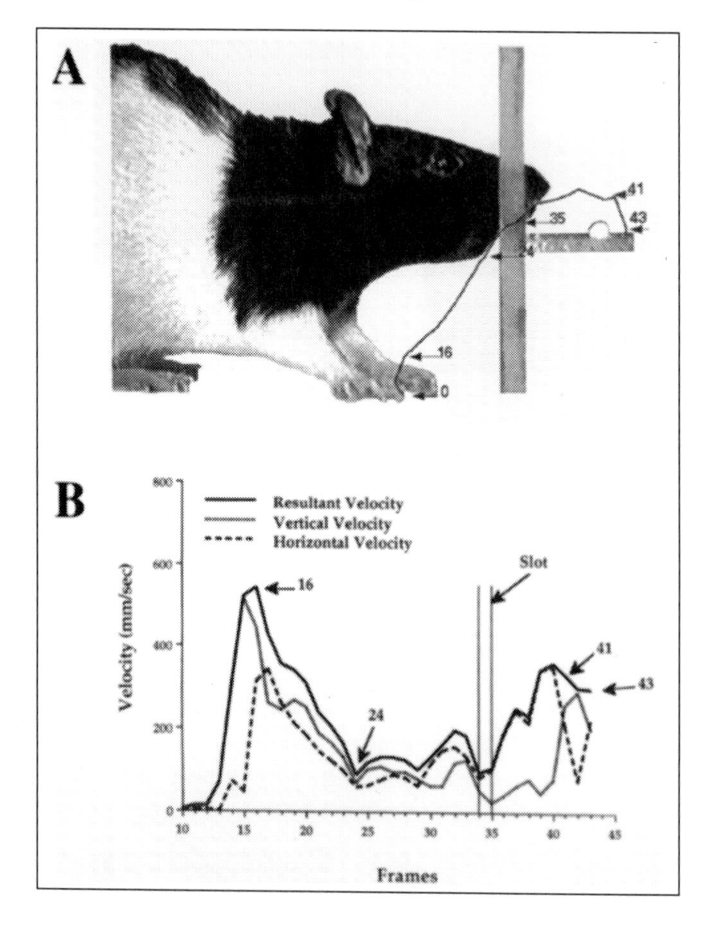

Fig. 8.7. (A) the location of a rat prior to initiating a reach and the trajectory that the tip of digit 3 takes as the paw is transported to the food. Numbers are frames from a video sequence that gave 120 fields per second: thus advancing the limb takes approximately one third of a second. Note that the trajectory of the paw carries it above and beyond the location of the food pellet. (B) Velocity curves for the trajectory of the reach illustrated in A. The curves show the velocity of the vertical and horizontal displacement of the limb as well as the combined or resultant velocity. Numbers indicate digit position as shown in A. We have found substantial variation in velocity profiles in individual rats even though the trajectories are quite similar.

longitudinal axis, gravity, or body wise in relation to the next proximal or distal segments.[66-68] Since a rat can make many body rotations while at the same time advancing a limb, a way of disentangling the limb movements from movements of other body parts is essential.

It is time consuming to notate every instance of a movement using EWMNS. Once the movement is described it usually becomes readily recognized to visual observation and thus can be documented using simpler recording procedures.[1] Some of the typical features of a reach identified by movement notation can be seen in Figures 8.8 and 8.9: (1) When the rat lifts its limb, the digits are semiflexed and the paw is rotated so that it faces the midline of the body, with the tips of the digits aligned along the axis of the midline of the body. This component is the high velocity component of the movement. (2) The elbow is then adducted so that it too is aligned along the midline of the body. To adduct the elbow the digits must be "fixed" to maintain their midline position, which actually requires that the forearm be abducted in relation to the movement of the elbow. This movement positions the limb so that it is "aimed" toward the target. (3) The limb is then advanced along the midline axis of the body (the snout is lifted to allow the limb to advance) and as it advances the digits are opened. (4) As the paw approaches the target, the elbow is abducted to pronate the paw over the food. Adduction of the elbow also extends the paw above and beyond the food (the reach exceeds the grasp). The paw then catches the food as the limb is withdrawn. (5) The food is grasped by the digits (see below). (6) Once the food is grasped the wrist is extended and supinated by movements around the wrist and adduction of the elbow so that palm of the paw faces medially. (7) The paw is withdrawn from the slot to a position just beneath the snout and then it is passively carried as the rat sits back on its haunches. (8) To eat, the rat supinates the paw at the wrist to place the food in its mouth or to partially transfer the food to the other paw for eating.

We would like to emphasize that the richness of descriptive technique is that not only does it provide a reliable way of describing movement, it is the best tutor we know for learning how to watch behavior. Once the topography of a movement is established by EWMNS, a number of the movement features can be measured and documented using a Cartesian coordinate system with initial and terminating components of the movements as reference points. Also, once certain features of the movements are identified, they can be quantified with simple rating scales.

DIGIT MOVEMENTS

The digits are numbered from 1 to 5, medial to lateral (Fig. 8.1) Digit 1, the equivalent to the human thumb, is quite small and has a nail while the other digits are larger and have claws. The relative size

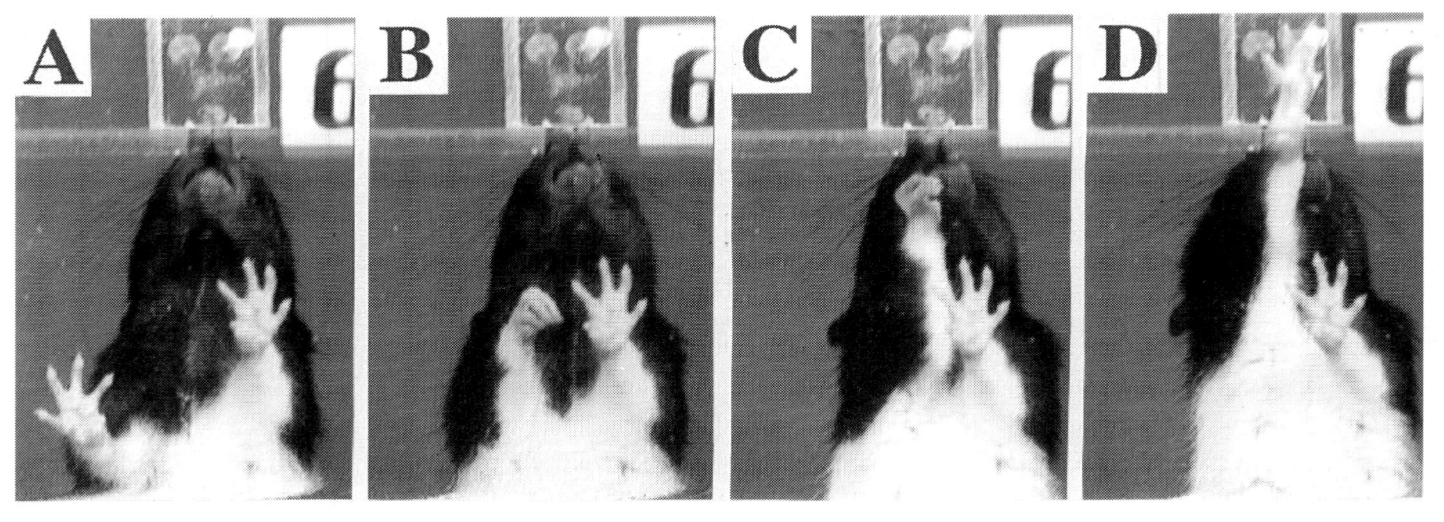

Fig. 8.8. Component movements involved in transporting the paw to the food in a typical reaching act. (A) The rat initiates the reach by aligning its body with the food slot and sniffing for the food pellet. (B) The paw is lifted so that the palm is turned medially and the tips of the digits are brought to the the midline of the body. (C) The elbow is brought to the midline of the body while the tips of the digits are held at their position on the body midline. This movement aims the paw at the food slot. (D) After the paw is advanced through the slot so that it is at the level of the food pellet, the paw is pronated by adduction of the elbow and rotation of the paw at the wrist. Adduction of the elbow not only aids in pronating the paw but extends the limb fully so that the digits extend beyond the food pellet.

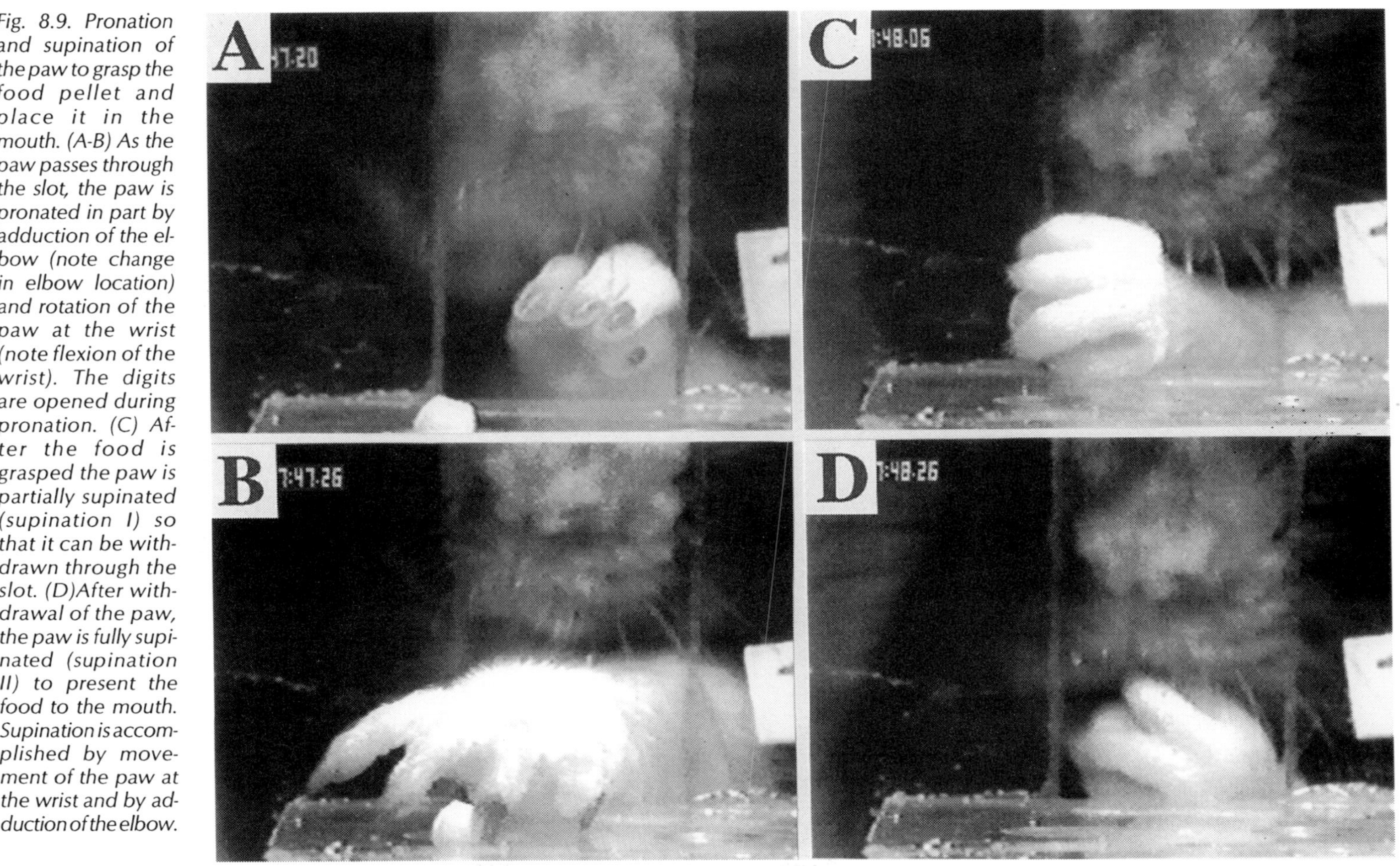

Fig. 8.9. Pronation and supination of the paw to grasp the food pellet and place it in the mouth. (A-B) As the paw passes through the slot, the paw is pronated in part by adduction of the elbow (note change in elbow location) and rotation of the paw at the wrist (note flexion of the wrist). The digits are opened during pronation. (C) After the food is grasped the paw is partially supinated (supination I) so that it can be withdrawn through the slot. (D) After withdrawal of the paw, the paw is fully supinated (supination II) to present the food to the mouth. Supination is accomplished by movement of the paw at the wrist and by adduction of the elbow.

of the digits are somewhat like that of humans. Little description has been made of digit movements, largely because the movements are so quick. For example, during a single reach the grasp will take place in less than 2/30th of a second, about two video frames. Description of digit movements are also encumbered by another problem: as yet no descriptive system for them has been devised. Thus, our descriptions are limited to movements during a particular act and digit shaping when an object is grasped.

We have examined the movements of the digits using high speed video recording that gives 60 frames/sec on normal replay and 120 fields/sec on replay.[31] This doubles the resolution of conventional video recording and can provide 8 to 12 frames of digit action during the approach to food and the grasp. We have found that as the paw is pronated to grasp a food pellet from a shelf, the 5th digit is placed onto the shelf first, followed in succession by digits 4, 3, and 2 in what we call an arpeggio pattern (Fig. 8.10). As each digit is placed onto the shelf, it is spread away from the preceding digit so to cover a wide area of the shelf. The paw is then pushed down onto the shelf in a palpating motion. If food is not present, the paw is withdrawn without flexure of the digits and then replaced. When food is present, the pattern of grasping depends in part on the size of the food pellet. Larger pieces of food are contacted by the pad of digit 3 and grasped between digits 3 and 4. Smaller food pellets are contacted by the pad of digit 4 and grasped between digits 4 and 5 (Fig. 8.11).

There is some degree of independent digit movement during grasping. When larger food pellets are grasped, flexure of digits 3 and 4 appears to precede flexion of the other digits and when smaller food pellets are grasped, flexure of digits 4 and 5 appears to precede flexure of the other digits. The most striking independent digit movement is made by digit 5, which is turned medially to grasp, thus playing the role of the human thumb. There are many other situations in which independent digit movements might occur, including climbing, handling prey or food, and grasping the fur when grooming but there are no studies of these movements.

Rats may also use a grasp movement that is comparable to a human pincer grasp (Fig. 8.12). When eating a thin long item such as pasta, rats hold one end of the pasta to their mouth using a grip in which the pasta appears to be held between digit 1 digit 2. The digits may even hold the pasta using the pads of one or both digits (since the digits are against the mouth the exact grasp is difficult to see). Although digit 1 is short and digit 2 is long, when digit 2 flexes it can be pressed against digit 1.

NEURAL CONTROL OF REACHING

It is beyond the scope of this chapter to describe how the brain controls limb and digit movements nor is it possible to provide a theo-

Fig. 8.10. The arpeggio movement used by the rat to locate food. The complete pattern is seen when there is no food present. The paw is pronated so that digit 5 touches the surface of the shelf (A) followed by digit 4 (B), digit 3 (C) and digit 4 (D). The rat then presses the paw down onto the surface of the shelf in searching for the pellet. When the food is not found the paw is slowly withdrawn, with the digits open and with one of the digits passing through the food indentation, to feel for the food.

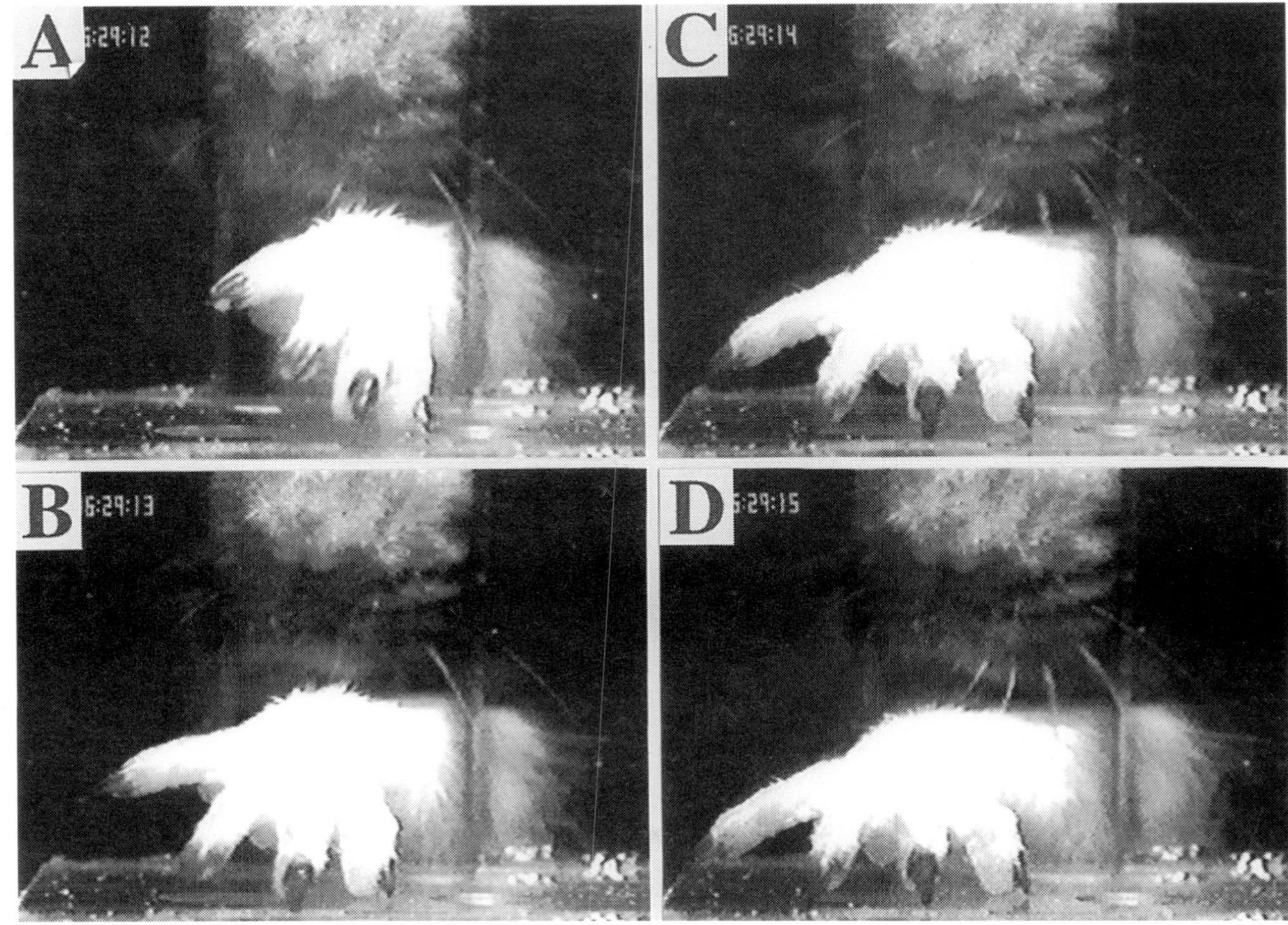

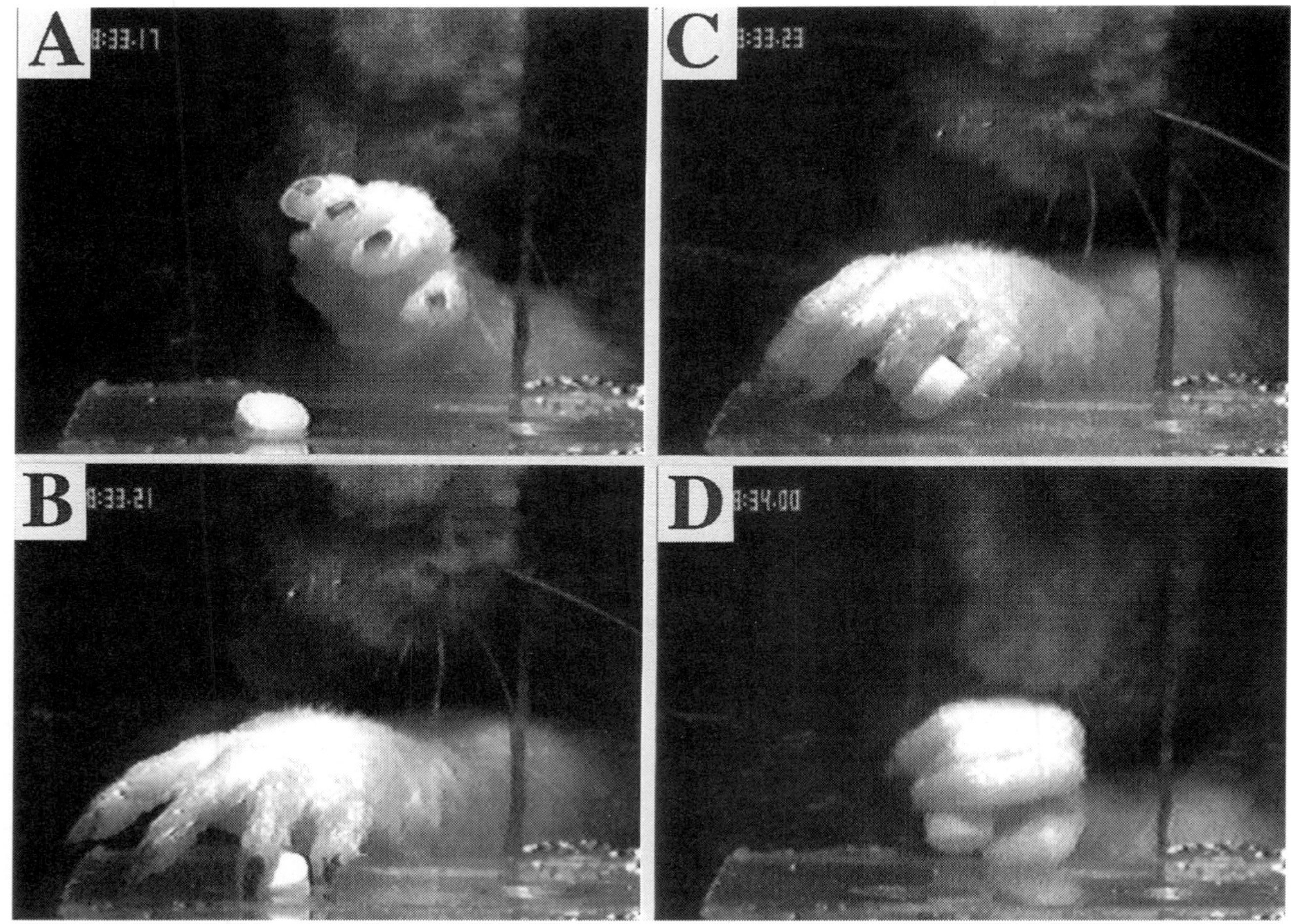

Fig. 8.11. Relatively independent use of the digits in grasping a 20 mg food pellet. After the paw is pronated over the food pellet (A) the arpeggio movement brings digit 4 into contact with the food pellet (B). The food is then grasped between digit 4 and digit 5 with digit 5 moving medially in a relatively independent movement as might a primate thumb. As the paw is supinated the other digits eventually close (D). Larger food pellets are usually grasped between digits 3 and 4 or less frequently between digits 2 and 3.

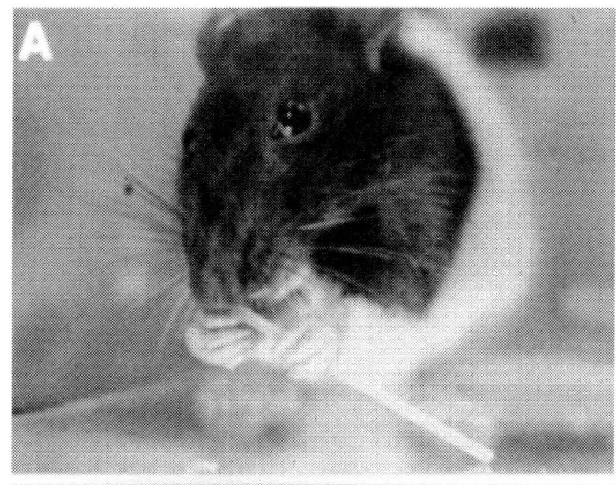

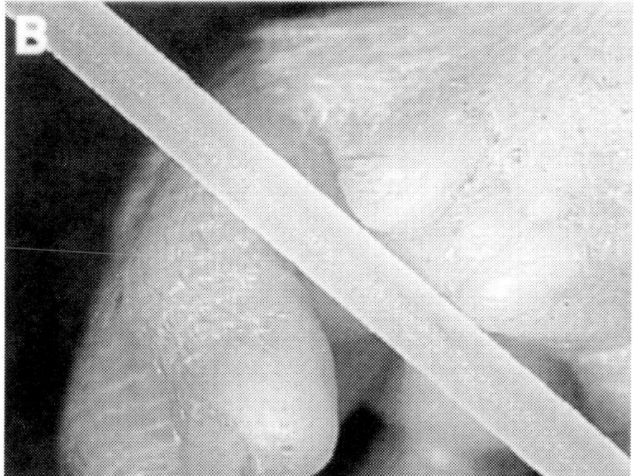

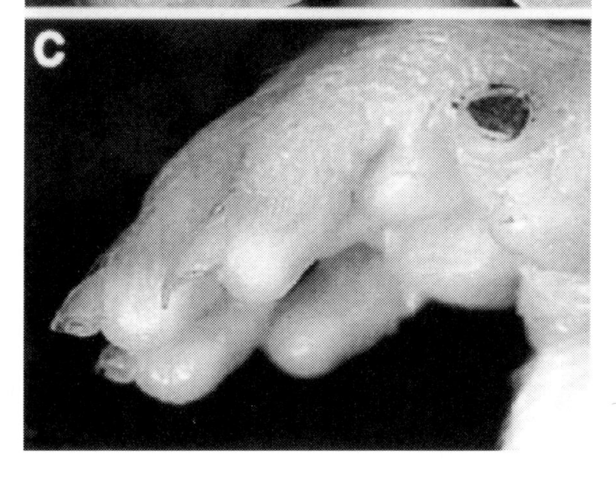

Fig. 8.12. Grasp patterns during pasta eating in the rat. (A) The rat is presenting the pasta to its mouth with its right paw. The other paw is used to push the food to the mouth as eating progresses and the grip pattern of left paw is different from that of the right paw. (B) The grasp pattern displayed by the right paw involves holding the pasta between the pads of digit 1 (thumb) and digit 2. (C) Digit 1 has a nail whereas digits 2 through 5 have claws. The presence of a nail on digit 1 suggests that it may receive considerable use in grasping objects.

retical framework for the movements. It is appropriate to provide a brief description of how brain damage can change movements, and to illustrate how the procedures described here can be used to detect elements of reaching and to show how they can change after different kinds of brain damage. We emphasize that single measures of a behavior can be misleading when used alone but can be very informative when used in conjunction with other measures.

Motor Cortex: Two Kinds of Recovery

Lesions of the motor cortex change limb preference[69] and produce acute and chronic deficits in limb use in reaching.[28,70] We have examined the basis of these deficits by conducting studies in which we have made various sized lesions to the motor cortex of well-trained rats.[71] One of the most curious features of the performance of rats with motor cortex damage is that their asymptotic performance is not closely related to lesion size. Rats with lesions that removed all of forelimb motor cortex and a good deal of surrounding cortex performed about as well as rats in which forelimb motor cortex was largely spared.

This initially very puzzling finding was resolved when we examined the behavior of the animals using slow motion video techniques and behavioral analysis using EWMNS. This analysis demonstrated that the rats with small lesions displayed genuine motoric recovery. Their ability to aim their limb, pronate the paw to grasp, and supinate the paw to withdraw the food and place in their mouth appeared quite normal. This was not true of the rats with the large lesion. They seemed unable to make any of these limb movements. Rather they substituted rotary movement of the body to replace lost limb movements, or stated differently, they used their body as a crutch to help them get the food. To aim they rotated their body ipsilateral to the limb to align the limb with the food slot. To pronate the paw they continued this rotation so that they frequently slid their paw under the food. To withdraw their paw, they counter-rotated their body (thus pronating the paw when control rats were supinating) and continued this counter-rotation so that they could bring their snout under the paw to aid in removing the food.

Thus in this study, using two kinds of measurement, we demonstrate two different kinds of recovery following forelimb damage. These behavioral and neural changes are very similar to what be expected following damage to motor cortex in primates. Real recovery following small lesions is likely mediated by spared motor cortex. Apparent recovery following large lesions is likely due to compensatory movements produced under the influence of the remaining motor cortex. Clearly, if either success scores or observation had been used alone, neither genuine recovery nor the effectiveness of substitution of movement could have been demonstrated.

Pyramidal Tract: Deficits Without Loss and Recovery on End Point Measures

The pyramidal tract has its origins not only in the forelimb area of the cortex, but in a wide area of the frontal and parietal cortex. This anatomical arrangement suggests that damage to the tract might produce deficits that are greater than those produced by motor cortex lesions. We have examined the effects of pyramidal tract lesions on reaching ability and found some quite surprising differences in these rats' performance as contrasted with the performance of rats with motor cortex lesions.[63] On the food tray test, the animals displayed almost no impairment. On the single food pellet test they showed a very marked reduction in performance. Surprising, the severe decline in performance followed by recovery, characteristic of motor cortex lesions, was not observed. The performance that an animal displayed on the day following surgery remained unchanged over a very long postoperative recovery period. Kinematic analysis, however, did indicate that in the immediate period following the damage, reaches were slowed and then recovered over the first two postoperative weeks. Video analysis indicated an enduring impairment in aiming, pronating, and supinating the limb and releasing the food. Rotational movements of the body and other compensatory actions are used, as is the case for rats with motor cortex lesions, to substitute for lost movements.

Thus, some of the impairments do resemble those of motor cortex, as might be expected, but the severe immediate postoperative impairment so characteristic of motor cortex lesions is not obtained, suggesting that this impairment may be uniquely related to neocortex damage. The notion that the pyramidal tract is involved mainly in distal movements was not supported either, since the movements that were impaired were both proximal and distal movements.

Red Nucleus: The Search Continues

Anatomical evidence suggests a role for the red nucleus in limb movements. Lawrence and Kuypers,[46] using the monkey, have suggested that the red nucleus has a role in the control of arm and hand movements. Electrophysiological studies have suggested that the red nucleus is involved in digit use, especially digit opening.[72] We have removed the cells of the red nucleus using the neurotoxin ibotenic acid. We have found within a day or two of surgery that the animals are performing at preoperative levels on the food tray test.[61] To visual observation they also appear to have little movement impairment, having only some mild impairments in aiming the limb.[73] We also found, however, that superior cerebellar peduncle, which passes through the red nucleus, was likely slightly damaged by the lesions. Thus, we could not unequivocally rule out the possibility that the mild behavioral deficits had their origin from damage to these fibers of passage.

Recently, we have reanalyzed reaching following red nucleus lesions by filming the movement with a high speed camera. We have found that when the rats grasp food, the arpeggio movement is absent and the grasp consists of a rapid flexion of the digits.[74] This suggests to us that the red nucleus may function to maintain extensor posture in the paw while the cortex produces the more fractionated movements of pronation and digit modification for grasping.

Basal Ganglia: Making Two Movements at Once

Damage to the basal ganglia, either by ibotenic acid lesions of the cell bodies, or by depletion of dopamine, produces a profound decline of performance in rats in end point tests of performance. These declines in performance are not characterized by the decline and recovery of performance seen after cortex lesions, but are immediate and enduring.[28,75-80]

To understand the basis of this impairment, we have examined reaching in rats depleted of dopamine (DA) bilaterally neonatally or unilaterally in adulthood.[42,41] End point measures showed that the neonatally depleted animals were severely impaired in using either limb. The adult animals had an enduring severe impairment in the use of the limb contralateral to the lesion. They were also impaired in the use of the ipsilateral limb but they showed some recovery in the use of this limb.

An examination of the performance of the neonatally DA depleted animals suggested that they had at least two impairments. The neonatally depleted rats were impaired in making limb movements, including aiming, pronating and supinating the limb. They were also impaired in adjusting their posture to compensate for weight changes produced by their limb movements. Their behavior was characterized by first making a postural adjustment, then making a reaching movement, then making a postural adjustment, etc. These alternating movements continued until they were successful in grasping a piece of food and they continued as the rat attempted to retrieve the food and eat it.

The animals depleted in adulthood are also impaired in making limb movements. They do adduct the limb to aim it, and they are impaired in pronating and supinating the limb. Thus, they seldom grasp the food and if they do grasp it, they are impaired in bringing the food to the mouth. They also do not use their affected (contralateral to the lesion) limbs to adjust posture. Consequently, when reaching with the bad forelimb, they support weight and move on their two good limbs (rather than using a diagonal couplet). When reaching with their good forelimb, they stand and adjust posture using only their good (ipsilateral) hindlimb.

The results of these studies suggest that the impairments underlying various kinds of brain damage in rats may be more complex than has been thought. If only end point measures are used, then it appears that basal ganglia damage produces effects similar to those of motor cortex. When end point measures are combined with observation, however, additional deficits are seen. These may also involve many changes in posture and reaching strategies.

RESTORATION OF FUNCTION

There have been a number of attempts to minimize the impairments in skilled limb movements either by making the lesion early in life, so that brain reorganization may take place, or by grafting tissue into damaged areas so that lost functions can be restored.

Damage to the motor cortex in infant rodents results in anatomical changes that can mediate deficits that might otherwise be expected to occur. For example, when the pyramidal tract is cut, as yet undescended fibers will grow around the cut and these will mediate seemingly normal behavior in adulthood. When the origin of the fibers, the motor cortex, is removed, fibers will descend from the contralateral motor cortex as an ipsilateral pyramidal tract pathway and this will mediate improved behavior in adulthood,[59] see Castro[81] for a review. Some features of this plastic remodeling are also obtained with cats[82] but apparently not with primates.[83]

Attempts to restore function with brain grafts have been marked by some failures and some promising outcomes. In a number of studies, in which suspension of DA-rich cells have been injected into the caudate-putamen after the DA system has been damaged, no improvement of performance has been obtained.[84-87] Other studies do report improvements,[88] suggesting that the nature of the graft is important for the outcome. When the cells in the caudate-putamen have been lesioned, however, some functional improvement has been obtained with grafts of tissue into the caudate putamen.[87,89] In has also been reported that grafts of cortical tissue given to neonatal rats after motor cortex lesions can make connections with the spinal cord and are electrophysiologically active[81] and can mediate improved performance in adulthood.[90] The latter finding, although interesting, is difficult to interpret given the extensive reorganization and accompanying behavioral improvement observed after neonatal motor cortex lesions.[59]

As promising as some of the results are, two cautionary statements must be made. In the studies in which neonatal rats are used there is substantial "rewiring" normally after damage so that it is unclear as yet how improvements mediated by rewiring can be distinguished from those conferred by the grafts of neural tissue. In addition, for most of the studies, the major measure of performance has been end point measures. Future studies will have to use multiple measures of end point success, behavioral observation, and kinematics to distinguish improvements in the use of compensatory processes from those of true recovery of function.

CONCLUSION

Although the use of multiple measures of performance is central to our research, its conceptual origins lie elsewhere. Philip Teitelbaum has repeatedly emphasized to his students and coworkers that behavioral research finds its strength in the use of multiple measures. He in turn acknowledges that this was a lesson taught to him by Georg von Békésy.[91] This chapter has been directed toward describing the methods and the results that we have obtained in the study of skilled limb movements in the rat. Importantly, we want to stress that it is unlikely that any single descriptive procedure will capture the richness and complexity of movement, the changes in movement that follow brain damage, or the changes that follow attempts to restore function. Until such a time when the "laws of movement" are understood, we think the simultaneous use of a number of descriptive measures will be necessary to represent the richness of movement.

ACKNOWLEDGMENTS

This research was supported by grants from the Natural Sciences and Engineering Council of Canada and by the National Centers of Excellence for Recovery of Function. Elena Miklyaeva was supported by a postdoctoral fellowship from the Alberta Heritage Foundation for Medical Research.

REFERENCES

1. Whishaw IQ. The decorticate rat. In: Kolb B, Tees RC, eds. The Cerebral Cortex of the Rat. Cambridge, MA: MIT Press, 1990a: 237-67.
2. Lassek AM. The Pyramidal Tract. Springfield, IL: Charles C. Thomas, 1954.
3. MacNeilage PF. Grasping in modern primates: the evolutionary context. In: Goodale MA, ed. Vision and Action: The Control of Grasping. Norwood, NJ: Ablex Publishing Corp., 1990:1-32.
4. Passingham R. The Human Primate. Oxford: Freeman, 1982.
5. Kuypers HGJM. Anatomy of the descending pathways. In: Brookhart, JM, Mountcastle, VB, eds. Handbook of Physiology: The Nervous System, Vol. 2, Part 1. Baltimore: Williams and Wilkins Company, 1981: 579-666.
6. Nudo RJ, Masterton RB. Descending pathways to the spinal cord, IV. Some factors related to the amount of cortex devoted to the corticospinal tract. J Comp Anat 1990; 296:584-97.
7. Gioanni Y, Lamarche M. A reappraisal of rat motor cortex organization by intracortical microstimulation. Brain Res 1985; 344:49-61.
8. Neafsey EJ, Bold EL, Haas G et al. The organization of the rat motor cortex: a microstimulation mapping study. Brain Res Rev 1986; 11:77-96.
9. Rouiller EM, Liang F, Moret V et al. Trajectory of redirected corticospinal axons after unilateral lesion of the sensorimotor cortex in neonatal rat: a phaseolus vulgaris-leucoagglutinin (PHA-L) tracing study. Exp Neurol 1991; 114:53-65.

10. Valverde F. The pyramidal tract in rodents. A study of its relations with the posterior column nuclei, dorsolateral reticular formation of the medulla oblongata, and cervical spinal cord (Golgi and electron microscopic observations). Zeitschrift für Zellforschung 1966; 71:297-363.
11. Kolb B, Whishaw IQ. Dissociation of the contributions of the prefrontal, motor, and parietal cortex to the control of movement in the rat: an experimental review. Can J Psychol 1983; 37:211-32.
12. Wise SP, Donoghue JP. Motor cortex of rodents. In: Jones EJ, Peters A, eds. Sensory-Motor Areas and Aspects of Cortical Connectivity: Cerebral Cortex. Vol 5. New York: Plenum, 1986:243-65.
13. Lashley KS. Brain Mechanisms and Intelligence. Chicago: University of Chicago Press, 1929.
14. Peterson GM. Mechanisms of handedness in the rat. Comp Psychol Monogr 1932-1937; 9:21-43.
15. Peterson GM, Fracarol C. The relative influence of the locus and mass of destruction upon the control of handedness by the cerebral cortex. J Comp Neurol 1938; 68:191-96.
16. Peterson GM, McGiboney DR. Reeducation of handedness in the rat following cerebral injuries. J Comp Physiol Psychol 1951; 44:191-96.
17. Peterson GM, Barnett PE. The cortical destruction necessary to produce a transfer of a forced-practice function. J Comp Physiol Psychol 1961; 54:382-85.
18. Peterson GM, Devine JV. Transfers in handedness in the rat resulting from small cortical lesions after limited forced practice. J Comp Physiol Psychol 1963; 56: 752-56.
19. Bures J, Brácha V. The control of movements by the motor cortex, In: Kolb B, Tees RC, eds. The Cerebral Cortex of the Rat. Cambridge, MA: The MIT Press, 1990:213-38.
20. Evenden JL, Robbins TW. Effects of unilateral 6-hydroxydopamine lesions of the caudate-putamen on skilled forepaws in the rat. Behav Brain Res 1984; 14:61-68.
21. Montoya CP, Campbell-Hope LJ, Pemberton KD et al. The "staircase test": a measure of independent forelimb reaching and grasping abilities in rats. J Neurosci Meth 1991; 36:219-28.
22. Price AW, Fowler SC. Deficits in contralateral and ipsilateral forepaw motor control following unilateral motor cortical ablations in rats. Brain Res 1981; 205:81-90.
23. Whishaw IQ, Dringenberg HC, Pellis SM. Spontaneous forelimb grasping in free feeding by rats: motor cortex aids limb and digit positioning. Behav Brain Res 1992b; 48:113-25.
24. Whishaw IQ, Coles BLK. Varieties of paw and digit movement during spontaneous food handling in rats: Postures, bimanual coordination, preferences, and the effect of forelimb cortex lesions. Behav Brain Res 1995; in press.
25. Ellard CG, Stewart DJ, Donaghy S et al. Behavioural effects of neocortical and cingulate lesions in the Mongolian gerbil. Behav Brain Res 1990; 36:41-51.

26. Kalil D, Schneider GE. Motor performance following unilateral pyramidal tract lesions in the hamster. Brain Res 1975; 100:170-74.
27. Greenough WT, Larson JR, Withers GS. Effects of unilateral and bilateral training in a reaching task on dendritic branching of neurons in the rat motor-sensory forelimb cortex. Behav Neural Biol 1985; 44:301-14.
28. Whishaw IQ, O'Connor RB, Dunnett SB. The contributions of motor cortex, nigrostriatal dopamine and caudate-putamen to skilled forelimb use in the rat. Brain 1986; 109:805-43.
29. Mihalik V, Saling M. Continual monitoring of reaching in rat using magnetic induction law. Physiol Behav 1989; 45:351-54.
30. Saling M, Sitarova T, Vejsada R et al. Reaching behavior in the rat: absence of forelimb peripheral input. Physiol Behav 1992; 51:1151:56.
31. Whishaw IQ, Gorny B. Arpeggio and fractionated digit movements used in prehension by rats. Behav Brain Res 1993.
32. Whishaw IQ, Pellis SM, Gorny BP Skilled reaching in rats and humans: Evidence of parallel development or homology. Behav Brain Res 1992d; 47:59-70.
33. Whishaw IQ, Pellis, SM. The structure of skilled forelimb reaching in the rat: A proximally driven movement with a single distal rotatory component. Behav Brain Res 1990; 41:49-59.
34. Whishaw IQ, Tomie J. Olfaction directs skilled forelimb reaching in the rat. Behav Brain Res 1989; 32:11-21.
35. Whishaw IQ. Time estimates contribute to food handling decisions by rats: Implications for neural control of hoarding. Psychobiology 1990b; 18:460-66.
36. Goodale MA, Milner AD, Jakobson LS et al. A neurological dissociation between perceiving objects and grasping them. Nature 1991; 349:154-57.
37. Ioffe ME, Ivanova NG, Frolov AA et al. On the role of motor cortex in the learned rearrangement of postural coordinations. In: Gurfinkel, VS, Ioffe, ME, Massion J et al, eds. Stance and Motion. New York: Plenum Press, 1988:213-26.
38. DeLong M. Motor functions of the basal ganglia: single-unit activity during movement. In: Schmitt FO, Worden FG, eds. The Neurosciences: Third Study Program. Cambridge, MA: The MIT Press, 1974:319-25.
39. Fukuda T. Statokinetic Reflexes in Equilibrium and Movement. Tokyo: University of Tokyo Press, 1984.
40. Martin JP. The Basal Ganglia and Posture. London: Pitman Medical Publishing Co., Ltd., 1967.
41. Miklyaeva EI, Whishaw IQ. Skilled reaching deficits in unilateral dopamine-depleted rats: Impairments in movement and posture and compensatory adjustments. J Neurosci 1994; 14:7148-58.
42. Whishaw IQ, Gorny B, Trau-Nguyen LTH et al. Making two movements at once: Impairments of movement, posture, and their integration underlie the adult skilled reaching deficit of neonatally dopamine-depleted rats. Behav Brain Res 1994; 61:65-77.
43. Jackson J, ed. Hughlings, Selected Writings of John Hughlings Jackson (2 vols.) New York: Basic Books, Inc., 1956.

44. Schieber MH, Hibbard LD. How somatotopic is the motor cortex hand area? Science 1993; 261:489-92.
45. Jeannerod M. The Neural and Behavioral Organization of Goal-directed Movements. Oxford: Clarendon Press, 1988.
46. Lawrence DG, Kuypers HGJM. The functional organization of the motor system in the monkey. I. The effects of bilateral pyramidal lesions. Brain 1968; 91:1-14.
47. Green EC. Anatomy of the Rat. New York: Hafner Publishing, 1963.
48. Hyland BI, Reynolds JN. Pattern of activity in muscles of shoulder and elbow during forelimb reaching in the rat. Human Movement Sci 1993; 12:51-70.
49. Eisenberg JF, Golani I. Communication in metatheria. In: Seboek, TA, ed. How Animals Communicate. Bloomington, IN: Indiana University Press, 1977.
50. Whishaw IQ. Lateralization and reaching skill related: results and implications from a large sample of Long-Evans rats. Behav Brain Res 1992; 52: 45-8.
51. Miklyaeva EI, Ioffe ME, Kulikov MA. Innate versus learned factors determining limb preference in the rat. Behav Brain Res 1991; 46:103-16.
52. Brácha V, Zhuravin IA, Bures J. The reaching reaction in the rat: a part of the digging pattern? Behav Brain Res 1990; 36:53-64.
53. Miklyaeva E I, Varlinskaya EI, Ioffe ME. et al Differences in the recovery rate of a learned forelimb movement after ablation of the motor cortex in right and left hemisphere in white rats. Behav Brain Res 1993; 56:145-54.
54. Miklyaeva EI, Bures J. Reversal of "handedness" in rats is achieved more effectively by training under peripheral than under central blockade of the preferred forepaw. Neurosci Lett 1991; 125:89-92.
55. Tsai LS, Maurer S. "Right handedness" in white rats. Science 1930; 72:436-38.
56. Yoshioka JG. Handedness in rats. J Genet Psychol 1930; 39:471-74.
57. Wentworth KL. Some factors determining handedness in the white rat. Genet Psychol Monogr 1942; 26:55-117.
58. Collins RL. Toward an admissible genetic model for the inheritance of the degree and direction of asymmetry. In: Harnad S, Doty RW, Goldstein L et al. Lateralization in the Nervous System. New York: Academic Press, 1977:137-150.
59. Whishaw IQ, Kolb B. Sparing of skilled forelimb reaching and corticospinal projections after neonatal motor cortex removal or hemidecortication in the rat: support for the Kennard doctrine. Brain Res 1988; 451:97-114.
60. Whishaw IQ, Pellis SM, Gorny BP. Medial frontal cortex lesions impair the aiming component of rat reaching. Behav Brain Res 1992c; 50:93-104.
61. Whishaw IQ, Tomie J, Ladowsky RL. Red nucleus lesions do not affect limb preference or use, but exacerbate the effects of motor cortex lesions on grasping in the rat. Behav Brain Res 1990; 40:131-44.

62. Castro-Alamancos MA, Borrell J. Reversal of paw preference after ablation of the preferred forelimb primary motor cortex representation of the rat depends on the size of the forelimb representation. Neuroscience 1993; 552:636-44.
63. Whishaw IQ, Pellis SM, Gorny B et al. Proximal and distal impairments in rat forelimb use in reaching follow unilateral pyramidal tract lesions. Behav Brain Res 1993; 56: 59-76.
64. Eshkol N, Wachman A. Movement Notation. London: Weidenfeld and Nicholson, 1958.
65. Golani I, Wolgin DL, Teitelbaum, P. A proposed natural geometry of recovery from akinesia in the lateral hypothalamic rat. Brain Res 1979; 164:237-67.
66. Ganor I, Golani I. Coordination and integration in the hindleg step cycle of the rat: Kinematic synergies. Brain Res 1980; 195:57-67.
67. Golani I. Homeostatic motor processes in mammalian interactions: a choreography of display. In: Bateson, PPG, Klopfer, PH, eds. Perspectives in Ethology, Vol. 2. New York: Plenum, 1976:69-134.
68. Pellis SM Development of head and foot coordination in Australian magpie *Gymnorhina tibicen*, and the function of play. Bird Behav 1983; 4:57-62.
69. Peterson GM, Barnett PE. The cortical destruction necessary to produce a transfer of a forced-practice function. J Comp Physiol Psychol 1961; 54:382-85.
70. Castro AJ. The effects of cortical ablations on digital usage in the rat. Brain Res 1972; 37: 173-85.
71. Whishaw IQ, Pellis SM, Gorny BP et al. The impairments in reaching and the movements of compensation in rats with motor cortex lesions: an endpoint, videorecording, and movement notation analysis. Behav Brain Res 1991; 42: 77-91.
72. Houk JC, Gibson AR, Harvey CF et al. Activity of primate magnocellular red nucleus related to hand and finger movements. Behav Brain Res 1988; 28:201-06.
73. Whishaw IQ, Pellis SM, Pellis VC. A behavioral study of the contributions of cells and fibers of passage in the red nucleus of the rat to postural righting, skilled movements, and learning. Behav Brain Res 1992; 52:29-44.
74. Whishaw IQ, Gorny B. Does the red nucleus provide the tonic support against which fractionated movements occur?: A study on forepaw movements used in skilled reaching by the rat. Behav Brain Res 1995; In press.
75. Pisa M. Motor functions of the striatum in the rat: critical role of the lateral region in tongue and forelimb reaching. Neurosciences 1988; 24:453-63.
76. Pisa M. Motor somatotopy in the striatum of rat: manipulation, biting and gait. Behav Brain Res 1988; 27:21-35.
77. Pisa M, Cyr J. Regionally selective roles of the rat's striatum in modality-specific discrimination learning and forelimb reaching. Behav Brain Res 1990; 37:281-92.
78. Sabol KE, Neill DB, Wages SA et al. Dopamine depletion in a striatal subregion disrupts performance of a skilled motor task in the rat. Brain Res 1985; 335:33-43.

79. Schneider JS, Olazabal UE. Behaviorally specific limb use deficits following globus pallidus lesions in rats. Brain Res 1974; 308:341-46.
80. Whishaw IQ, Castañeda E, Gorny BP. Dopamine and skilled limb use in the rat: more severe bilateral impairments follow substantia nigra than sensorimotor cortex 6-hydroxydopamine injection. Behav Brain Res 1992; 47: 89-92.
81. Castro AJ. Plasticity in the motor system. In: Kolb B, Tees RC, eds. The Cerebral Cortex of the Rat. Cambridge, MA: The MIT Press, 1990: 563-88.
82. Armand J, Kalby B. Critical timing of sensorimotor cortex lesions for the recovery of motor skills in the developing cat. Exp Brain Res 1993; 93:73-88.
83. Passingham RE, Perry VH, Wilkinson F. The long-term effects of removal of sensorimotor cortex in infant and adult rhesus monkeys. Brain 1983; 385:675-705.
84. Abrous DN, Wareham AT, Torres EM et al. Unilateral lesions in neonatal, weanling and adult rats: comparison of rotation and reaching deficits. Behav Brain Res 1992; 51: 67-75.
85. Abrous DN, Shalot A, Torres EM et al. Dopamine-rich grafts in the neostriatum and/or the nucleus accumbens: effects on drug-induced behaviours and skilled paw reaching. Neuroscience 1993; 53:187-97.
86. Dunnett SB, Whishaw IQ, Rogers DC et al. Dopamine-rich grafts ameliorate whole body motor asymmetry and sensory neglect but not independent limb use in rats with 6-hydroxydopamine lesions. Brain Res 1987; 415:63-78.
87. Montoya CP, Astell S, Dunnett SB. Effect of nigral and striatal grafts on skilled forelimb use in the rat. Progress in Brain Res 1990; 82:459-66.
88. Nikkhah G, Duan WM, Knappe U. et al. Restoration of complex sensorimotor behavior and skilled forelimb use by a modified nigral cell suspension transplantation approach in the rat parkinson model. Neurosciences 1993; 56: 33-44.
89. Dunnett SB, Isaacson O, Sirinathsinghji DJS et al. Striatal graft in rats with unilateral neostriatal lesions. III. Recovery from dopamine-dependent motor asymmetry and deficits in skilled paw reaching. Neuroscience 1988; 24:813-20.
90. Plumet J, Cadusseau J, Roger M. Skilled forelimb use in the rat: amelioration of functional deficits resulting from neonatal damage to the frontal cortex by neonatal transplantation of fetal cortical tissue. Rest Neurol Neurosci 1991; 3: 134-37.
91. von Békésy G. Experiments in Hearing. New York: McGraw-Hill, 1960.

CHAPTER 9

Measurement of Swimming Kinematics in Small Terrestrial Mammals

Frank E. Fish

INTRODUCTION

Virtually all mammals can swim,[1,2] but the sophistication and development of this important locomotor activity varies. While swimming by small mammals has been investigated for its own intrinsic merit to determine the mechanics and energetics of thrust generation,[3-7] various researchers used mammalian swimming as an experimental technique.

Swimming allows the maintenance of constant activity over a prolonged time period.[8] Swimming endurance was used as a test of survivability for fossorial species faced with floods in their natural habitats.[9-12] Physiological changes associated with bone remodeling and muscle metabolism were examined after prolonged swimming bouts.[13-16] Prolonged swimming trials in rats were employed as a model for human depression associated with drug effects.[17] Although antidepressant drugs were observed to reduce immobility and increase swimming time, the appropriateness of the model is to be viewed cautiously because the response of the rat to prolonged immersion could be an adaptive response to a stressful situation.[18]

Swimming is ideal for studies of motor response and development, because during swimming coordinated movements are required of the limbs and trunk.[19] Because swimming is less demanding in terms of postural and gravitational constraints,[20] this locomotor mode is less mechanically stressful for the experimental animal. Comparisons between swimming and stepping were performed to investigate neural

Measuring Movement and Locomotion: From Invertebrates to Humans, edited by Klaus-Peter Ossenkopp, Martin Kavaliers and Paul R. Sanberg.

organization.[21,22] Changes in locomotor movements between swimming and walking are due possibly to differences in sensory feedback which modify pre-programmed locomotor commands.[21,23] Experiments on the development of coordination may be undertaken on mammals, such as the rat, which are born in a relatively immature state.[24-26] Studies of movement disorders were investigated using swimming to test drugs that induce or reverse motor impairment.[19,27] Recently, swimming was used to assess behavioral adaptation to gravitational alterations with application to space flight.[28,29]

Precise information regarding the swimming motion of the body and limbs of a small mammal may be ascertained through kinematic analysis. This method is preferable to simplistic descriptions of the gross movements of the body. Descriptions of swimming motions, such as "dog paddle,"[1,12] are not only imprecise but erroneous. The complexity of the coordinated swimming movements requires analytical techniques that accurately measure movement and characterize the principle determinants for movement. While it has been suggested that kinematic analysis is limited,[20] kinematic analysis is relatively simple to perform and can supply more data on animal movement than techniques individually using electromyographics, goniometers, accelerometers, strain gauges, or force transducers. However, few studies have reported on the kinematic properties of the locomotor patterns in small mammals.

This chapter discusses some of the basic techniques and considerations for kinematic analysis in swimming by small terrestrial mammals. Included in this discussion are semiaquatic mammals which exhibit morphologies and behaviors related to the aquatic environment,[30] but show similar swimming patterns with their terrestrial relatives. Indeed, Wall[31] recognized only two groups of mammals, aquatic and terrestrial.

KINEMATICS

Kinematics is the study of motion which deals with position, displacement, velocity, and acceleration.[32] In this regard, kinematics provides a mathematical description of motion in time and space irrespective of the dynamic forces that produce the motion. Kinematic analysis has been applied to examinations of humans in regard to athletic performance, neuromotor function, and developmental changes. However, the roots of kinematic analysis in the biological system are grounded in the studies of animal locomotion. Eadweard Muybridge[33] began his studies of gait in racehorses in 1872. Muybridge was able to capture individual images of the horse over a gait cycle using a battery of still cameras. With the advent of cine cameras, video technology, high-speed strobes, and computers, kinematic analysis for the study of animal locomotion has become simpler and more precise to perform.[32,34-37]

Cine and Video Analysis

Although subjective observations can be used to judge animal performance, the motion of the limbs of small mammals is too rapid for the observer to record detailed kinematics. High-speed cinematography can be used to quantitatively evaluate swimming motions. Numerical data can be compared, ranked, and analyzed statistically.[36] Hildebrand[34] listed various advantages of cinematography for motion analysis, including: (1) the motion of animals that in life are far too fast and complex to be observed with the unaided eye can be slowed down, (2) each frame of film can be studied independently as a still picture, (3) each frame can be recorded at a discrete time interval, (4) variations in the durations of periodic cycles can be measured, and (5) the various motions which combine to compose an animal's activity can be examined with respect to one another both temporally and spatially. Additional advantages of cinematography include that films can be stored for further study in the future, the application of cinematography does not restrict the motions of the animal due to recording equipment or wiring, and the technique is non-invasive, requiring no surgery.[38]

Cinematographic examination of the swimming motions of small mammals is undertaken easily with two-dimensional (2D) analysis, because the major motions of the limbs during the paddling stroke are confined to the sagittal or vertical plane.[39] As a spatial reference, the animal and its movements should be placed in a Cartesian or rectangular coordinate system (Fig. 9.1). Therefore it is helpful to place a reference grid of equal squares of known size in the field of view. Such a grid acts as a scale to determine actual distances and to correct for the aspect ratio of the camera. The grid should be aligned with the horizontal and vertical axes of the coordinate system, with the vertical axis aligned with gravity.[32]

A camera placed laterally and at right angles to the plane of movement of the limbs can record major propulsive movements. Use of cine (i.e., super 8 mm, 16 mm) or video cameras can provide sharp images at regular timed intervals for a high level of resolution during analysis. Loeb and Gans[32] list the relative advantages of film and videotape for motion analysis and they provide technical information about the use of each medium.

An important concern for motion analysis is the framing rate of the camera. Hildebrand[34] recommended that events be recorded with at least 20 frames per cycle with 30 frames per cycle as optimal. In general, a filming rate of 50-200 frames per second is required for motion of less than 6 Hz,[35] which is within the frequency range for steadily swimming small mammals.[1,4-6] Standard filming rate for cine cameras is 24 frames per second, although variable speed cameras can go up to 64 frames per second, and medium and high speed cameras have filming rates of 500 and 10,000 frames per second, respectively.[32]

However, such high filming rates require large amounts of illumination, which may alter the behavior of the animal. Another drawback of using high speed cameras is the time required to analyze the vast amount of film generated.[35] Standard video cameras generate only 30 frames per second. Each video frame is composed of two interlaced image fields which are 16.7 msec apart. Special video systems (e.g. Peak Performance Technologies) are available which can separate and enhance the image fields to provide a rate of 60 images per second. Kodak produces a video system that can generate up to 12,000 digital pictures per second (Kodak Ecta Pro High Speed Video).

Individual frames of film can be displayed for analysis using a stop-action projector and video images can be analyzed using a video recorder. From film projections, position changes of the body and movements of the animal's limbs are obtained from sequential tracings. The tracings can be reduced to stick figures to display relevant motions (Fig. 9.2). The joints may be assumed to have fixed centers of rotation so long as the limb motion remain planar.[39] The superimposition of multiple images over a full cycle of motion assists in measuring displacement and clearly shows the changes in position between time intervals. A similar approach for video is to trace sequential images onto a sheet of clear acetate overlaying the video monitor or multiple images can be superimposed electronically.

Although tracings provide a pictorial representation, an additional step is required to obtain numerical data. Digital information on position

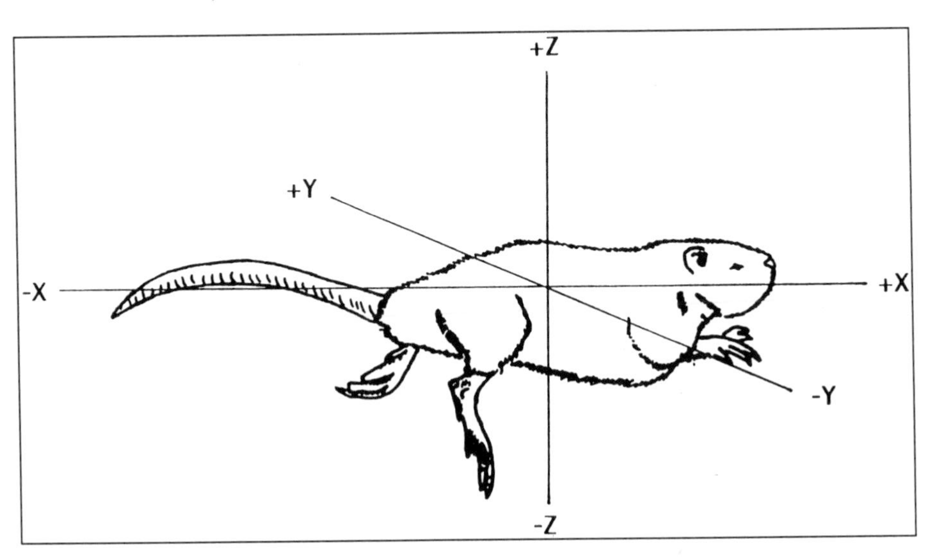

Fig. 9.1. Swimming mammal within Cartesian or rectangular coordinate system. The direction of motion is labelled as the x-axis, the vertical axis is the z-axis, and the y-axis is the directed mediolateral. Each axis is perpendicular to the other two. Conventions for labelling axes vary between researchers and animals studied (see refs. 53 and 57).

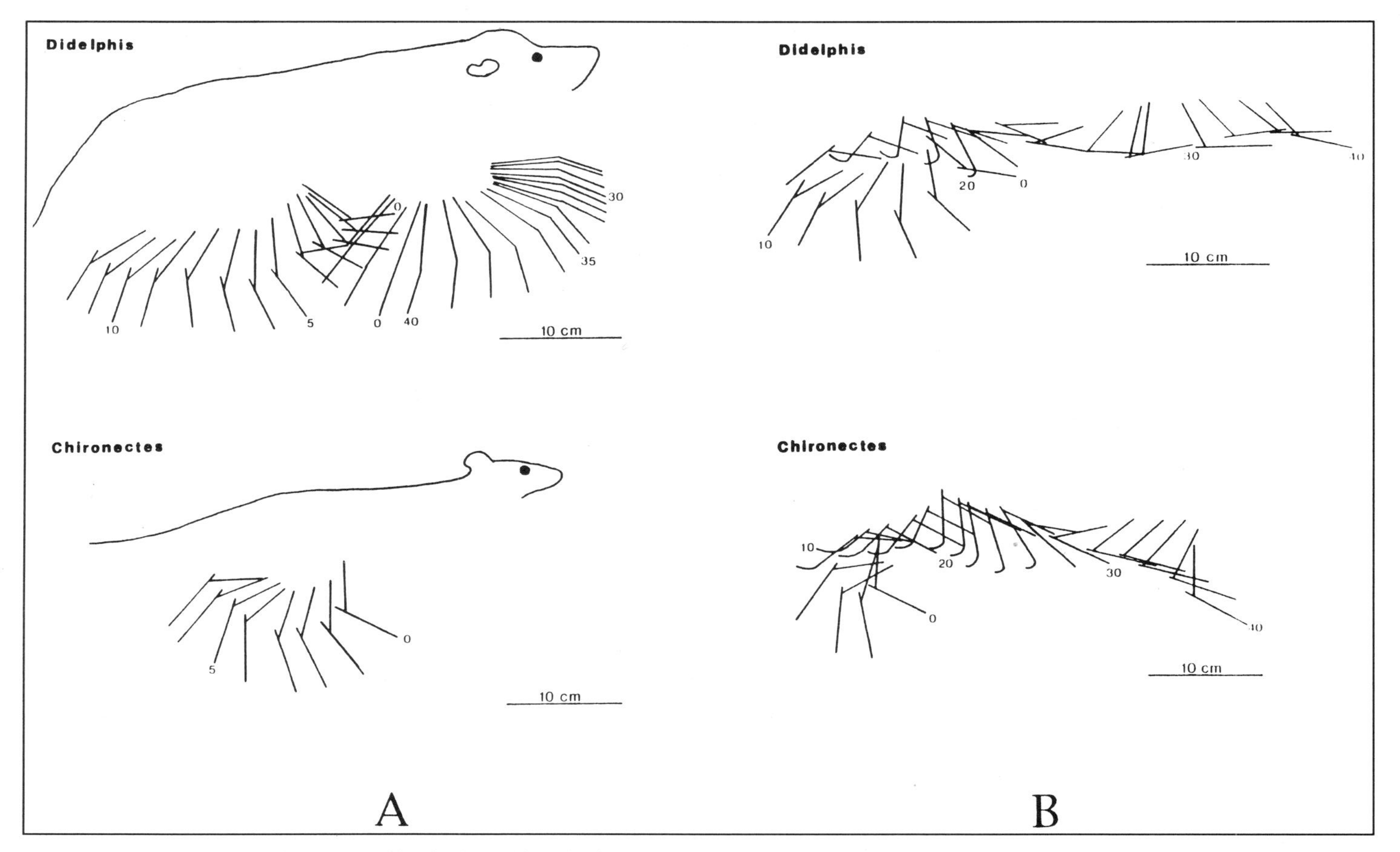

*Fig. 9.2. Sequential tracings from films of forelimbs and hindlimbs of swimming Virginia opossum (*Didelphis virginiana*) and yapok or water opossum (*Chironectes minimus*). Swimming speed was 0.43 m/s for Didelphis and 0.45 for Chironectes. Filming rate was 64 frames per second. Numbers indicate film frames through the stroke cycle, where frame 0 indicates the start of the power phase for the hind limb. (A). The power phase of the paddling cycle with the body position held constant as a fixed frame of reference. (B.) Movement of the hindlimb is shown through power and recovery phases with body position not held constant. Figures were originally published from Fish.[6]*

may be directly obtained by film projection onto a digitizer tablet interfaced to a computer. The data for discrete points on the body are selected and stored as X and Y coordinates which can be manipulated for calculation of kinematic variables and statistical parameters. Advances in video and computer technology have made digitizing video images available as a measurement technique in animal locomotion. Computer hardware, such as a frame-grabber board, can import an analog video image recorded on videotape into a computer (Peak Performance Technologies). Besides converting and storing the image digitally, the computer can control the video recorder for playback.

Various errors occur in the application of cinematography in studies of locomotion.[32,34,36,38,40] The periodic motion of the limbs will vary between consecutive strokes. Variations will be greater for small animals than large animals and relatively greater for immature animals than adults.[34] Such errors are controlled by averaging the kinematics of at least three consecutive strokes. Errors due to parallax are avoided by using a telephoto lens with the camera positioned at a distance from the subject.[32] To maintain precision and accuracy in digitizing points on the body, a shuttered camera is necessary to provide sharp images for digitizing. In addition, markers should be placed on primary features to be analyzed (i.e., joints, limb segments). In water, painted markers are preferable to markers attached by adhesives. I have found that correction fluids such as "Liquid Paper" (Gillette Company, Stationary Products Divisions) perform well because correction fluids do not wash off in water, are quick drying after application, and contrast well with the skin when viewed from videotape. Control errors due to skin movement artifact can be avoided by painting markers on segments where the skin movement is small enough to be neglected.[36]

An alternate approach to cinematographic data collection on propulsive movements is to use multiple flash photography.[41] A pulsed electronic strobe in conjunction with a still camera can provide multiple images for motion analysis (Fig. 9.3). Although this method is relatively inexpensive compared to film and video analysis, there is a large amount of trial-and-error required to coordinate the flash rate with the periodic motions of the animal subject and exposure time of the camera.

Swim Tanks and Flow Tanks

The simplest apparatus for observing swimming motions in small mammals is an observation tank. Glass-walled aquaria, which are manufactured in a variety of sizes, can be purchased for use as observation tanks, or a tank can be fabricated with acrylic plastic (e.g., Plexiglas, Lucite). The tank should be long enough to allow the animal to accelerate up to and maintain a constant velocity within the field of observation. The depth of the tank must be sufficiently deep to avoid interference with the motion of the feet. A desirable feature to have in

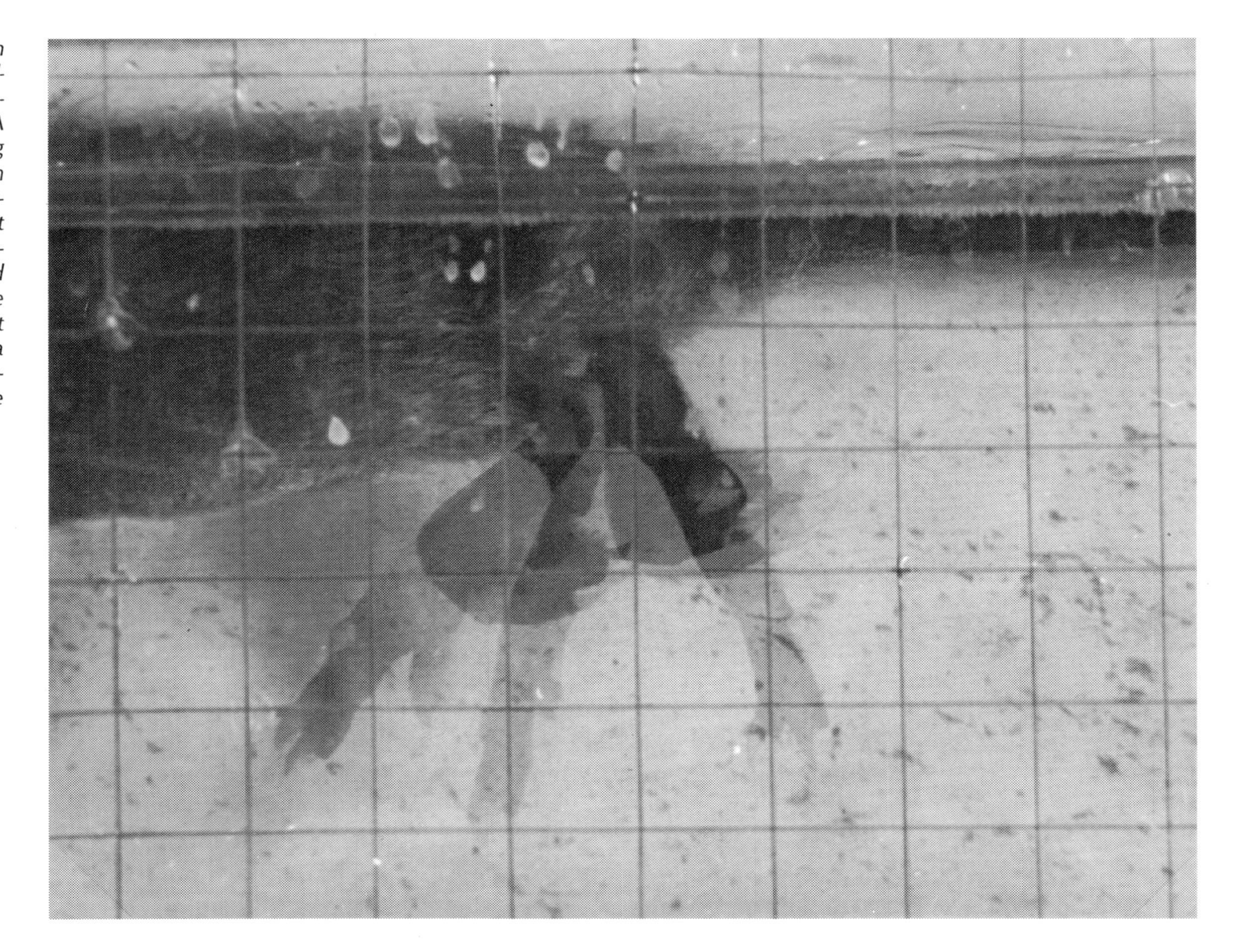

Fig. 9.3. Multiple flash photograph of the hind-feet of a muskrat swimming in a flow tank. A complete paddling cycle is shown with power phase (toes extended and foot swept to the right) and recovery phase (toes flexed and foot swept to the left). It can be seen that the foot experiences a large acceleration during the latter part of the power phase.

the observation tank is a transparent floor. A mirror positioned at a 45° angle below the floor will allow simultaneous observations of ventral and lateral views of the swimming mammal. This arrangement is particularly helpful in noting deviations of the limb movements from the vertical plane which are demonstrated in submerged swimming moles[12] and muskrat.[42]

The disadvantage of using observation tanks for kinematic analysis is the minimal control over the motions and swimming effort of the animal. A small mammal may not swim steadily or rectilinearly across the field of vision. Bekoff and Trainer[24] observed young rat pups (1-14 days) to often swim in circles in a square tank. Furthermore, the field of vision required for the camera may be so large in order to capture successive cycles of propulsive movements that resolution is sacrificed.

Studies on animal swimming have been facilitated greatly by the use of flow tanks or swimming flumes. Such apparatuses, which act like an aquatic treadmill, provide the animal with a steady current of water to swim against, and allow the experimenter to control the animal's swimming velocity, position, and effort.[3,4,7] By eliminating the translational movements of the animal, the movements of the appendages can then be easily dissected out from the gross movements of the body. In addition with the subject swimming in a fixed position, the field of view needed for cinematography can be reduced for maximum resolution of the pictorial records.

Designs for inexpensive, simple flow tanks are provided by Vogel and LaBarbera,[43] Vogel,[44] and Denny.[45] In brief, recirculating flow tanks consist of an observation section, return channel, and motor (Fig. 9.4). The observation section, where the animal swims, can be constructed as a long, horizontal, rectangular trough from acrylic plastic, and should be large enough to accommodate the animal without interference from the walls or floor. Flow grids of plastic tubes or straws should be placed in the upstream end of the working section to straighten water flow and remove turbulence which may affect animal swimming. For the return channel, plastic piping is desirable because it is easy to make water-tight and is available in a variety of sizes in both straight and curved sections. It is recommended that the observation section be located above the return channel to minimize turbulence and wave formation from the exposed air-water interface.[44]

To drive water through the flow tank, a small electric motor can be used to turn a propeller situated in a vertical section of the return channel. A constant-speed motor can produce different flow speeds by driving the propeller shaft through a series of pulleys.[43] A more expensive alternative is to use commercially available high-torque, variable-speed laboratory stirrers.[46]

Whether working with subjects in an aquarium or flow tank, filming through water and a transparent wall present problems with respect to illumination. Photographic flood lights must not be positioned directly perpendicular to the observation area, because of the resulting reflective glare. Lights should be positioned at an angle to the observation area. This will reduce glare and reduce shadows in the background. However, stronger illumination is required because much of the light is reflected and refracted as it travels through the different media.

KINEMATIC VARIABLES

Qualitatively, the paddling motion of the limbs can be divided into two phases: power and recovery.[4,47] The beginning of the power phase is indicated by the farthest anterior extension of foot before it is accelerated posteriorly through an arc. The end of the power phase is indicated by the farthest extension of the foot before it is moved anteriorly. Alternatively, power phase has been defined as the extension of the limb from minimum to maximum hip angle.[21] The posterior sweep of the foot is produced by extension of the joints of the limb and accompanied by abduction of the digits of the foot. These actions generate a propulsive thrust force to the animal as the foot pushes posteriorly on the water.[4,48] Maximum thrust is attained when

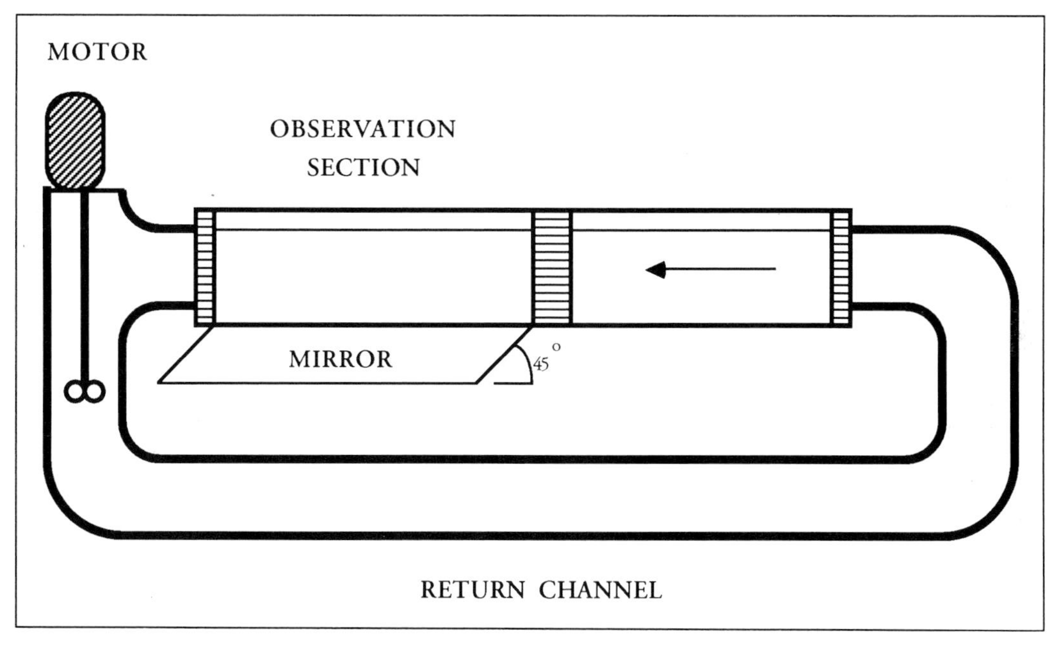

Fig. 9.4. Schematic diagram of a recirculating flow tank. The observation section, where the animal swims, is rectangular in cross-section and constructed with transparent walls and floor. A mirror can be positioned below the observation section and canted at a 45° angle for simultaneous viewing of lateral and ventral aspects of the animal. The water speed is controlled by a variable speed electric motor which drives a propeller in the vertical section of the return channel. Water direction is indicated by the arrow. Flow straightening grids are located at the up- and downstream ends of the observation section.

the foot is oriented 90° to the direction of movement of the body.[48] No thrust is generated during the recovery phase of the stroke, which is associated with repositioning the foot for the next power phase. During recovery, the foot is swept anteriorly by flexion of the limb joints. The digits of the foot are adducted to reduce resistance and prevent a reduction of net thrust production as the foot is repositioned.

Movement of the limbs during the paddling stroke cycle can be described by simple physical parameters related to oscillatory motion. The key physical parameters that affect the velocity and the power output are:

1. Frequency—the number of stroke cycles per second (Hz). For small mammals, frequency ranges from 2.5 Hz for the muskrat, *Ondatra zibethicus*,[4] to 25 Hz for the smaller house mouse, *Mus musculus*.[1] The frequency of paddling generally remains constant in relation to swimming speed. However, the opossum, *Didelphis virginiana*, which swims using all four limbs, increases stroke frequency with speed.[6]

2. Phase times—elapsed time of power and recovery phases of the stroke cycle. Contrary to terrestrial locomotion in which the recovery phase is shorter than the power phase,[49,50] paddle propulsion requires a relatively long recovery phase. The recovery phase for terrestrial locomotion is "wasted" time for repositioning the limb, and a shorter recovery phase would maximize the time that the limb contacts the substrate for more efficient propulsion.[50] A short recovery phase during swimming, however, would give the limb a large relative velocity. The increased velocity would greatly increase the drag on the limb and reduce propulsive efficiency.[2,4,48]

3. Relative Phase—indicates the stage in the paddling cycle in which the foot begins the power phase. The cycle starts when one arbitrarily chosen foot begins its power stroke. Relative phase for the starting foot is zero, and the initiation of the power phases of each of the other feet which are used is indicated as a fraction of the total cycle time.[51]

4. Amplitude—distance traversed by the limb element over the duration of the power phase. The foot is used typically as the limb element to describe amplitude. The amplitude can be obtained directly by measuring the distance that the foot moves between successive frames of film from the beginning to the end of the power phase. Alternately, indirect indicators of amplitude are obtained by measuring the linear displacement of the foot or angular displacement of the foot between the beginning and the end of the power phase. The angular displacement method may be used when the major propulsive motions of the limb are rotational rather than translational. Varying degrees of rotational and translational components of movements by the

paddling limbs are observed in semiaquatic and terrestrial mammals.[4,6,7] In addition, amplitude increases directly with swimming speed.[4,6]

5. Joint angles—measured angles between segments of the limb (Fig. 9.5). Flexion is a decrease in angle between the longitudinal axes of two limb segments; extension is an increase in angle and hyperextension is an increase greater than 180°. An alternative method to measure joint angle is provided by Hoy and Zernicke[52,59] whereby the angle is measured between the limb segment an a horizontal reference line oriented through the center of rotation of the joint. Leach[53] suggested that precise and repeatable joint angle measurements could be collected from markers placed at the instant center of rotation (ICR). The ICR is the point which has zero velocity at any specific time during joint movement and coincides with the extreme ends of the limb segments in line with the long-bone axis. In addition, such points are easily palpable from the skeleton. Joint phase relationships are ascertained by examining simultaneous changes over a flexion/extension cycle between joints in the same limb.[28]

AN APPLICATION OF KINEMATIC ANALYSIS

The use kinematic analysis to study swimming is illustrated in a comparison of the swimming modes of terrestrial and semiaquatic

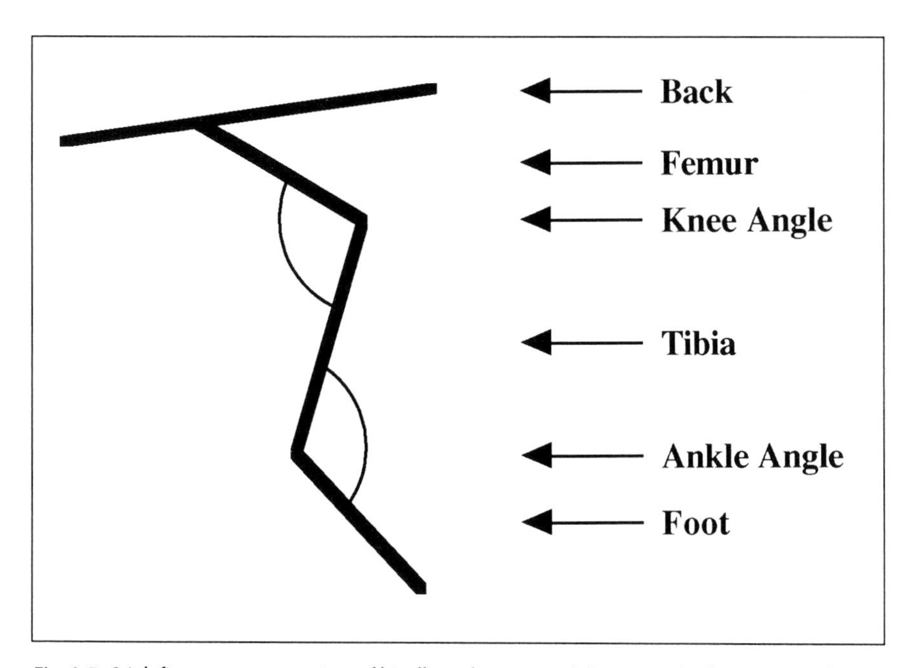

Fig. 9.5. Stick figure representation of hindleg of a mammal illustrating limb segments (femur, tibia, foot) and joint angles (knee, ankle). The anterior direction is oriented to the right.

mammals. Although such comparisons are performed to elucidate the evolution of aquatic adaptations, the swimming patterns observed and type of data collected are indicative of other studies which examine swimming kinematics.

The terrestrial Virginia opossum, *Didelphis virginiana*, and semi-aquatic yapok or water opossum, *Chironectes minimus*, are closely related New World marsupials.[54] While both species are capable of swimming, *Chironectes* displays a number of adaptations (i.e., webbed feet, non-wettable fur) and a hindlimb-paddling mode of swimming similar to other semiaquatic mammals; whereas, *Didelphis* swims with a quadrupedal paddling stroke similar to a terrestrial slow to fast diagonal sequence run.[6] Sequential tracings of foot movements for both species of opossum are shown in Figure 9.2. Tracings were produced from films taken with a cine camera at 64 frames per second as animals swam rectilinearly in an aquarium.

Despite the difference in swimming mode (hindlimb vs. quadrupedal paddling), the paddling frequency was the same at 1.6 Hz for nearly identical swimming speeds. Differences, however, were observed for other kinematic variables (Table 9.1). Amplitudes were greater for *Didelphis* compared to *Chironectes*. Times of the power phase and re-

Table 9.1. Kinematic parameters for two species of opossum from Figures 9.2 and 9.7

Parameter		Species	
		Didelphis	Chironectes
Frequency (Hz)		1.6	1.6
Time Power Phase (s)		0.188	0.109
Time Recovery Phase (s)		0.438	0.516
Amplitude (cm)			
	Hindfoot	32.4	23.4
	Forefoot	31.2	
Amplitude (degrees)			
	Hindfoot	130.8	104.5
	Forefoot	152.6	
Relative Phase			
	Left Hindfoot	0	0
	Right Hindfoot	0.52	0.49
	Left Forefoot	0.79	
	Right Forefoot	0.29 (RF)	

covery phase were respectively shorter and longer for *Chironectes* compared to *Didelphis*. This trend is indicative of semiaquatic mammals (see above).[4,48]

Changes in the ankle angle through the stroke cycle showed similar patterns for both species (Fig. 9.6). *Chironectes* exhibited smaller angles than *Didelphis* throughout the power phase. The larger angles for *Didelphis* reflect increased translation movements by the foot. Such movements are necessary to maintain thrust through the power phase; thereby compensating for the small mass of water accelerated due to the absence of webbing and the small size of the feet. During recovery, *Didelphis* showed greater flexion at the beginning of the phase and increased extension in the end of the phase compared to *Chironectes*. Increased extension aids *Didelphis* in increasing stroke amplitude. The relative phases of the paddling hind limbs are approximately the same for the two species (Table 9.1). Such findings suggest that *Chironectes* maintained the same pattern of limb coordination with *Didelphis* despite the shift to exclusive use of hind limbs for swimming.

Limb coordination can be graphically illustrated using a technique employed in terrestrial gait analysis. The gait diagram indicates when a foot supports the body by contact with the ground against a time scale.[55,56] For swimming, the length of time that the feet are in the power phase of the stroke is displayed (see ref. 6, Fig. 9.7). One complete

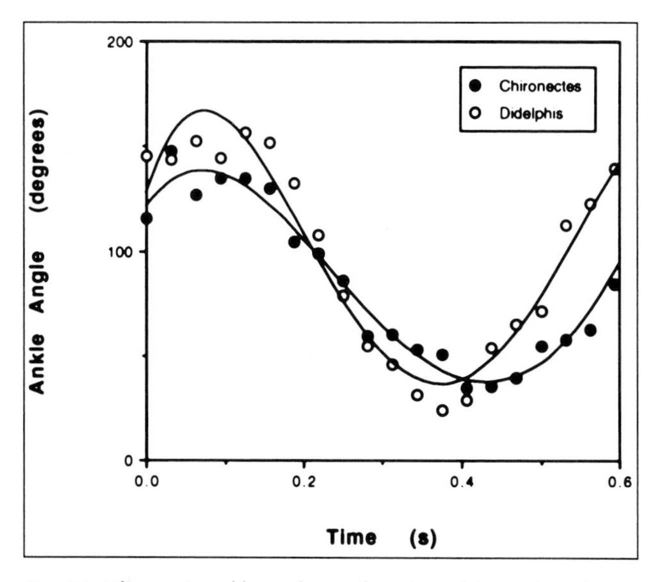

Fig. 9.6. Change in ankle angle as a function of time plotted over one complete stroke cycle. Data were obtained from Figure 9.2. Lines are drawn from fourth-order polynomials fitted to the data.

stroke cycle is shown in each diagram starting with the instant that the left hindfoot begins its power phase.

CONCLUSIONS

Kinematic analysis provides the opportunity to elucidate neuromotor patterns of limb usage during swimming in small mammals. These patterns, once defined, can be used in experiments to test effects due to drugs, microgravity, developmental stage, locomotive disorders, or phylogenetic differences. While the equipment and techniques used in kinematic analysis may be expensive and complex, inexpensive and simple alternatives can be used that provide sufficient resolution. The cyclical nature of the propulsive stroke permits application of physical parameters related to oscillatory motion. As swimming becomes more attractive as a medium to study behavior and the neurological basis of behavior, kinematics will serve as a valuable technique.

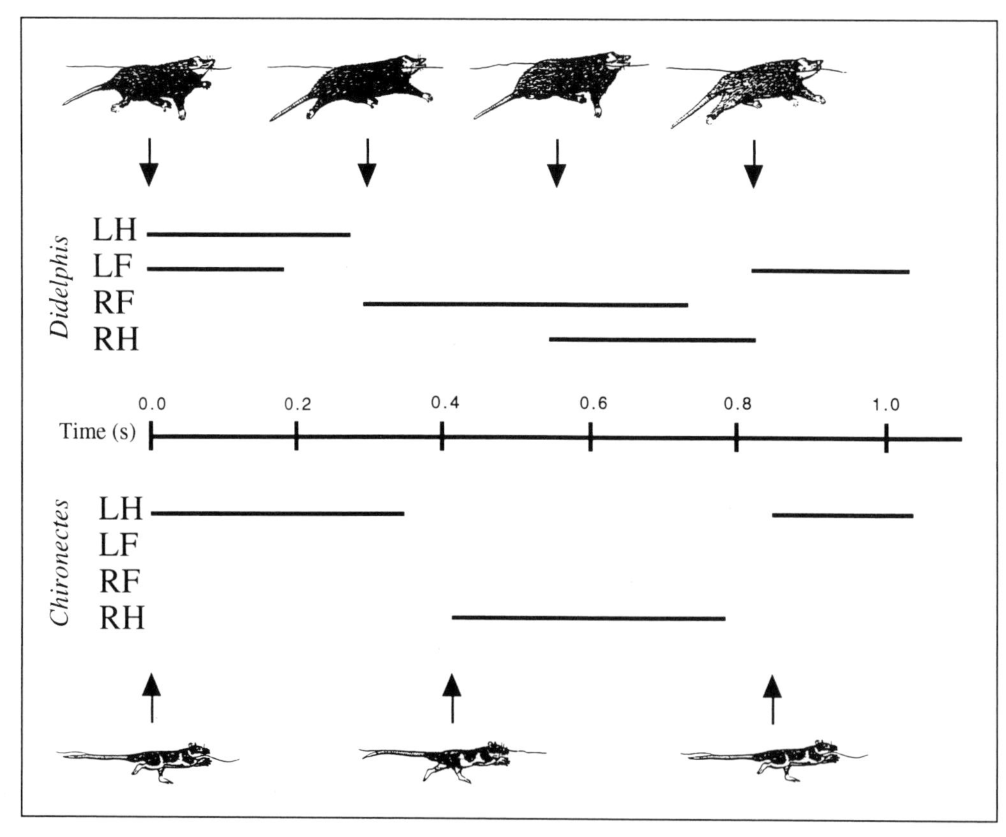

Fig. 9.7. Gait diagrams comparing swimming opossums. Horizontal bars indicate time of power phase for left hindfoot (LH), left forefoot (LF), right forefoot (RF), and right hind foot (RH). Vertical arrows correspond to time of limb position shown by cartoons. Swimming speeds for Didelphis *and* Chironectes *were 0.24 m/s and 0.26 m/s, respectively. Redrawn from Fish.*[6]

ACKNOWLEDGMENTS

I wish to thank K.-P. Ossenkopp, M. Kavaliers, and P.R. Sanberg for the opportunity to contribute to this edition. I also wish to thank T.L. Aigeldinger, B.D. Clark, K. Liem, and J. Smelstoys for information incorporated into this text, W. Bastings for the drawings, and M.J. Sheehan for reviewing an earlier version of this manuscript. This work was supported in part from grant DCB-9117274 from the National Science Foundation.

REFERENCES

1. Dagg AI, Windsor DE. Swimming in northern terrestrial mammals. Can J Zool 1972; 50:117-130.
2. Fish FE. Aquatic locomotion. In: Tomasi TE, Horton TH, ed. Mammalian energetics: interdisciplinary views of metabolism and reproduction. Ithaca, New York: Cornell University Press, 1992:34-63.
3. Fish FE. Aerobic energetics of surface swimming muskrats *Ondatra zibethicus*. Physiol. Zool. 1982; 55:180-189.
4. Fish FE. Mechanics, power output and efficiency of the swimming muskrat (*Ondatra zibethicus*). J Exp Biol 1984; 110:183-201.
5. Fish FE. Swimming dynamics of a small semi-aquatic mammal. Amer Zool 1985; 25: 13A.
6. Fish FE. Comparison of swimming kinematics between terrestrial and semiaquatic opossums. J Mamm 1993; 74:275-284.
7. Williams TM. Locomotion in the North American mink, a semiaquatic mammal. I. Swimming energetics and body drag. J Exp Biol 1983; 103:155-168.
8. Friedman WA, Garland T, Jr, Dohm MR. (1992) Individual variation in locomotor behavior and maximal oxygen consumption in mice. Physiol Behav 1992; 52:97-104.
9. Best TL, Hart EB. Swimming ability of pocket gophers (Geomyidae). Tex J Sci 1976; 27:361-366.
10. Hickman GC. Swimming behavior in representative species of the three genera of North American geomyids. Southwest Nat 1977; 21:531-538.
11. Hickman GC. Burrows, surface movement, and swimming of *Tachyoryctes splendens* (Rodentia: Rhizomyidae) during flood conditions in Kenya. J Zool 1983; 200:71-82.
12. Hickman GC. Swimming ability of talpid moles, with particular reference to the semi-aquatic *Condylura cristata*. Mammalia 1984; 48:505-513.
13. Simkin A, Leichter I, Swissa A et al. The effect of swimming activity on bone architecture in growing rats. J Biomech 1989; 22:845-851.
14. Bollaert PE, Gimene, M, Robin-Lherbier B et al. Respective effects of malnutrition and phosphate depletion on endurance swimming and muscle metabolism in rats. Acta Physiol Scand 1992; 144:1-7.
15. Bourrin S, Ghaemmaghami F, Vico L et al. Effect of a five-week swimming program on rat bone: A histomorpometric study. Calcif Tissue Int 1992; 51:137-142.

16. Varrik E, Viru A, Oopik V et al. Exercise-induced catabolic responses in various muscle fibres. Can J Spt Sci 1992; 17:125-128.
17. Porsolt RD, Le Pichon M, Jalfre M. Depression: a new animal model sensitive to antidepressant treatment. Nature 1977; 266:730-732.
18. Hawkins J, Hicks RA, Phillips N et al. Swimming rats and human depression. Nature 1978; 274:512-513.
19. Marshall JF, Berrios N. Movement disorders of aged rats: Reversal by dopamine receptor stimulation. Science 1979; 206:477-479.
20. Cazalets JR, Menard I, Cremieux J et al. Variability as a characteristic of immature motor systems: an electromyographic study of swimming in the newborn rat. Behav Brain Res 1990; 40:215-225.
21. Gruner JA, Altman J. Swimming in the rat: Analysis of locomotor performance in comparison to stepping. Exp Brain Res 1980; 40:374-382.
22. Johnson RM, Bekoff A. Constrained and flexible features of rhythmical hindlimb movements in chicks: Kinematic profiles of walking, swimming and airstepping. J Exp Biol 1992; 171:43-66.
23. Miller S, van der Burg J, van der Meche FGA. Coordination of movements of the hindlimbs and forelimbs in different forms of locomotion in normal and decerebrate cats. Brain Res 1975; 91:217-237.
24. Bekoff A, Trainer W. The development of interlimb co-ordination during swimming in postnatal rats. J Exp Biol 1979; 83:1-11.
25. Tamaki Y, Kameyama S-IOY. Postnatal locomotion development in a neurological mutant of rolling mouse Nagoya. Dev Psychobiol 1986; 19:67-77.
26. Walton KD, Lieberman D, Llnas A et al. Identification of a critical period for motor development in neonatal rats. Neuroscience 1992; 51:763-767.
27. Bass MB, Lester D. Swimming as a measure of motor impairment after ethanol and pentobarbital in rats. J Studies Alcohol 1978; 39:1618-1622.
28. Daunton N, D'Amelio F, Fox R et al. Investigating neural adaptation to altered gravity. NASA Technical Memorandum 1990; 103850:341-342.
29. Fox RA, Daunton N, Corcoran, M et al. Time-course of behavioral adaptation to hyper-gravity. In: Woolacott M, Houk F, ed. Posture and gait: control mechanisms. Portland: University of Oregon Books, 1992:178-181.
30. Fish FE, Stein BR. Functional correlates of differences in bone density among terrestrial and aquatic genera in the family Mustelidae (Mammalia). Zoomorphology 1991; 110:339-345.
31. Wall WP. The correlation between high limb-bone density and aquatic habits in recent mammals. J Paleontol 1983; 57:197-207.
32. Loeb GE, Gans C. Electromyography for experimentalists. Chicago: University of Chicago Press, 1986.
33. Muybridge E. Animals in motion. New York: Dover Publ, 1957.
34. Hildebrand M. Cinematography for research on vertebrate locomotion. Research Film 1964; 5:1-4.

35. Bennett MB. Empirical studies of walking and running. In: Alexander RMcN, ed. Advances in comparative & environmental physiology, Vol. 11. Berlin: Springer-Verlag, 1992:141-166.
36. Schamhardt HC, van den Bogert AJ, Hartman W. Measurement techniques in animal locomotion analysis. Acta Anat 1993; 146:123-129.
37. van den Bogert AJ, Schamhardt HC. Multi-body modelling and simulation of animal locomotion. Acta Anat 1993; 146:95-102.
38. Fredricson I, Drevemo S, Dalin G et al. The application of high-speed cinematography for the quantitative analysis of equine locomotion. Equine Vet J 1980; 12:54-59.
39. Hoy MG, Zernicke RF. The role of intersegmental dynamics during rapid limb oscillations. J Biomech 1986; 19:867-877.
40. Harper DG, Blake RW. A critical analysis of the use of high-speed film to determine maximum acceleration of fish. J Exp Biol 1989; 142:465-471.
41. Edgerton HE. Electronic flash, strobe. 2nd ed. Cambridge, Massachusetts: MIT Press, 1979.
42. Mizelle JD. Swimming of the muskrat. J Mamm 1935; 16:22-25.
43. Vogel S, LaBarbera M. Simple flow tanks for research and teaching. Bioscience 1978; 28:638-643.
44. Vogel S. Life in moving fluids. Boston: Willard Grant Press, 1981.
45. Denny MW. Biology and the mechanics of the wave-swept environment. Princeton: Princeton University Press,1988.
46. Fish FE, Fegeley J, Xanthopoulos CJ. Burst-and-coast swimming in schooling fish (*Notemigonus crysoleucas*) with implications for energy economy. Comp. Biochem. Physiol 1991; 100A:633-637.
47. Blake RW. The mechanics of labriform locomotion. I. Labriform locomotion in the angelfish (*Pterophyllum eimekei*): an analysis of the power stroke. J Exp Biol 1979; 82:255-271.
48. Fish FE. Influence of hydrodynamic design and propulsive mode on mammalian swimming energetics. Aust J Zool 1993; 79-101.
49. Goslow GE, Jr, Reinking RM, Stuart DG. The cat step cycle: hind limb joint angles and muscle lengths during unrestricted locomotion. J Morph 1973; 141:1-41.
50. Edwards JL. A comparative study of locomotion in terrestrial salamanders. Ph.D. dissertation, University of California, Berkeley, 1976.
51. Alexander RMcN. Terrestrial locomotion. In: Alexander RMcN, Goldspink G, eds. Mechanics and energetics of animal locomotion. London: Chapman and Hall, 1977:168-203.
52. Hoy MG, Zernicke RF. Modulation of limb dynamics in the swing phase of locomotion. J Biomech 1985; 18:49-60.
53. Leach D. Recommended terminology for researchers in locomotion and biomechanics of quadrupedal animals. Acta Anat 1993; 146:130-136.
54. Stein BR. Comparative limb myology of two opossums, *Didelphis* and *Chironectes*. J Morph 1981; 169:113-140.

55. Hildebrand M. Analysis of tetrapod gait: general considerations and symmetrical gaits. In: Herman RM, Grillner S, Stein PSG et al eds. Neural control of locomotion. New York: Plenum Press, 1976:203-236.
56. Hildebrand M. The adaptive significance of tetrapod gait selection. Amer Zool 1980; 20:255-267.
57. Kreighbaum E, Barthels KM. Biomechanics: a qualitative approach for studying human movement. Minneapolis: Burgess Publishing Co, 1985.

CHAPTER 10

Quantitative Analyses of Equine Locomotion

Henk C. Schamhardt

INTRODUCTION

Extensive research on equine locomotion has been carried out over the last 20 years by the Equine Biomechanics Research Group, Faculty of Veterinary Medicine of the Utrecht University, The Netherlands. It was started by Prof. D.M. Badoux, who published several papers on theoretical biomechanics, applied to the equine locomotor system. Furthermore, the foundation was put in place for electromyographical studies. The combination of these techniques led to several theoretical papers on muscle function and applied biomechanics of the horse. From 1980 onwards a more experimental branch developed, in which the recording and analysis of ground reaction forces and bone strain was the central theme. Slightly later, studies on equine tendon functioning began, both from an experimental and a theoretical viewpoint. Dutch Studbooks donated funds to purchase a computer-assisted kinematic analysis system (CODA-3), which formed the basis of an extensive and successful line of research on equine kinematics. All experimental techniques were applied simultaneously during the development of a computer model of the locomotor system of the horse. The most recent development is the start of a research project on skeletal muscle modeling.

Over the years the Equine Biomechanics Research Group changed with several participants leaving and new ones joining the group. One particular quality was kept: the group is still multidisciplinary, with veterinarians, researchers with a technical background, and electro-technicians closely working together. This type of collaboration makes the group successful.

Results of the above mentioned research topics have been published in international journals. A vast amount of experience has been

Measuring Movement and Locomotion: From Invertebrates to Humans, edited by Klaus-Peter Ossenkopp, Martin Kavaliers and Paul R. Sanberg.

gained over the years, both in experimental design and data analysis, and tools were developed to avoid possible bear clamps and other pitfalls.[1,2] Only the successful solutions tend to appear in the literature. However, descriptions of the experience gained on several aspects of research is rarely published. Therefore, this chapter focuses on the methodology and experimental rationale, while results will be presented as illustrations only.

DESIGN OF EXPERIMENTS

Qualitative Analysis

In daily life, almost everybody uses gait analysis. While walking in a shopping center, it takes only a fraction of a second to determine whether a person is male or female, or someone familiar or a stranger. The human eye, which captures the image, and the human brain, which processes this information, appear to be a surprisingly powerful system for recognition and identification. After a little training the human observer is also able to judge the quality of gait. One can determine whether a particular walking pattern is supple and graceful, or whether it is more rough and the result of real power development. The statement given above holds not only for man moving in various activities (e.g., walking or running, dancing or sport), but also for judging animal performance. However, this kind of "gait analysis" and the judgment as mentioned above, are essentially subjective, with all of the risk for dispute inherent in such subjectivity.

A well known example, where qualitative gait analysis is applied successfully, is the diagnosis of lameness in the horse. An experienced clinician will rarely need quantitative information for diagnosis and identification of the gait disturbing disorder. However, when locomotor performance has to be evaluated over time, more sophisticated tools for the quantification of gait are required to support findings, such as satisfactory response to treatment in a patient.

Qualitative observation has the advantage of being simple and rapid, and when carried out by one observer, of being reproducible. In an experiment where carpal lameness was induced in one limb of the horse by injecting lipopolysaccharide (LPS),[3] it was found that the lameness, scored on a scale from not visible at all (0), not visible at the walk, and slightly lame at the trot (1), to non-load bearing (5), differed less than 0.2 points when scores of two independent observers were compared. This semi-quantitative attempt to score lameness objectively illustrated that the human observer is consistent in his or her judgments, and that two different observers may derive the same score, even though they are using only visual observation. However, this scoring technique, although proven to be useful for several purposes, remains essentially subjective.

Quantitative Analysis

As soon as tools are used for objective recording of movement, one can speak of quantitative gait analysis. Of many possible examples, I will deal with the recording of kinematics. Capturing the movement of an animal on high speed film or video is still qualitative, but as soon as one attempts to localize joint centers of rotation and to plot a joint angle-time diagram, one can speak of a quantitative analysis. Quantitative analyses can have large advantages. The resulting data are objective, they can be mutually compared, ranked and analyzed, and all kinds of statistical analyses can be performed.[4] However, numerical data may also have serious disadvantages. The major one is that data tend to be considered absolutely true, while the inaccuracy which is essentially part of any quantification of observations is not critically evaluated, or even worse, omitted. Therefore, numerical data are only then superior to results of subjective observations when they give answers to precisely defined questions in well-designed experiments.

Quantitative analysis is not always better than qualitative analysis. It may even be impossible to perform certain kinds of quantitative analyses with the accuracy required for a particular purpose. An example may illustrate this point. Let us consider the influence of a particular bandage material on the kinematics of the equine lower limb. It might be expected that the bandaging will affect the angulation pattern of the fetlock joint. If equipment is available to quantify kinematics on the basis of markers applied to the skin of the moving animal, two questions have to be answered before it can be determined whether any bandage-induced influences can be recorded at all. First, how reproducible is the placement of a skin marker on or close to the joint center of rotation with and without bandaging. If an inaccuracy of several millimeters is inevitable, the error in joint angle due to this positioning fault may already be as large, or even larger, than the effects of the bandaging itself. Furthermore, the resolution of the kinematic analysis system must be better than several millimeters to be able to detect these differences. Finally, the frame rate of the system must be high enough to "freeze" the moving image, otherwise a movement glare impairs accuracy of the data.

There are situations in which data have to be collected under conditions in which they are not as carefully controlled as they would be in the laboratory. These data still can be quite valuable, due to the fact that they are unique, or that it is simply not possible to collect them under laboratory conditions. In this case, an even more careful evaluation and interpretation of the data is obligatory before the value of the data can be judged.

Repeated Measurements from One Subject

Although it is widely recognized that a certain variability is inherent in data obtained from repeated measurements on biological material, little is said as to how to treat these data correctly. Let us consider the ground reaction force (GRF) measurements as an example. When a horse is guided over the force plate, the chance of a correct hit of at least one hoof on the plate is about 50%. However, nothing is said about the chance of the hit being from a right or left limb. Consequently, after several runs the number of correct hits from each limb will differ. When calculating the mean and the standard error of the mean (SEM) of a certain variable by averaging the data of these runs, the mean of the data obtained from the limb with the higher number of correct hits usually has a lower SEM. Are data from that limb "more correct?" Obviously not, but it is hard to define a universal, statistically correct recipe to cope with this problem, other than by deleting data points until the same minimum number is obtained from each limb. In our laboratory we collect data until a sufficient number of correct hits are recorded from each limb (i.e., at least five). Thereafter, the data from each limb are averaged and considered to be "representative" for the GRF-pattern of that limb, and treated as a single hit in further analysis. So, the fact that the average is constructed from a different number of runs for each limb is disregarded.

Statistical Analysis

In all living subjects a certain variability will be found in data resulting from measurements of a variable under "similar" experimental conditions. Also, the response to a certain manipulation (e.g., drug treatment, shoeing) may be qualitatively and quantitatively different when comparing different animals. Impressive libraries of statistical routines have been developed to extract trends in the data, to detect differences between groups, or to identify a "statistically significant" response to a certain treatment. Unfortunately, the prerequisites for these statistical tests are not always met. For example, data may not be normally distributed, or data consisting of different variables collected at the same time may not be independent. Therefore, it is very important and rather difficult to treat the data in a statistically correct manner. Actually, before any experiment should be carried out, a thorough evaluation of the problem must be carried out. Subsequently, a hypothesis should be formulated, and an appropriate statistical test selected. It frequently appears that after collection of data, there are factors, such as dependency within a series of data, which disqualify a particular statistical test. Because many researchers are not familiar with all of these pitfalls and problems associated with statistical tests, incorrect analyses appear frequently in the literature and many times a certain test is used because of its availability, and not because it is the most appropriate one for that particular purpose.

There are other comments that can be made about statistical analysis. First, a statistical test answers the question of whether a certain hypothesis can be accepted or has to be rejected. It must be noted, however, that the answer is not absolute, but a statement of probability. Having selected an uncertainty level of, for example, $p < 0.05$, "accept" or "reject" has a chance of 95% of being true. Consequently, it also has a 5% chance of being wrong. It is absolutely impossible to "prove" any statement with any kind of statistical test. Only the chance for a certain statement to be true can be indicated. As another consequence of the statistical uncertainty, it has to be accepted that (with $p < 0.05$) 5 out of 100 observations differ from the other 95, or that one "statistically significant" relationship in 20 is found completely due to chance.

A final remark on statistics is the importance attributed to "statistically significant." In many papers attention is focused on the statistically significant differences or relationships only. Trends are sometimes indicated, but most of the time only when the author would like them to be significant. However, the biological relevance of the particular observation is usually not mentioned at all. For example, if the heart rate in a group of animals should increase significantly after administration of a certain drug by 5 beats/min, while the range in normal functioning is between 30 and 200 beats/min, it might be hard to defend that the significant increase found after treatment has any biological relevance. However, the opposite may also be true. If in a sample a trend is clearly visible, but the level of significance is not reached due to the fact that only one or a few subjects behave differently, then the observed trend may be important from a biological point of view.

In summary, statistical analysis of biological data is quite important, but rather hard to carry out correctly. Due to the complexity and the large number of tests available, it might be even more difficult to select the most appropriate test for a particular purpose. However, the results of any statistical test must be interpreted not only on the basis of "statistical significance" but also on the basis of biological relevance.

ANALYSIS OF KINEMATICS

Horses are kept primarily because of their outstanding locomotor performance. In judging equine performance the analysis of movement, or *kinematics*, is rather important. When an objective comparison has to be made between the locomotor performance of different horses, tools are necessary to capture the image of the moving horse and to analyze it afterwards. Well known examples are high-speed film or video, and a subsequent frame-by-frame analysis and quantification of movement. In our research group we use the high-speed, computer-assisted kinematic analysis system CODA-3.[5] This produces 3-dimensional (3D) coordinates of 12 markers, 300 times per second, with an accuracy in the transverse plane of about 0.3 mm at a measuring distance of 8 m. The CODA-3 system uses a rigid and portable scanner, and does not need a complex calibration prior to each use (as is required in camera based systems), because the three light sources are fixed to the steel frame of the scanner and the 3D-coordinates are calculated with respect to this frame.

Kinematic data can be analyzed in several ways. Stride variables, such as stride length, stride duration and stride frequency, are all related to the pace of the horse.[6,7] A limitation of kinematic stride variables is that no information is available on the changes in joint angles in the limbs. These might be more descriptive for a certain abnormality in the locomotor pattern than the kinematic stride variables.[3] However, the determination of joint angles from kinematic data can be rather laborious, especially when they have to be calculated after (manually) digitizing high-speed film or video.[8] Practically, only computer assisted equipment is suitable for this kind of analysis (Fig. 10.1). When joint angular changes are used as input to a subsequent biomechanical analysis, they have the potential to reveal real cause-effect relationships between forces and moments loading internal structures in the body. This kind of modeling of the locomotor system usually gives more insight into the way it functions.[9]

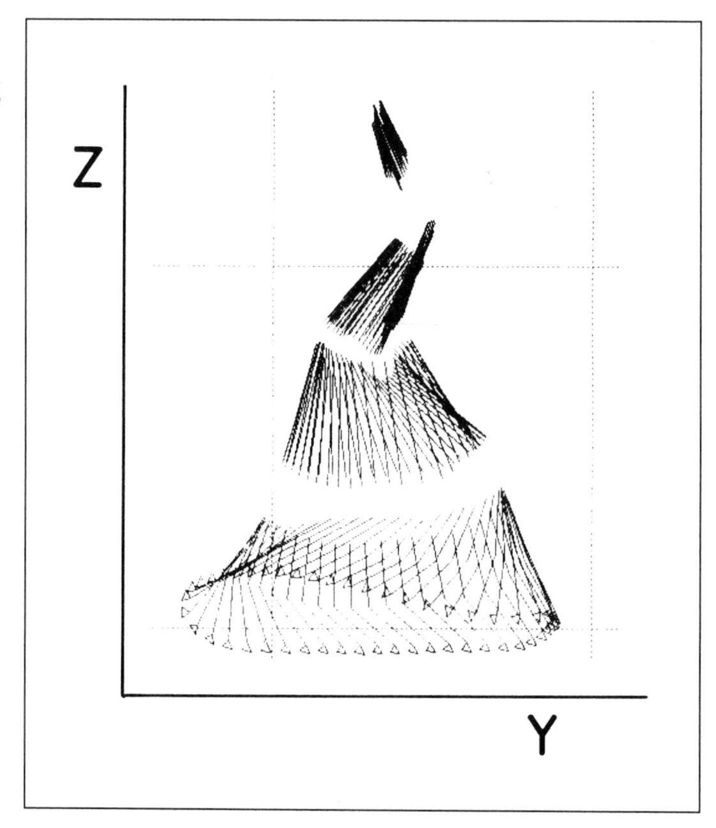

Fig. 10.1. "Stick diagram" of the kinematics of the forelimb of a trotting horse (4 m/s) on a treadmill. The markers on anatomical landmarks are connected to construct a stick diagram.

Factors Affecting the Accuracy of Kinematic Data

Kinematic stride variables can be calculated from the kinematics of the hooves alone. These data are rather easily collected and the interpretation of the data is straightforward. In horses moving at faster gaits (horses can move as fast as about 20 m/s) the resolution in time must be rather high to achieve sufficient accuracy. For example, if a horse moves at 10 m/s and the stride frequency is 2 s^{-1} then the time for a complete stride cycle is 0.5 s which can be divided into a stance phase of about 0.2 s and a swing phase of about 0.3 s. The placement of the hoof and the lift-off after the stance phase, taking about 1/10 of the swing time each, last about 0.03 s. A kinematic analysis system with a frame rate of 50 s^{-1} is, thus, not capable of collecting more than about 1 frame during the entire transition from swing to stance phase. Furthermore, the hoof has moved about 30 cm during that time. Inevitably, a "blur" or "glare" of 30 cm, or an uncertainty in positional data of that magnitude, will occur when a high-speed shutter is used. Even the 300 s^{-1} CODA-3 system is frequently not fast enough to capture the movements of the fast moving parts of the horse with sufficient accuracy. Finally, the process of hoof landing and lift-off is rather smooth. To capture the movements and to be able to answer the simple question of whether the horse lands with the heels or the toes first require extremely fast and accurate equipment.

The analysis of kinematics of locomoting animals is always based on the use of markers, applied to the skin covering palpable skeletal landmarks.[10] During movement the skin will move with respect to the underlying bony landmarks.[11-13] This will lead to differences in movement when comparing movements recorded from skin markers as compared to those of the bony landmarks. The movement of a marker may also have an oscillatory component, especially when connective tissue is loose and soft tissue lies between the skin and the bones. These oscillations are essentially tied to the movements themselves, and thus never can be removed by any kind of data processing. For several particular kinds of movements of the Dutch Warmblood horse, algorithms for skin movement correction have been developed. These are based on simultaneous recording of skin and bone movement using light emitting diodes in the distal bones or transcutaneous pins in the proximal parts of the limbs.[12-15] It appeared that the skin movement could be as large as 12 cm in the proximal parts of the thigh in a riding horse. In the forelimb distal to the elbow joint and in the hindlimb distal to the stifle the skin movement usually can be neglected.

Skin movement might have a dramatic influence when interpreting kinematic data. In the horse, the coupling between the movements of the stifle and hock joints by the M. peroneus tertius seemed to be far from complete, as determined from kinematics. However, after correction for skin displacement, the difference in joint angular changes almost vanished (see Fig. 10.2).

The final comment to be made on the use of skin markers concerns the reproducibility in the positioning of the markers themselves. Usually, markers are applied in the standing horse. When the animal is not loading the limb completely, or when it is not sufficiently cooperative, it might be rather difficult to attach the markers with an accuracy better than about 0.5 cm. Inevitably, this has consequences for repeated measurements in a particular horse, where the markers have to be removed between sessions. A possible way to avoid this problem is to standardize joint angular measurements to those obtained in the standing horse (see Fig. 10.3).[16] Only changes from this square standing position will be reported. Unfortunately, these angles are different from those obtained without this particular standardization, which impairs comparison of data from different laboratories.

When only one camera is used to collect kinematic data, the variables calculated from this 2-dimensional (2D) image are straightforward. A calibration is not necessary and all variables, such as joint angles, are completely defined. However, if the horse should have been

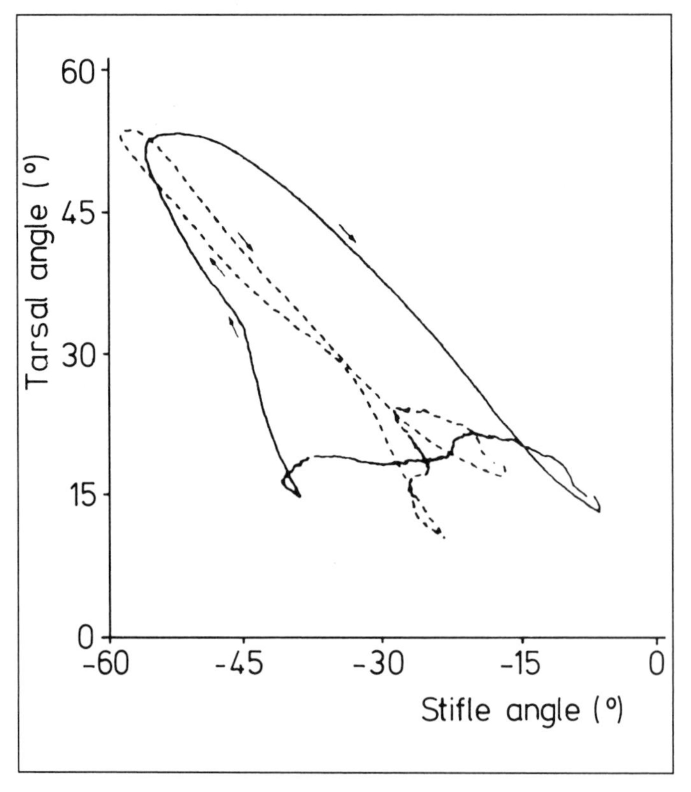

Fig. 10.2. Angle-angle diagram of the stifle and tarsal joints of a horse at the walk. The continuous line is obtained using skin markers and the broken line after correction for skin displacement.

slightly further away from the camera in a subsequent run, it will appear smaller in the camera image, and the linear dimensions will have changed. An erroneous conclusion could be that the stride length had decreased. Fortunately, correction for this kind of error by scaling the measurement, is relatively simple. If the horse did not move completely perpendicula to the camera, the same problem as stated above will also occur and the calculated joint angles will contain an error due to image distortion. For length measurements in the longitudinal direction, this distortion is rather small, because it is proportional to the cosine of the angle under which the horse moves with the desired direction. As long as this "oblique movement angle" is less than about 15°, this error is smaller than 5%. However, if a transverse distance also plays a role (i.e., the advanced placement comparing left and right limbs), the error is proportional to the sine of the "oblique movement angle." Assuming the same angle of 15°, this error can be as large as 26% (Fig. 10.4). If more than one camera is available, another 2D-image can be obtained, which facilitates interpretation of the data. It also can be used to correct for the above mentioned errors in one 2D-image.

Several kinematic analysis tools, including the CODA-3 system, produce 3D-coordinates of markers fixed to the horse. In camera-based systems (film, video) a laborious calibration is required prior to measurements. The accuracy in this calibration completely determines the accuracy of the final 3D-data set.[17] This stresses the importance of investing much effort in the calibration of the volume of space in which measurements will be taken. The real advantage of 3D-data collection is that the positions in space of the markers fixed to the

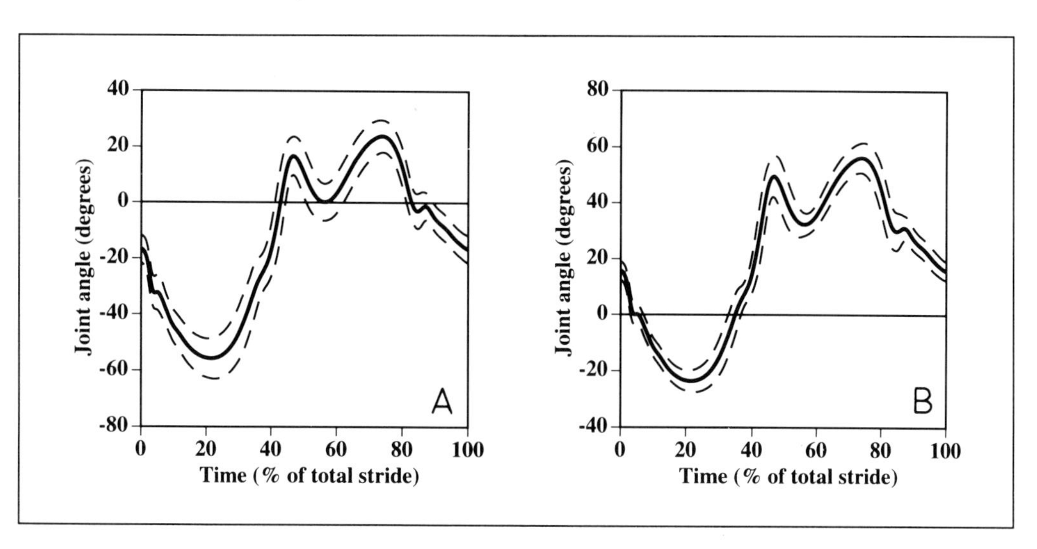

Fig. 10.3. (A) Angle-time diagram of the fetlock joint of the forelimb of a trotting horse (4 m/s) on the treadmill. (B) The same diagram, after standardization of the joint angles to those at square stance.

horse are calculated. Even if the horse should have moved obliquely through the measurement space, the position data are calculated correctly. All linear and angular variables in any desired direction can be determined by using appropriate software.

The accuracy of kinematic analysis equipment is limited. This implies that all data will contain a certain amount of random noise. Sometimes, this can be eliminated effectively by using data smoothing algorithms,[18,19] which may also allow one to calculate time derivatives of the kinematic data, such as (angular) velocity and acceleration.[19,20] Data smoothing is a tricky process and will be successful only when carefully controlled and used with care. It should be mentioned once more that artifacts, such as skin movement, or oscillations of soft tissue underneath the skin, can never be eliminated by data smoothing. This is due to the fact that the tissue oscillates with exactly the same rhythm

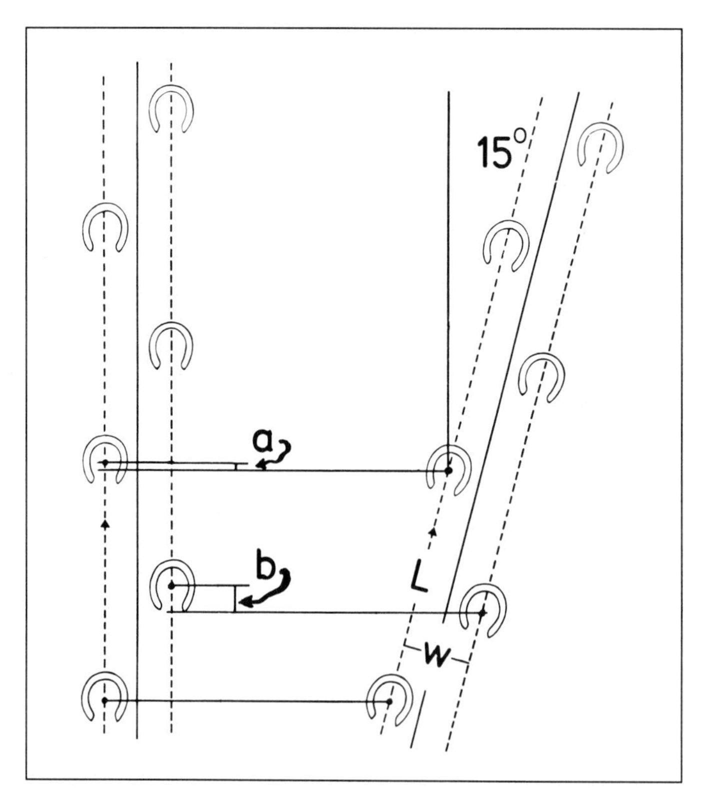

Fig. 10.4. Influence of oblique passing (15°) of a horse through the measurement field, top view of the footfall pattern. The erroneously calculated stride length equals L • cosine (α), or 0.95 • L. The difference from the actual length L is marked a. The calculated placement of the right limb in front of the left limb is much more affected (marked b), because b is proportional to w times the sine of α (about 0.26 • w).

as the real signal. Smoothing will only be successful when the frequency of the "noise" and the signal are sufficiently different.

Presentation of Kinematic Data

Even when the data are correctly obtained from a moving horse, there are several possibilities for presentation and analysis, which will raise serious conflicts when comparing data from different sources. In 2D-analysis standardization is usually not a problem. The only discrepancy one may encounter may originate from joint angles, either defined at the dorsal or the palmar/plantar aspect of the limb, or the presence or lack of square stance standardization.

In 3D-analysis the problems of standardization are much more complicated. First, each length measurement has three components in space, and the orientation in space of a body can be characterized by a minimum of 6 numbers. Also joint angles can only be described uniquely in a rather complex way.[19] The most practical approach is to project angles onto planes tied to the laboratory coordinate system, which degrades the 3D-analysis to a quasi-2D one. An acceptable compromise might be to use multiple projections. However, projecting angles onto planes may cause the "oblique movement" error as stated above. Furthermore, there are many planes to project angles onto, and each plane has its own advantages and disadvantages. As well, interpretation of 3D-joint angular changes is usually too complex for routine applications beyond the gait lab. This may be one of the reasons why powerful kinematic analyses have not yet become popular in the clinical setting.

At present, many different methods are used in kinematic data presentation. Because the dispute on this topic is considerable, it is not very likely that a consensus will be found in due course. Therefore, it seems most practical to use a method of presentation that works and to pay sufficient attention to the explanation for choice of data analysis procedure and method of data presentation.

TREADMILL

In many cases it is tempting to study the gait of the moving horse at full speed. This is usually not possible in the field. However, the introduction of treadmills for use in equine gait analysis was a big step forward.[21] Although treadmill locomotion does not differ from over ground locomotion from a theoretical point of view,[22] differences in kinematic stride variables were reported.[21,23] Also, the time required for a horse to adapt to treadmill locomotion was not known. Therefore, we carried out a study in our laboratory to establish the number of training sessions required to obtain a stable locomotion pattern.[24] More rapid habituation appeared to occur at faster gaits, but a minimum of three sessions of at least 5 min were required before a stable locomotion pattern developed. We also attempted to find possible differences between treadmill and overground locomotion[25] and found that the differences were small but significant. The duration of the retraction phase was longer and the vertical movements of the withers were smaller on the treadmill than overground.

An explanation for the differences between treadmill and overground locomotion is difficult to provide. As Ingen Schenau[22] stated, there should be no (mechanical) difference, as long as the speed of the treadmill belt is rigidly constant and one is allowed to neglect air resistance. However, due to limitations in the treadmill speed control, and the friction induced between the treadmill belt and the gliding surface, a minimal change in belt speed may occur. This translates into a net energy transfer from the treadmill engine to the horse and may explain, at least in part, the observed differences.

GROUND REACTION FORCES

A force plate is used for ground reaction force measurement. The forces developed by muscles in the body of an animal are transformed into rotations of limb segments, causing movement. The reaction to

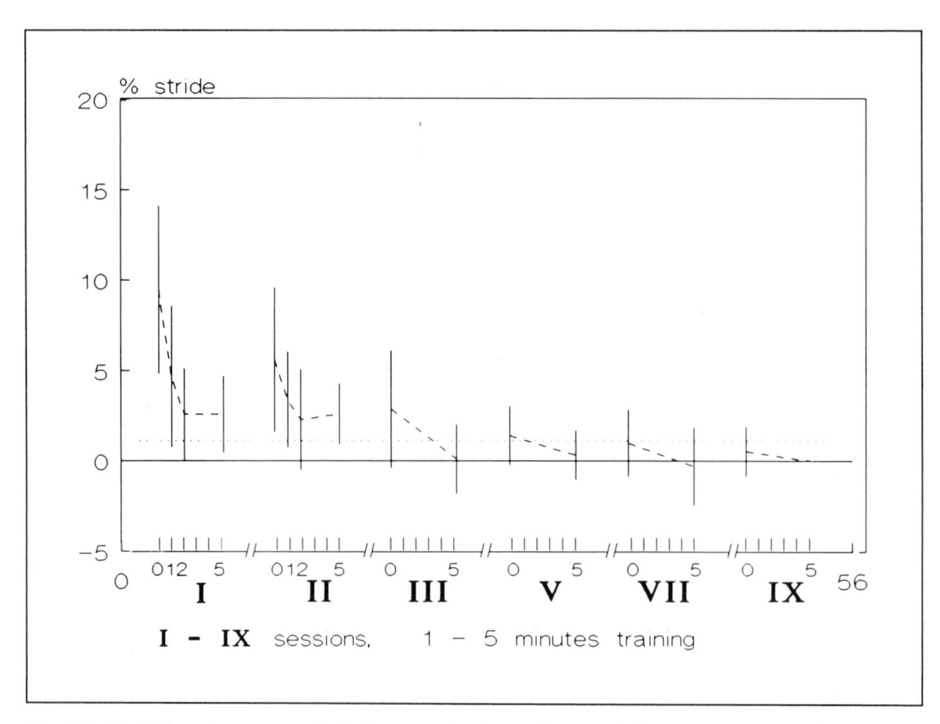

Fig. 10.5. Habituation to treadmill locomotion in 10 horses; influence on stance duration as percentage of total stride duration. Horizontal axis: number of training sessions of 5 min each. Vertical axis: Relative stance duration. The vertical lines indicate the standard deviation of the 10 horses. The horizontal line indicates the "habituation limit," based on data of the final recording session.

gravity, and the braking and propelling forces occurring during locomotion, can be recorded as ground reaction forces (GRF) using a force plate.[26,27] GRF analysis is carried out either to quantify the GRF and use this information to characterize gait, or to use the GRF as input for further biomechanical analyses, such as to estimate intrinsic forces in parts of the locomotor system.

During force plate data collection, the horse is guided by an assistant in a straight path over the force plate. The probability of recording a correct hit can be adjusted by altering the distance between the starting point of the run and the force plate. A success rate of 1 out of 2-3 attempts could be obtained in horses at a walk, trot and canter.[28-31] In our laboratory we also made measurements of horses jumping a vertical fence of 0.8 to 1.55 m in height. After adjusting the distance from the fence to the force plate, we obtained success rates similar to those at other gaits.[32]

The peak amplitudes of the GRFs appear to be speed dependent, as shown for greyhounds.[33] It also might be expected that in horses the GRF amplitudes are larger at faster gaits. However, this relationship differs in each horse and is certainly not linear. This implies that the experimenter should try to keep the speed as constant as possible in each subsequent run. This may be a significant problem, since the assistant guiding the horse may have difficulties in keeping speed constant, especially at faster gaits. We standardize the GRF amplitudes to the body mass of the horse. This allows for a comparison of GRF amplitudes between horses of different body mass. We also standardize stance time to the duration of the stance phase, to account for slight differences in loading time between subsequent trials.

When a horse passes over the force plate at an angle with respect to the force plate's coordinate system the resulting transverse horizontal (Fx) and the longitudinal horizontal (Fy) GRF amplitudes are not reliable because cross-talk between the Fx and Fy signals will occur (see Fig. 10.6). In our laboratory we routinely use standard video equipment to record every trial. This "scratch book" enables us to identify the limb actually loading the force plate (this is especially difficult when the horse has similarly colored limbs). These recordings also allow us to determine during which runs the horse loaded the force plate close to, or just on, an edge. Finally, we also can easily identify deviations from normal gait or oblique crossings of the plate.

Quantification of GRF Patterns

In order to compare data from different horses, quantification of GRF patterns is required. This approach was used to identify peak amplitudes and inclinations characterizing the patterns. This also allowed us to devise a procedure to combine the amplitudes and times of occurrence of these peaks within the patterns. The result is a H(orse)INDEX, which combines over 90 numbers obtained from each individual horse.[34-36]

Although this method is valid, it has the limitation that it only uses signal peak-amplitudes, peak-time positions, and force "impulses" (calculated as area under the force-time curves), which are selected by the user and essentially are signal shape dependent. It does not quantify the real pattern of the curve. Other techniques, such as correlations characterizing the resemblances between curves, should also be considered.

ELECTROMYOGRAPHY

Muscle contraction is preceded by electrical activation and this can be recorded both by using wire or needle electrodes inserted into the muscle,[37] or by surface electrodes placed on the skin covering the muscle of interest. Although there is a so-called electro-mechanical delay between activation and mechanical contraction, the electromyographic (EMG) signals are frequently used to indicate the period of activity of a muscle.[38,39] The amplitude of the EMG-signal is dependent on a number of factors. These include the dimensions of the electrodes,

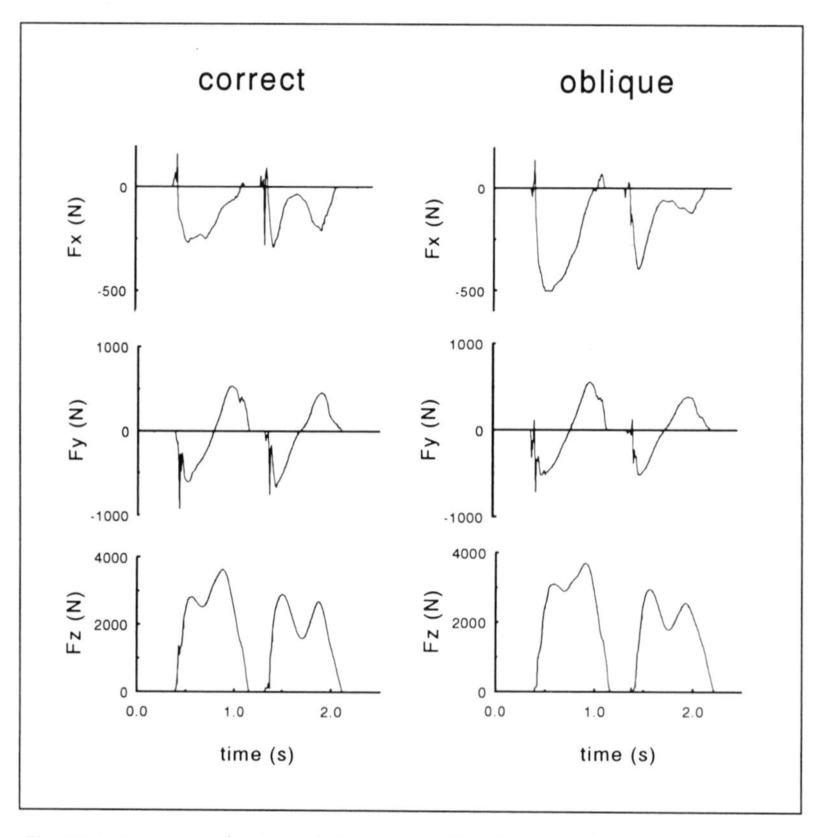

Fig. 10.6. Transverse horizontal (Fx), longitudinal horizontal (Fy), and vertical (Fz) ground reaction forces obtained from the hindlimb of a horse at the walk, crossing the force plate correctly, or oblique.

their electrical contact with the muscle, and the type of electrode used. Signal amplitudes from in-dwelling wire electrodes are usually much lower than those obtained from surface electrodes. However, the major influence on EMG-signal amplitude is the degree of activation of the muscle. When it is completely activated, the EMG-signal will reach a maximum. This relationship enables us to use the EMG-signal amplitude as a measure of the degree of activation, and thus indirectly, for muscle force development.[40]

EMG-signal analysis has lots of applications. On the basis of the presence of EMG-activity, Wentink[37] identified several muscles in the hind limb of the horse to be active at times which were different from what was expected on the basis of their topography. In combination with a biomechanical analysis, he was able to shed new light on the function of these muscles during locomotion. Following more complicated EMG-signal processing, it appeared possible to use the muscle's "active state" as a better estimate of muscle force development. Using this approach, the function of a number of muscles in the forelimb and the hindlimb of the horse have been evaluated in a semi-quantitative manner.[41] It was found that muscles which are assumed to be extensors of a particular joint were also active during the period when the joint appeared to flex. Actually, the muscle acted to prevent excessive flexion. In the example illustrated in Figure 10.7 (M. extensor carpi radialis), the bi-articular nature of this muscle may explain why activity is found during flexion of the carpus: due to its origin at the distal humerus, it will support flexion of the elbow joint at the beginning of the swing phase.

Until now, it has not been possible to devise a reliable estimate for muscle force development on the basis of EMG-signal analysis alone. A sophisticated muscle model needs to be developed in which the muscle architecture, the force-length and force-velocity relationships of the muscle fibers, and the activation of the muscle (possibly from EMG-signal analysis) are incorporated. However, it will take several years before this model is developed to the point where it can be validated in experimental animals.

STRAIN IN HARD AND SOFT TISSUE

Definition of Strain

When a tensile force is applied to a solid material, its length increases, while bending of the structure causes both increases and decreases in length. In ideally elastic materials the deformation is proportional to the applied force and the material will restore its original shape as soon as the deforming force vanishes. The deformation of the material, usually expressed in terms of *strain* (ε), is defined as:

$$\varepsilon = \frac{l_1 - l_0}{l_0}$$

where $l_1 - l_0$ is the change in length of the material comparing condition 1 and the starting condition where the length of the material is l_0. Usually, this *resting length* is defined to be the length at zero loading force. Strain is a relative measure, being a length change of 1 m per m of original material length, and is expressed as a percentage or in the unit "strain."

Measurement and Analysis of Bone Strain

Strain on the surface of long bones of sheep, horses and goats is small (with an upper value of about 2 x 10^{-3} m/m), but large enough to be recorded *in vivo*, even at fast gaits.[42-45] Following a complex preparation procedure to allow the strain gauges to survive in the aggressive medium formed by the living body, they are bonded to the bones using tissue glue. In this application strain gauges appear to last for several weeks. This facilitates the study of bone response to changes in the loading regime.[46] It was found that bones are loaded during bending and torsion in normal locomotion. A practical problem in quantifying bone strain is that the resting length of bone is

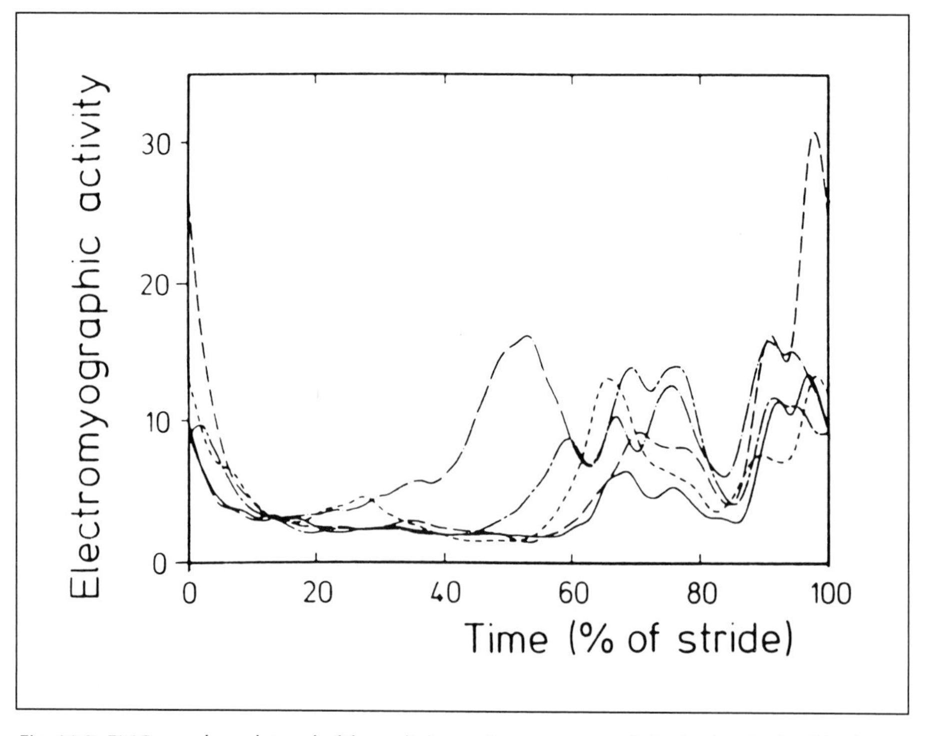

Fig. 10.7. EMG-enveloped signal of the radial carpal extensor muscle in the forelimb of the horse. Considerable EMG-activity is visible when the carpus is flexing, at the beginning of the swing phase (between 55 and 65% stride duration). Apparently, the radial carpal extensor muscle supports flexion of the elbow joint.

difficult to determine. When the animal is standing quietly with the limb lifted from the ground, the loading may be assumed to be small. However, a certain muscular contraction cannot be excluded completely, and the influence of gravity may affect the "zero"-strain determination. Software has been developed to calculate a "zero-strain compensation" in in vivo strain gauge data of horses at the walk, using the assumption that the strain will be minimal during the middle of the swing phase, when the limb is moving forward with an almost constant velocity.[47]

Surface strain is related to forces loading the bone. However, the relationship between surface strain and load is very complicated, especially in non-homogeneous, non-linear, visco-elastic structures such as bones. Roszek et al[45] presented an elegant technique to quantify the loading forces from a *post-mortem* calibration using multiple strain gauges and known bending and torsional loading forces. Without the availability of this kind of calibration capability, bone strain recordings nevertheless remain a valuable, although qualitative, estimate of bone loading.

Tendon Strain Measurements

The long tendons found in the lower limb of the horse can be considered as elastic, more or less homogeneous, cables. When loaded their length increases. However, strain in tendons is not as well defined as in bones. An unloaded tendon will shrink in length, whereby the tendon fibers become wrinkled. When elongated, the fibers are first straightened out with only minimal force development. At greater lengths the tendon fibers themselves are gradually stretched and a more pronounced increase in force occurs. It appears that the "resting length," or the "length at zero force" of tendons, can only be approximated. Consequently, tendon strain is only meaningful if the conditions under which the tendon is assumed to have this "reference length" is accurately described.

In vivo tendon strain can be measured using implanted, highly compliant transducers such as liquid metal filled elastic tubes.[48,49] These transducers have to be custom made, and are difficult to manufacture, but appear to function correctly, even in vivo. A problem associated with this technique is that the length changes of the tendon, which have to be recorded by the transducer, are rather small. A tendon strains maximally about 10%, and assuming a typical transducer length of 15 mm, the corresponding transducer length change is only 1.5 mm. This implies that the attachment of the transducer to the tendon must be so rigid that length changes of only fractions of a millimeter can be recorded correctly. Even the smallest change in the transducer-tendon interface may seriously interfere with the possibility of correctly calibrating tendon length changes to tendon force.[50]

The definition of "zero-length" in tendons has already been mentioned. Unfortunately, it appears that there is almost no objective and applicable method that can identify this length in vivo. The shape of the tendon length-time signal does not always suffice (Fig. 10.8). Also, the method of recording the length when the limb is not loaded, as carried out in bone strain measurements, is not applicable in tendons due to their ability to shrink in length. Finally, the compliance of the tendon strain transducer will cause an apparent reduction in length, seemingly corresponding with a further reduction in the length of the tendon.

The final comment to be made about tendon strain transducers is that they record only length changes in their direct vicinity. When the transducer is connected to the outside of the tendon the resulting signals may be influenced by contact of the transducer with surrounding tissue, causing false signals. However, when implanted, the local tendon properties may have changed as a result of the surgery. It is therefore rather dangerous to extrapolate the recorded local tendon strain to the behavior of the entire musculo-tendinous structure (MTS).

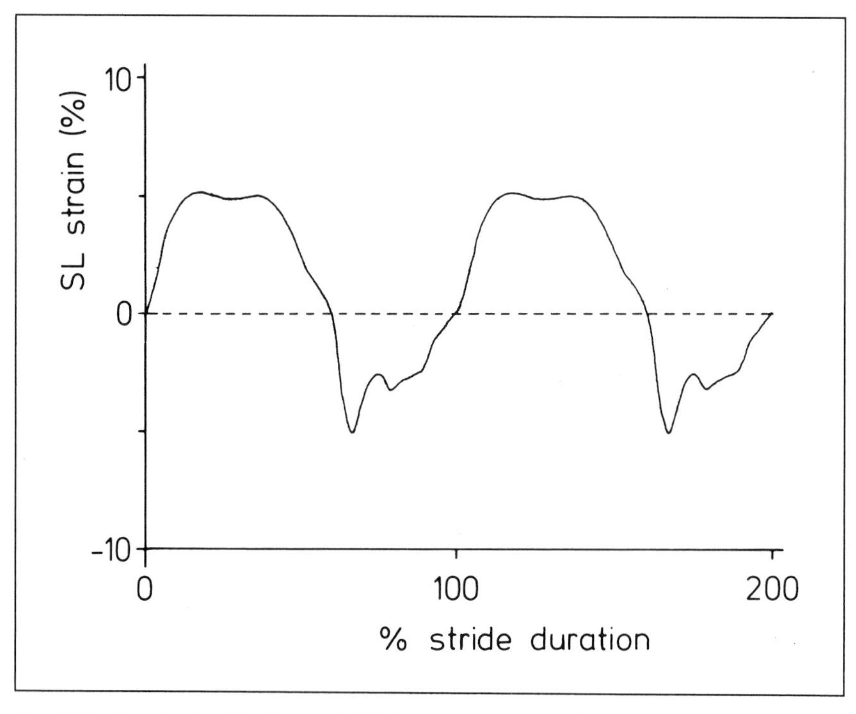

Fig. 10.8. Signal of a liquid metal filled strain gauge implanted into the suspensory ligament of a horse at the walk. A fast change in signal amplitude is visible close to the onset of ground contact (determined using an accelerometer).

As an alternative to recording tendon length via tendon strain transducers, the length of the entire MTS can be determined from the change in length between origin and insertion, using the geometry of the limb and the angles between bones determined from kinematics.[51] This method is very sensitive to the exact location of the sites of origin and insertion of the tendon, and models are required to describe the path of the tendon where bony surfaces have to be passed. However, it has the advantage that instrumentation of the tendons of interest is not necessary. A disadvantage might be that contraction of the muscle belly, in series with the tendon, cannot be accounted for.

Tendon Force Measurement

Tendon forces have been estimated indirectly from the signal of tendon strain transducers, using a post-mortem force-length calibration. This procedure uses a materials-testing machine, and requires isolation of the tendon and, thus, the sacrifice of the experimental animal. Except for a rather complex correction for shift in the signal due to tendon isolation and clamping,[50] this calibration is straightforward. Several other devices have been developed for direct in vivo tendon force measurement, but these have not been tested in our laboratory.

MODELING OF THE EQUINE LOCOMOTOR SYSTEM

The complex interaction between control of the musculoskeletal system by the central nervous system, muscle force development, tendon elongation, and accelerations of body segments leading to movement, cannot be studied using each of the techniques as described above separately. Knowledge gained in experiments studying each of these components has to be integrated. For this purpose mathematical models of the musculoskeletal system are required.[7,52] In such a model the bony segments are usually considered as rigid segments, connected by simple joints. The movements of each segment are governed by Newton's Laws. Muscles are considered as force or torque generators, and the tendons either transfer muscle force from the muscle belly to the insertion, or act as passive springs where a dominant muscle belly is absent. The kinematics of the horse, as recorded in vivo, can be used as input to the model where this information is used to determine segment accelerations by twice differentiating positional data. Subsequently, internal forces and moments are calculated ("inverse dynamics"). In a "forward dynamics" approach the muscle forces are prescribed, and the model computes the overall movements. Kinematics than functions as a check on the validity of the model predictions.

Such mathematical models are not yet sufficiently sophisticated to produce reasonable estimates of equine movement. Also, the predicted loads on parts of the locomotor system are not accurate enough to be

33. Riggs CM, DeCamp CE, Soutas-Litte RW et al. Effects of subject velocity on force plate-measured ground reaction forces in Greyhounds at the trot. Am J Vet Res 1993; 54:1523-1526.
34. Schamhardt HC, Merkens HW. Quantification of equine ground reaction force patterns. J Biomech 1987; 20:443-446.
35. Merkens HW, Schamhardt HC. Evaluation of equine locomotion during different degrees of experimentally induced lameness. I. Lameness model and quantification of ground reaction force patterns of the limbs. Equine Vet J Suppl 1988; 6:99-106.
36. Merkens HW, Schamhardt HC, Hartman W et al. The use of Horse (INDEX), a method of analyzing the ground reaction force patterns of lame and normal gaited horses at the walk. Equine Vet J 1988; 20:29-36.
37. Wentink GH. Biokinetical analysis of the movements of the pelvic limb of the horse and the role of the muscles in the walk and trot. Anat Embryol 1978; 152:261-272.
38. Korsgaard E. Muscle function in the forelimb of the horse. An electromyographical and kinesiological study. Ph.D. Thesis, Kopenhagen, Denmark, 1982.
39. Tokuriki M, Osamu A, Niki Y et al. Electromyographic activity of cubital joint muscles in horses during locomotion. Am J Vet Res 1989; 50:950-957.
40. Hof AL. EMG and muscle force: an introduction. Human Movem Sci 1984; 3:119-153.
41. Jansen MO, Raaij JAGM van, Bogert AJ van den et al. Quantitative analysis of computer-averaged electromyographic profiles of intrinsic limb muscles in ponies at the walk. Am J Vet Res 1992; 53:2343-2349.
42. Lanyon LE. The measurement of bone strain in vivo. Acta Orthop Belg Suppl 1, 1976; 42:98-108.
43. Hartman W, Schamhardt HC, Lammertink JLMA et al. Bone strain in the equine tibia: An in vivo strain gauge analysis. Am J Vet Res 1984; 45:880-884.
44. Davies HMS, McCarthy RN, Jeffcott LB. Strain in the equine metacarpus during locomotion. Acta Anat 1993; 146:148-153.
45. Roszek B, Loon P van, Weinans H et al. In vivo measurements of the loading conditions on the tibia of the goat. Acta Anat 1993; 146:188-192.
46. Schamhardt HC, Hartman W, Lammertink JLMA. In vivo bone strain in the equine tibia before and after transection of the peroneus tertius muscle. Res Vet Sci 1985; 39:139- 144.
47. Schamhardt HC, Hartman W. Automatic zero strain compensation of *in vivo* bone strain recordings. J Biomech 1982; 15:621-624.
48. Riemersma DJ, Schamhardt HC, Hartman W et al. Kinetics and kinematics of the equine hind limb. In vivo tendon loads and force plate measurements. Am J Vet Res 1988; 49:1344-1352.
49. Jansen MO, Bogert AJ van den, Riemersma DJ et al. *In vivo* tendon forces in the forelimb of ponies at the walk, validated by ground reaction force measurements. Acta Anat 1993; 146:162-167.

50. Riemersma DJ, Lammertink JLMA. Calibration of the Mercury-in-Silastic strain gauge in tendon load experiments. J Biomech 1988; 20:469-476.
51. Bogert AJ van den, Hartman W, Schamhardt HC et al. In vivo relationship between force, emg and length change in the deep digital flexor muscle of the horse. In: de Groot G, Hollander AP, van Ingen Schenau GJ, eds. Biomechanics XI. Amsterdam: Free University Press, 1988: 68-74.
52. Schryver HF, Bartel DL, Langrana N et al. Locomotion in the horse: Kinematics and external and internal forces in the normal equine digit in the walk and trot. Am J Vet Res 1978; 39:1728-1733.

PART III

Experimental Design and Data Analysis

CHAPTER 11

Single-Subject Design for Measuring Locomotor Activity

G.T. Pollard and J.L. Howard

INTRODUCTION

Locomotor activity in rodents is usually measured by assigning each treatment condition and the control condition to separate groups of subjects and submitting the results to between-subjects statistical analysis. Treatment groups are compared *post hoc* to the control group and to each other. Each subject is used once and discarded.[1-4] The left-hand column in Table 11.1 gives some advantages and disadvantages of this paradigm.

Repeated measurement of locomotor activity over weeks or months in individual subjects is usually done as part of a battery of behaviors, or as an adjunct to another behavior such as choice in a radial arm maze,[5] or as a noncontingent but schedule-induced behavior in an operant preparation.[6] It has been used in toxicology[7] and ethopharmacology.[8] However, spontaneous behaviors in general, which are distinguished from operant behaviors by the absence of programmed consequences that strengthen or weaken their occurrence,[9] are rarely chosen for experimental laboratory preparations in which the control is a long-term asymptote. (For an example of an asymptotic baseline of spontaneous cork gnawing used to distinguish $5\text{-}HT_{1A}$-agonist anxiolytics from other drugs, see ref. 10.)

ACUTE VS. MAINTAINED SUBJECTS IN LOCOMOTOR ACTIVITY

There is no intrinsic factor that precludes the use of asymptotic spontaneous behaviors such as locomotion in the single-subject design

---

Measuring Movement and Locomotion: From Invertebrates to Humans, edited by Klaus-Peter Ossenkopp, Martin Kavaliers and Paul R. Sanberg.

discussed by Sidman for the experimental analysis of behavior,[11,12] although there are practical factors. As lever-pressing for food can be brought under stimulus control and made to occur reliably within a range of values from day to day, as the change in heart rate that occurs upon placement of a subject in a test apparatus will habituate out with repeated exposure, so a spontaneously emitted behavior should come to occur at a predictable rate in each individual in a given context; and it should be possible to observe a change in this rate when a treatment such as a drug is applied, and then a return to baseline rate when the effect of the treatment has dissipated. The right-hand column of Table 11.1 gives some advantages and disadvantages of the within-subject paradigm:

Table 11.1. Some positive (+) and negative (–) aspects of between-subjects and within-subject designs for measuring locomotor activity in animals

Between (used once)	**Within (maintained)**
+ Rapid results	- Slower results
+ Simultaneous testing of all treatment conditions (comparisons unconfounded by age, experience, weather)	- Serial testing (possible confounding by temporally related factors)
+ Lethal end-point allowed	- Lethal end-point restricted
- Between-subjects variation (treatment group vs. control group)	+ No between-subjects variation (treatment condition vs. baseline condition)
- Many animals	+ Few animals

Rapidity of Results

A major initial advantage for the acute preparation is temporal. Acute subjects can be ordered from a supplier, conditioned to the laboratory for 1 to 2 weeks, and then used to measure the effects of a treatment such as a drug. If the experimenter has 12 activity chambers, is satisfied with 1 hour of activity (emitted at a high rate during initial exploration in the first 15 minutes of testing, a transitional rate in the second 15 minutes, and a low but still declining rate in the last 30 minutes) and a sample size of 6 subjects per dose level, believes that there will be no diurnal variation during a 4-hour part of the day (we have found a difference between 3 hours in the morning and 3 hours in the afternoon for rats on a regular light/dark cycle), is willing to clean chambers between runs or assume that the presence of scent from early runs will not affect activity in later runs with different subjects, and allows time for changing subjects and attending to other physical matters, then he can generate data for 6 dose levels (12 chambers ÷ 6 subjects per dose = 2 levels tested per hour x 3 runs per day). This would allow extensive initial examination of 1 drug (5 doses and vehicle) per day. Many variations are possible, but this scheme gives an idea of typical daily output for an acute preparation. A reasonable answer to the question "How does Agent X change locomotor activity?" could be received in perhaps 3 weeks from inception, or on the same day if a supply of subjects is kept on hand. The experiment would probably be repeated to yield a sample size of 12 subjects per dose to generate data of publication quality.

Chronically maintained subjects, in contrast, would require many weeks of daily 1-hour runs to achieve asymptotic activity levels, and they would then have to be accustomed to the injection procedure and possibly to the experience of being under the influence of some standard drugs before their individual baselines could be trusted. Several months would elapse before the question about Agent X's effect could be addressed. If 6 subjects were used with a Latin square design, some indication of effect would begin to emerge, but the 6-level dose-effect relationship mentioned above (5 doses and vehicle) would require 3 weeks (2 treatment days, 2 baseline days, and 1 other day per week). Six subjects should be sufficient, even if some baselines are occasionally unsettled. Six squads of 6 subjects each could be run each day, as with the acute preparation.

Once asymptotic baselines are achieved, output of publication-quality data from maintained subjects run once a day and treated twice a week would approach the output from acute subjects per unit of work time. Table 11.2 shows the comparative output from the acute preparation (subjects always on hand) and the maintained preparation (subjects conditioned to stable baselines) in 12 activity chambers with three 1-hour runs per day, Monday through Friday, for a drug with 5 dose levels and vehicle. When training time is factored in, the efficiency of the maintained preparation is modestly reduced, but many drugs can be tested over the useful life of a subject, which might be 18 months. In this hypothetical comparison, the acute preparation has a large temporal advantage in latency to initial results and some advantage in output per unit time when both preparations are fully operational. A technique that might shift the advantage to the maintained preparation—cumulative intra-run dosing—will be discussed below.

Control of Confounding Factors

The acute preparation has the advantage of behaviorally and pharmacologically naive subjects. Age is controlled. There is no previous exposure to drugs that might have produced long-term neurological or behavioral change (but naiveté reduces face validity if the results are extrapolated to humans, many of whom have been exposed to psychoactive substances). Weather probably does affect the level of locomotion; but because all doses are tested within a period of about 4 hours (with the sample size being doubled on another day), inter-dose comparison is relatively uncontaminated. Weather would be a factor in inter-drug comparison unless doses and drugs were counterbalanced over many days—a tedious procedure in comparison to the typical one of injecting 6 subjects (or all 12) with the same drug dose for a run. The maintained preparation, on the other hand, would be advantageous for inter-drug comparison because testing of a single drug would be spread over 3 weeks of weather conditions, though intra-drug, inter-dose comparisons would be subject to weather effects. Infra-sonic or ultra-sonic vibration would operate similarly. Interactions between environmental factors and treatment effects would be problematic for both acute and maintained preparations; interaction could be addressed in the former by increasing the sample size, in the latter by repeating the experiment in the same subjects.

Treatment Limitations

Acute subjects can be subjected to lesions, drugs, and toxins that produce permanent change or death. Testing these manipulations in maintained subjects would be, in many cases, prohibitively expensive. There are exceptions. The maintained preparation may be more economical if the object is to measure the effects of several agents in a lesioned subject: The surgery would be done once for many tests instead of for every test in acute subjects. The maintained preparation

Table 11.2. Hypothetical efficiencies of between-subjects and within-subject designs for assessing effects of drugs (or toxins) on locomotor activity in rats

Between (used once)
72 data points required (5 dose levels, 1 vehicle, $N = 12$)
36 data points per day (3 runs x 12 chambers)
1/2 drug per day (2 dose levels of $N = 6$ per run x 3 runs)
1 drug per 2 days ($N = 12$)
2 1/2 drugs per week
7 1/2 drugs per 3 weeks
Cost per drug: $990 for rats + $40 for labor = $1030

Within (maintained)
36 data points required (5 dose levels, 1 vehicle, $N = 6$)
36 data points per day (3 runs x 12 chambers)
6 squads with 6 subjects each (2 squads per run x 3 runs per day)
1 drug per squad (all subjects in a squad eventually receive all doses and vehicle)
2 treatment days per week (Tuesday and Friday), 2 baseline days, 1 other day
6 treatment days per 3 weeks (5 dose levels, 1 vehicle)
6 drugs per 3 weeks
Cost per drug: $293 for rats + $50 for labor = $343

would be appropriate for testing chronic treatments in an ABACADA... design, where A is baseline or washout and the other letters are different long-term treatment regimens.

Control of Variability

Inter-subject variability in the acute design requires a relatively large sample size and the use of inferential statistics based on probability. This source of unwanted variability is greatly reduced with the maintained design, where the effects are revealed to the eye in the form of orderly dose-effect curves in individual subjects. Within-subject data can be expressed as change from baseline or percent of baseline, and it can be submitted to within-subject analysis of variance and similar procedures if desired. In the acute design, the behavior of a subject is measured only once, for 1 hour, without regard for how it might differ if measured a day earlier or a week later. In the maintained design, the experimenter has direct data (from successive baseline days) to support a conclusion about the likelihood that a behavioral difference in the presence of an agent of interest is caused by the agent and not by an uncontrolled condition within the organism. This virtual elimination of a source of variance is a strength of the maintained design. If the dose-effect and time-effect patterns in most subjects are of similar shape, though the magnitudes differ (as they would in both designs), then the experimenter has strong confidence in his claim of cause and effect, and in his belief that a real effect has not been obscured by the overlap of subjects' qualitatively similar curves that differ in locus on the dose or time continuum.

A cautionary exemplum

Howard et al[13] tested 6 doses of β-phenylethylamine for effects on low baseline rates of lever-pressing for electrical stimulation of brain in a group of 6 rats. There was no statistically significant increase. Three doses were tested in another 6 rats. There was still no increase in the group data, even though β-phenylethylamine was known to be a stimulant and *d*-amphetamine produced a large increase in the same subjects. The results were published. Subsequently, still dissatisfied, we repeated the experiment, this time plotting the dose-effect curves of each subject. We discovered that the rapid onset and offset of the drug produced relatively brief spikes of high-rate lever pressing, with decreased rates preceding or following the spikes. When the data were analyzed on the basis of the group, the large differences between subjects and the complex temporal effects completely obscured the large rate increases.

Number of Animals and Cost

In response to recent public concern about the use of animals in research, some experimenters may wish to reduce the numbers. The maintained design does this. The acute design requires 72 rats per drug. The maintained design requires 36 rats tested 6 times per drug; they can be tested 140 times (twice per week for 18 months, less 10% for holidays, breakdowns, and the like), which, at 6 times per drug, is 23 drugs per rat per lifetime, or 1.5 rats per drug. Here, and in Table 11.2, is a rough estimate of the relative cost of subjects for testing one drug based on the hypothetical situation outlined above and the assumption that a rat can be bought for $10 and maintained for $0.25 per day. Acute: $10 + 0.25 per day x 15 days x 72 rats = $990. Maintained: $10 + 0.25 per day x 720 days x 36 rats ÷ 140 test runs x 6 test runs per drug = $293. With 4 hours of labor per day (three 1-hour runs and 1 hour of support time), the acute preparation yields 7 1/2 drugs and the maintained preparation yields 6 drugs per 3 weeks (20 hours), or 2.7 and 3.3 man-hours per drug. At $15 per hour, labor would cost $40 and $50 per drug. Total costs for rats and labor would be $1030 for acute, $343 for maintained. If the assumptions are roughly correct, the maintained design costs less than half as much as the acute design. With full replication, the maintained design would still cost less.

EXPERIMENT: EFFECTS OF THREE STANDARD DRUGS

The object was to establish stable baselines of locomotor activity by rats in daily 1-hour sessions, then to assess the sensitivity of baselines to disruption by a psychomotor stimulant, a depressant, and a sedative-hypnotic.

METHOD

Subjects were 12 ovariectomized Long-Evans rats from Charles River Breeding Laboratories (Wilmington, MA), housed 6 per cage in animal quarters on a reverse light/dark cycle (light on 1600-0400), with food and water available at all times except when subjects were in the laboratory. Mean body weight was 356 g when drug testing began.

Locomotion was measured in 12 doughnut-shaped activity chambers acquired in 1967 from Woodard Research Corporation, Herndon, VA. Each was 31 cm in diameter and 18 cm high, with 6 evenly spaced photocells around the outer wall, 1 cm from the wire mesh floor and a removable sheet-metal lid. The chambers were arranged 4 per shelf on a tier of 3 shelves in a dark room with white noise. Interruption of a photocell beam from a central light source (in the "hole" of the doughnut) was registered on a Data General NOVA 3/12 minicomputer via an InterAct interface. Each subject was assigned a specific chamber throughout the study.

Subjects were run 7 days a week, with minor exceptions, for the first 100 sessions, after which they were run every day but Saturday. They were brought to the laboratory either 10 minutes or 1 hour before the daily 1-hour session. Scatter plots revealed that 10 minutes in the laboratory produced higher activity counts than did 1 hour. In the 6-days-per-week regimen, Monday and Thursday were control days and Tuesday and Friday were drug days; on these days, subjects were brought to the laboratory 1 hour precession. *d*-amphetamine sulfate (Smith Kline & French), chlorpromazine hydrochloride (Smith Kline & French), and sodium pentobarbital (Sigma) were dissolved in 0.9% saline and injected p.o. 1 hour before testing in sessions 122, 125, 128, and 131; vehicle was given in sessions 112, 113, 124, and 130. Each drug was tested at 4 doses in a dose-doubling series. *d*-amphetamine was tested in subjects 1, 4, 7, and 10; chlorpromazine in subjects 2, 5, 8, and 11; pentobarbital in subjects 3, 6, 9, and 12.

For most of the first 109 sessions, locomotor counts were recorded in 5-minute bins. Thereafter, the sum of all counts in the 60-minute session was recorded and taken as the basic datum for baseline and drug testing. In addition to the plotting of individual data points, each subject's locomotion counts on a drug day were divided by the mean of its 4 saline days, and the values so derived for each of the 4 subjects assigned to a drug were subjected to the *t*-test for dependent samples.

Results

The left half of Figure 11.1 shows data for individual subjects: the last 10 baseline days, 4 saline days, and the effect of drug. In general, *d*-amphetamine produced dose-related increases in locomotion, and chlorpromazine and pentobarbital produced dose-related decreases. Data for pentobarbital 2.5 mg/kg in subject 6 were lost.

The right half of Figure 11.1 shows group data as percent of vehicle control, with standard errors and results of the *t*-test provided as descriptive statistics. *t*-values, in ascending order by dose, are as follows: for *d*-amphetamine, 0.816, 3.555, 3.970, 4.229; for chlorpromazine, 7.010, 6.084, 12.117, 5.561; for pentobarbital, 1.555 ($N = 3$), 11.588, 8.214, 4.871.

Inspection of data in 5-minute bins in session 1 revealed the expected spike in counts early in the session, followed by within-session habituation. In subsequent sessions, this spike declined; that is, between-session habituation occurred for the within-session spike as well as for the session total. Figure 11.2 shows the within-session habituation for sessions 1, 31, and 109. It also shows a low point at the 10-to-15-minute bin in sessions 31 and 109; inspection of data from other sessions run under the same conditions revealed this within-session pattern to be general.

Discussion

The results demonstrate that a maintained preparation for measuring locomotion is as valid and sensitive as a maintained preparation for measuring operant behavior. Drug effects in 1-hour sessions were orderly and consistent across subjects, and convincing group data were obtained with sample size of only 4. The cost of establishing stable baselines seems no higher for locomotion than for operant behavior: For several reasons, we allowed more than 100 sessions of training, but scatter plots suggested stable locomotion values by 30 sessions. There were peaks and valleys; possible seasonal variation should be kept in mind.

The productivity of an operant preparation for measuring the effects of rapid-onset agents can be greatly enhanced, with a modest loss of precision, by injecting successively higher doses at intervals in a single session, thereby generating a cumulative within-session dose-effect curve[14-16] that is analogous to the method used in an isolated tissue preparation.[17] This enhancement may be adaptable to locomotor activity. Following generation of the data in Figure 11.1, we put the

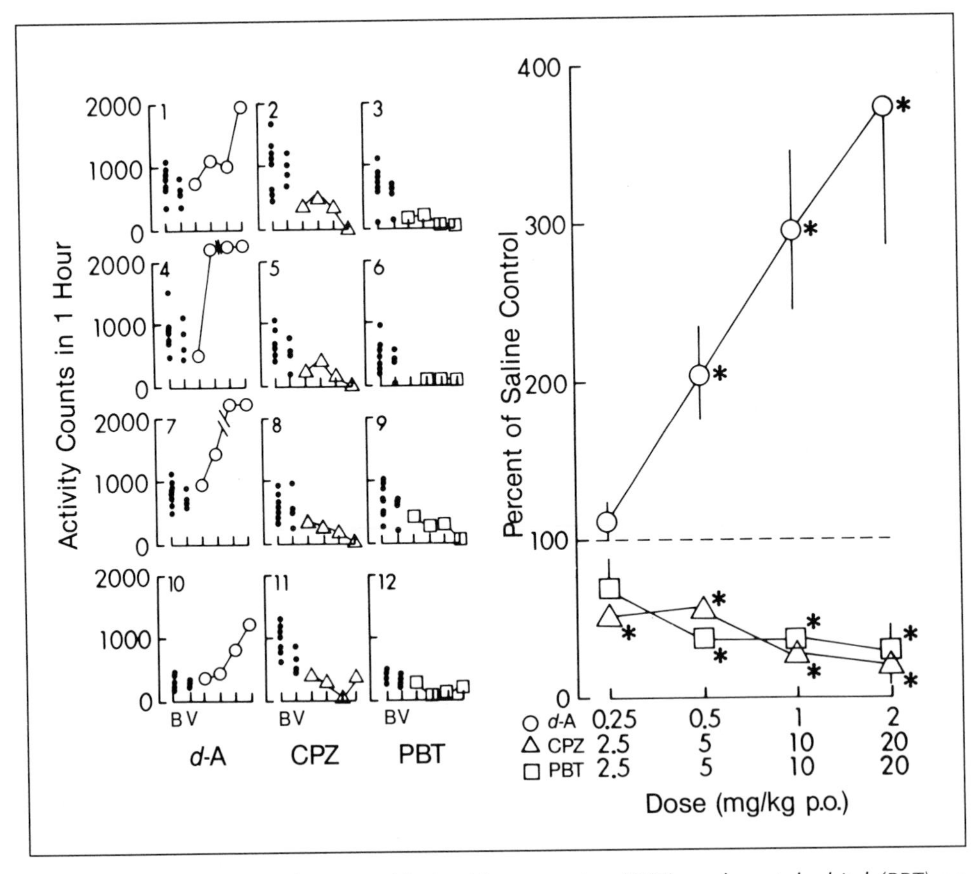

Fig. 11.1. Effects of d-amphetamine (d–a), *chlorpromazine (CPZ), and pentobarbital (PBT) on locomotion in rats. Left: Individual dose-effect curves of 12 subjects, 4 on each drug. Points above B are for 10 baseline sessions; points above V are for 4 saline vehicle sessions. Right: Group data expressed as percentage of saline control.* N = 4, *except for PBT 2.5 mg/kg, where* N = 3. * *indicates* p < .05, t-test. *Copyright by Wiley-Liss.*

subjects on a regimen of twice-weekly sessions for 4 weeks, then once-weekly sessions for 4 weeks, each session consisting of a 15-minute habituation period followed by five 15-minute test periods each of which was preceded by an injection of vehicle. Using the same drugs in the same subjects as before, we then attempted to generate cumulative dose-effect curves in a single session. The results were qualitatively similar to those in Figure 11.1 but less orderly. Variability was such that the lowest cumulative dose of *d*-amphetamine to increase locomotion significantly ($t \geq 3.182$) was 1.875 mg/kg, and the lowest cumulative doses of chlorpromazine and pentobarbital to decrease locomotion significantly were 18.75 and 38.75 mg/kg, respectively. It might be worthwhile to generate cumulative dose-effect curves on a baseline of daily rather than weekly sessions; the cumulative method, where it can be made to work, is a potent force multiplier.

The original intent was to establish a stable baseline for a 1-hour session to provide a window for measurement of the effects of drugs injected well before the session. We expected that, over weeks or months, the within-session variability of naive subjects would habituate out.

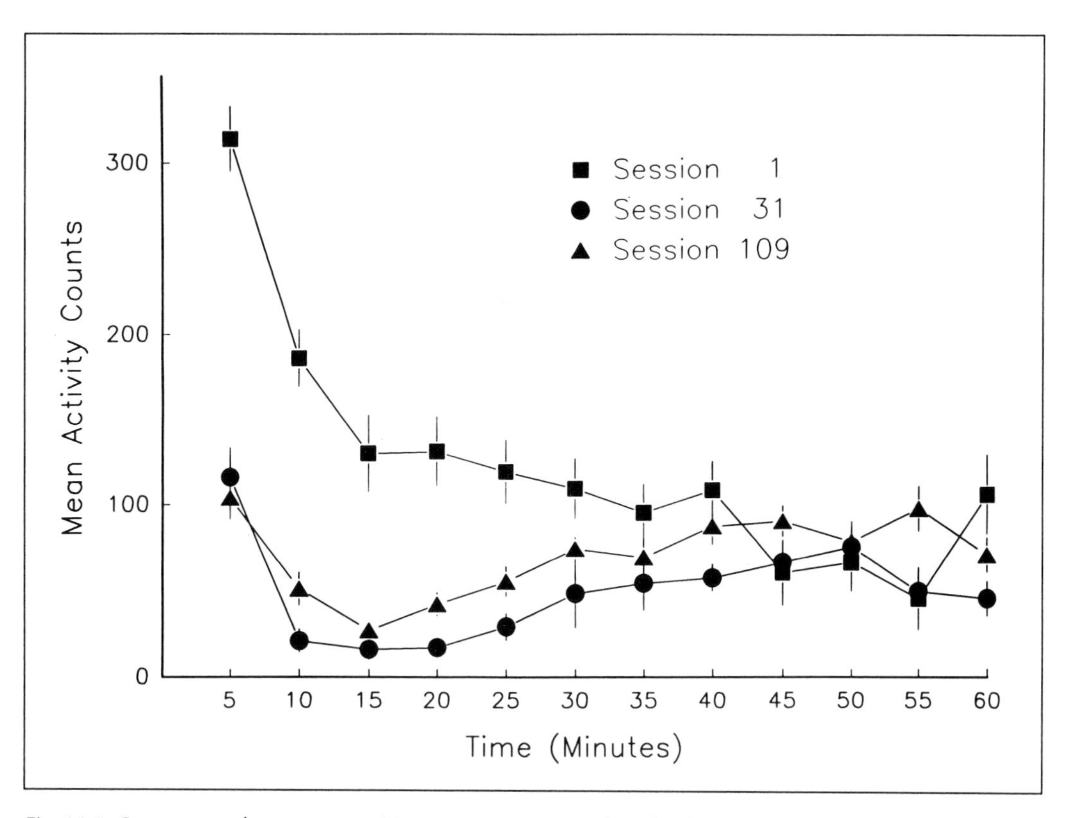

Fig. 11.2. Group mean locomotor activity counts in 5-minute bins for the 12 subjects when naive (session 1) and habituated (sessions 31 and 109).

To a large extent, that occurred, and the resultant baseline was sufficient for our purposes. However, subsequent inspection of data up to the point where we ceased to gather counts into 5-minute bins revealed a curious trough in the 10-15-minute bin. If the effects of drugs or toxins were to be measured in sufficiently fine temporal grain, this trough in the baseline would need to be considered.

The measuring device was 2 decades old and crude by present standards. It would be interesting to see the single-subject design applied in a sophisticated instrument such as the Digiscan, which can measure locomotion in several ways as well as other behaviors such as rearing.[18]

SUMMARY AND CONCLUSIONS

1. With repeated exposure to specified conditions, spontaneous behavior in individual subjects can reach asymptote and be managed by the methods of the experimental analysis of behavior.
2. Locomotor activity in the rat reaches a stable baseline in about the same number of sessions as does operant behavior, and the baseline is sensitive to disruption by standard psychoactive drugs.
3. The single-subject design for locomotor activity appears to have the same advantages and disadvantages as the single-subject design for operant behavior.
4. The single-subject design may be more economical than the acute between-subjects design in a laboratory with a constant need for testing.

ACKNOWLEDGMENTS

We thank Wiley-Liss, a division of John Wiley & Sons, Inc., for permission to use Figure 11.1 and several passages of text originally published in ref. 19. We thank Kevin P. Nanry for assistance with the manuscript preparation.

REFERENCES

1. Bunsey MD, Sanberg PR. The topography of the locomotor effects of haloperidol and domperidone. Behav Brain Res 1986; 19:147-152.
2. Sanberg PR, Henault MA, Hagenmeyer-Houser SH, et al. The topography of amphetamine-induced hyperactivity: toward an activity print. Behav Neurosci 1987; 101:131-133.
3. Howard JL, Pollard GT, Craft RM et al. Metoclopramide potentiates *d*-amphetamine-induced hypermotility and stereotypy in rat. Pharmacol Biochem Behav 1987; 27:165-169.
4. Crofton KM, Howard JL, Moser VC et al. Interlaboratory comparison of motor activity experiments: implications for neurotoxological assessments. Neurotoxicol Teratol 1991; 12:1-29.
5. Chrobak JJ, Napier TC. Delayed-non-match-to-sample performance in the radial arm maze: effects of dopaminergic and gabaergic agents. Psychopharmacol 1992; 108:72-78.

6. Reid AK, Staddon JER. Mechanisms of schedule entrainment. In: Cooper SJ, Dourish CT, ed. Neurobiology of stereotyped behavior. Oxford: Oxford University Press, 1990: 200-231.
7. Nachtman JP, Tubben RE, Commissaris RL. Behavioral effects of chronic manganese administration in rats: locomotor activity studies. Neurobehav Toxicol Teratol 1986; 8:711-715.
8. Miczek KA, ed. Ethopharmacology: primate models of neuropsychiatric disorders. New York: Alan R. Liss, 1983.
9. Ferster CB, Skinner BF. Schedules of Reinforcement. New York: Appleton-Century-Crofts, 1957.
10. Pollard GT, Howard JL. Cork gnawing in the rat as a screening method for anxiolytic drugs. Drug Develop Res 1991; 22:179-187.
11. Sidman M. Tactics of scientific research. New York: Basic Books, 1960.
12. Sidman M. Foreword. In: Iversen IH, Lattal KA, eds. Experimental analysis of behavior (vol. 6 of Techniques in the behavioral and neural sciences). New York: Elsevier, 1991: xi-xiv.
13. Howard JL, Pollard GT, Rohrbach KW et al. Effect of β-phenylethylamine and d-amphetamine on electrical self-stimulation of brain. Pharmacol Biochem Behav 1976; 5:661-664.
14. Kelleher RT, Goldberg SR. Effects of naloxone on schedule-controlled behavior in monkeys. In: Usdin E, Bunney WE Jr, Kline NS, eds. Endorphins in mental health research. New York: Oxford University Press, 1979: 461-472.
15. Howard JL, Rohrbach KW, Pollard GT. Cumulative dose-effect curves in a conflict test with incremental shock. Psychopharmacol 1982; 78:195-196.
16. Pollard GT, Howard JL. Cumulative dose-effect curves in rats run twice a week on an interresponse-time > 72-sec schedule. Drug Develop Res 1986; 7:233-244.
17. Van Rossum JM, Van den Brink FG. Cumulative dose-response curves. I. Introduction to the technique. Archives International de Pharmacodynamie et de Therapie 1963; 143:240-246.
18. Sanberg PR, Hagenmeyer SH, Henault MA. Automated measurement of multivariate locomotor behavior in rodents. Neurobehav Toxicol Teratol 1985; 7:87-94.
19. Pollard GT, Howard JL. Single-subject design for locomotor activity. Drug Develop Res 1989; 181-184.

CHAPTER 12

Reliability of Motor Activity Assessments

K.M. Crofton and R.C. MacPhail

INTRODUCTION

Motor activity is considered to be an 'apical' test of nervous system function, in that it reflects the integrated output of the nervous system.[1-3] Automated tests of motor activity are widely used to provide objective and quantitative pharmacological and toxicological data on chemical-induced changes in nervous system function.[1,2,4-6] Motor activity also has been used extensively in neuroscience to study the functional impact of experimentally induced neurodegeneration, as well as subsequent alterations in the effects of centrally acting chemicals.[5,7-10] Automated assessment of motor activity in humans also has proven to be an important technique for studying the effectiveness of drugs in human disease states such as psychiatric and arthritic disorders.[11] Motor activity also has been shown to be sensitive, reliable, and efficient.[2,12-16] Lastly, motor activity has been recommended by a number of national and international expert committees as an important component of screening batteries to evaluate the neurotoxic potential of chemicals.[17-23]

Because of its use in assessing neurotoxic chemicals, the US Environmental Protection Agency (EPA) recently published a revised guideline for motor activity assessments in both adult and developmental neurotoxicity studies.[24] These guidelines do not designate a 'standard' ap-

The research described in this article has been reviewed by the Health Effects Research Laboratory, U.S. Environmental Protection Agency, and approved for publication. Approval does not signify that the contents necessarily reflect the views and policies of the Agency nor does mention of trade names or commercial products constitute endorsement or recommendation for use.

Measuring Movement and Locomotion: From Invertebrates to Humans, edited by Klaus-Peter Ossenkopp, Martin Kavaliers and Paul R. Sanberg.

paratus or device for motor activity testing, but specify requirements for experimental design and testing proficiency. Also included in the guidelines are monitoring by an automated apparatus, the capability to "measure increases and decreases in activity," "reliability of operations across devices and across days," and a duration of testing adequate to "allow motor activity to approach asymptotic levels by the last 20% of the session for non-treated control animals."[24]

There have, however, been criticisms of the use of motor activity in neurotoxicity testing.[3,25,26] Critics have asserted that measures of motor activity have inherently large variability,[27-30] lack specificity for identifying neurotoxic agents,[3] and thus may not be reliable indicators of neurotoxicity. Previous work and reviews have already addressed these criticisms.[2,31]

The purpose of this review is to address the issues of variability in, and reliability of, motor activity data, to clearly define what they are, how they are measured and quantified, and to suggest how they help to define the characteristics of an appropriate device. Reliability is defined as the reproducibility of test results in terms of: (1) within laboratory sources of variability such as between-subject variability and reproducibility of control values across time; and (2) between-laboratory variability as assessed by reproducibility of qualitative and quantitative effects of xenobiotics.

RELIABILITY

Reliability of motor activity assessments within a laboratory may be assessed by examining the variability of data collected over time, both in terms of control values and the reproducibility of experimental results. There is an important relationship between the reproducibility of data over time and the control of within experiment variability, in that the former allows a critique of the latter. The primary sources of within-laboratory and between-experiment variability that must be understood and controlled are those arising from organismic and experimental variables. In the discussion that follows, these two factors and their role in motor activity assessments are discussed. Subsequent sections then assess the utility of historical data perspectives in evaluating the influence of these variables.

VARIABILITY WITHIN LABORATORIES

Tables 12.1 and 12.2 list the important organismic and experimental variables that can influence motor activity measurements.

Organismic Variables

Of the organismic variables, most experimenters carefully control the age of the subjects as well as the food availability, species, strain and gender (for reviews see ref. 1, 5, 6, 26). However, it is generally not clear from most publications whether testing may be confounded by the time of day in which testing occurs.

Table 12.1. Organismic factors that may influence motor activity measurements

Age
Gender
Species and Strain
Biological Rhythms
Previous Experience
Food Deprivation

Table 12.2. Experimental factors that may influence motor activity measurements

Multiple test chambers (box effects)
Method of detection
Social setting
Environmental conditions (lighting, noise, temperature, humidity, housing)
Length of test session
Environmental complexity

Motor activity is unquestionably affected by circadian rhythms,[32] and numerous pharmaceuticals[33] and toxicants[34,35] have been demonstrated to alter the circadian rhythm of motor activity. More importantly, as indicated in Table 12.3, levels of both horizontal and vertical activity can vary as much as 20-30% within the 'normal' work day. It is clear from these data that variability within an experiment could be lowered by excluding earlier and later times in the day. These data also point out the importance of balancing treatment groups across time of day.

Table 12.3. The effects of time of day on activity levels in rats

	Activity Levels (Mean ±SE)		
Time of day	**Horizontal**	**Vertical**	**N**
0700-0759	4040 ± 143	258 ± 14	36
0800-0859	4266 ± 193*	278 ± 14*	30
0900-0959	3825 ± 149	249 ± 12	30
1000-1059	3902 ± 118	219 ± 10	42
1100-1159	3717 ± 153	214 ± 16	36
1200-1259	4043 ± 160	251 ± 21	24
1300-1359	3724 ± 154	214 ± 19	24
1400-1459	3368 ± 167*	192 ± 13*	18

Animals were tested for 30 minutes using a Motron system (see ref. 31). Data are compiled from numerous experiments conducted over a 2-year period. All data are from control (non-treated) animals. Time of day indicates the start of the 30 minute sessions. * = for both horizontal and vertical data, counts at 0800 hr are significantly greater than counts at 1400 hr ($p < 0.05$) (unpublished data, ref. 36).

Previous experience in a test apparatus is another important factor that may impact variability in motor activity data. Vetulani et al[15,16] have shown for both mice and rats that group means decrease and at the same time variance increases when animals are tested a second time. Repeated testing on a daily basis has been shown to cause a between-session habituation after two or three days of testing (cf. ref. 37). The increasing use of motor activity tests in subchronic studies underscores the importance of understanding the effects of long-term repeated testing on levels of motor activity. For example, in a standard 13-week subchronic study animals may be tested prior to exposure, at a number of times during exposure, and at additional times following exposure for the purpose of assessing recovery. Recent data from a number of different laboratories suggest that the between-session habituation depends mostly on the time interval between testing.[38-42] Previous experience with other experimental conditions, especially previous drug and/or toxicant exposures, is also an important factor. For example, motor activity assessments of animals administered amphetamine result in higher activity levels when these animals are subsequently tested in a drug-free state (see also ref. 5, 6).[43] Therefore, care must be taken to match prior testing history across experimental groups when using animals that are not naive to the test apparatus.

Experimental Variables

There are also experimental variables that are important to recognize, and that, if not controlled, may lead to increased variability in motor activity data. The increasing use of multiple chamber systems underscores the need to insure compatability betweeen devices within a laboratory. Figure 12.1 illustrates the lack of any appreciable difference between sixteen figure-eight mazes used in one laboratory.[44] These mazes employ infrared photobeams that ensure ease of calibration. Devices that employ detection systems that are difficult to calibrate, such as those using infrared or capacitance detectors, may be especially susceptible to box-to-box variability.

The length of the test session used to measure motor activity is another important variable in determining the total activity level. Geyer[6] provides a pertinent review of this and concludes that short test sessions may be unduly influenced by factors such as handling and exploration of novel (or non-novel) environments. The degree of variabilty of activity measures can change during the course of the test session. Table 12.4 demonstrates that for two different devices the coefficient of variation (standard deviation expressed as a percentage of the group mean) actually increases throughout the test session. One reason for this finding is that animals may habituate or acclimate to the test apparatus at different rates. This observation underscores the need to understand the relationship between session length and data variance, and their potential interaction with the effects of an experimental treatment. If, for example, a chemical has a very short half-life (5-10 minutes), shorter sessions may be more appropriate. On the other hand, for a chemical that increases activity, through perhaps an inhibition of within-session habituation processes, longer sessions may be necessary (cf. ref. 45).

Proper control of environmental variables, such as noise, lighting, humidity and temperature may also play an important role in limiting data variability. Richter[46] first showed that ambient temperature influenced motor activity. Gordon and Fogelson[47] reported that increased ambient temperatures resulted in decreased motor activity (Fig. 12.2). Ambient noise levels have also been shown to influence activity, with higher activity levels associated with louder noise intensities.[48] There have also been a wide variety of studies describing the effects of illumination level on activity.[46,49-51] It should be clear that failure to maintain consistent test conditions in regard to environmental factors could increase the variability, and thus decrease the reliability, of motor activity data.

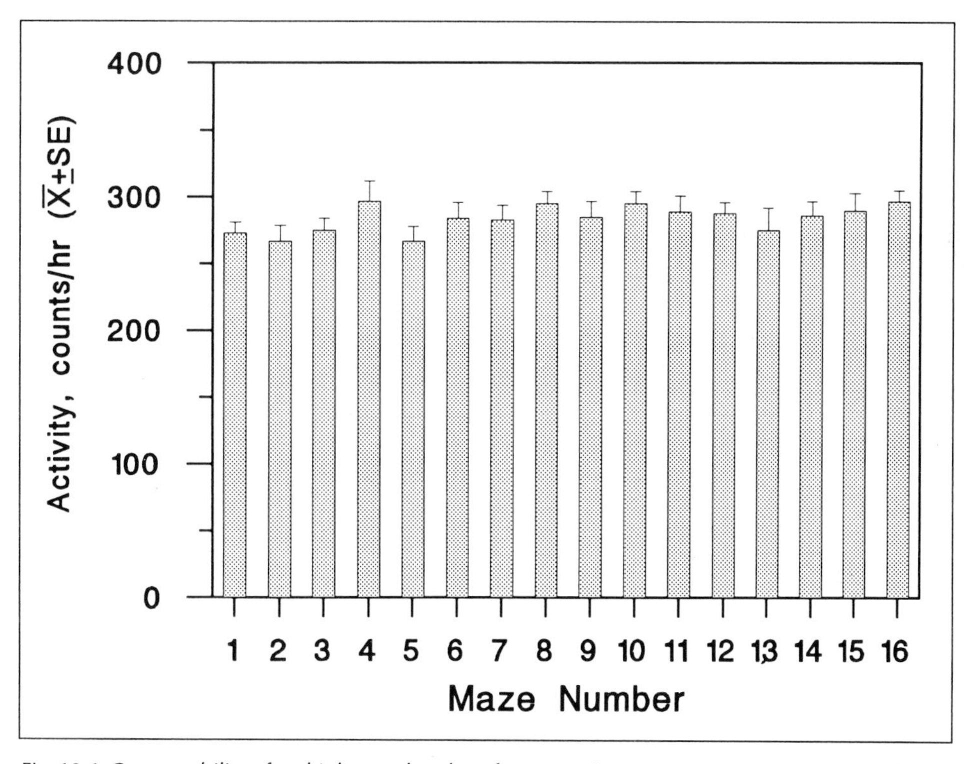

Fig. 12.1. Comparability of multiple test chambers for measuring motor activity. Data were collected in sixteen individual figure-eight mazes. Data represent control means (+ SE) from experiments conducted over a three-year period (n = 25 to 50 rats per maze). There is no statistically significant difference between any individual mazes (Data from Crofton and MacPhail.)[36]

Table 12.4. Effect of session length on coefficients of variations for motor activity data

Device	Time Interval	Activity counts	SD	CV
Figure-eight Maze	1	64.3	10.2	15.8
	2	53.1	10.9	20.5
	3	43.5	11.5	26.6
	4	36.1	11.7	32.3
	5	30.4	12.4	40.9
	6	26.3	12.8	48.8
	7	24.5	12.5	50.8
	8	21.6	12.1	56.2
	9	18.9	11.8	62.4
	10	17.5	12.2	69.6
	11	16.4	12.3	75.1
	12	15.4	12.1	78.7
Motron	1	1338	235	17.5
	2	958	238	24.8
	3	668	221	33.1
	4	524	225	42.9
	5	397	233	58.8

Data are from a total of 603 rats tested for one hour in figure-eight mazes, and 240 rats tested for 30 minutes in Motrons. Figure-eight maze data were collected from 1988 to 1994. Motron data were collected from 1990 to 1993. Time interval = successive 5-minute intervals for figure-eight maze data and 6-minute intervals for Motron data; Activity counts = mean total photocell interruptions per interval; SD = standard deviation of the mean, CV = (SD/Mean) * 100% (unpublished data, ref. 36).

In a review of experimental and organismic influences on motor activity Reiter and MacPhail[1] acknowledged that the '...failure to recognize, specify, and consider these factors is likely to result in equivocal studies that are open to multiple interpretations.' Similarly, Cohen[52] in a discussion of statistical power and random measurement error reminded researchers that "In general, anything which reduces the variability of observations by the exclusion of sources of variability which are irrelevant to the assessment of the phenomenon under study will serve to increase power." Clearly, careful control, to the extent feasible, of these factors will increase the likelihood of generating reliable results.

WITHIN-LABORATORY HISTORICAL DATA ANALYSES

In the previous section we discussed many of the sources of within-laboratory variability. In the present section we will attempt to demonstrate how analyses of data from a historical perspective can aid in evaluating the efficacy of efforts to control environmental and organismic variables. Considerable information on the reliability of a test methodology may be gleaned from retrospective studies of historical data.

Reproducibility of Control Data

One approach to evaluating the reproducibility of control data involves analyses of variability between test subjects in control groups. Figure 12.3 presents data on the between-subject variability of historical control motor activity values from several laboratories.[31] Each panel presents distributions of between-subject coefficients of variation based on relatively large numbers of experiments. Also shown in each panel is the mean coefficient of variation for each laboratory. Coefficients of variation ranged between 20-25% for four laboratories, while a slightly higher value (31%) was obtained in the fifth lab. These values are roughly comparable to those obtained by Vetulani et al[15] that are presented in the top portion of Table 12.5. The overall consistency of these values is remarkable, as no attempt was made to standardize across laboratories many of the variables mentioned above that could influence the measurement of motor activity.

Another approach to evaluating the reproducibility of control data is to determine the variablity of control group means across replications. One of the first attempts to gain an understanding of the reliability of control data in motor activity studies was made by Dews.[4]

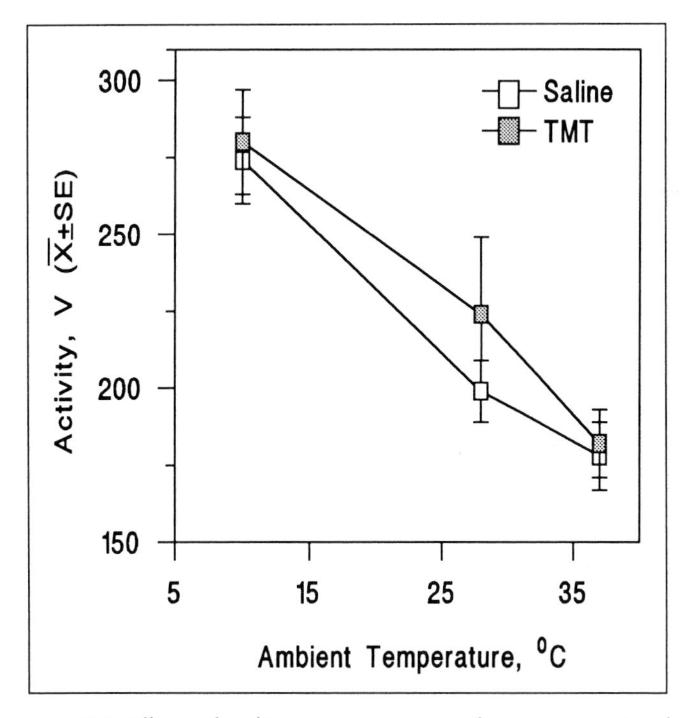

Fig. 12.2. Effects of ambient temperature on the motor activity of rats. Activity was monitored using a Doppler radar detection system in a temperature-controlled environmental chamber. (Data of Gordon and Fogelson;[47] adapted and reprinted with permission).

Reliability, assessed as the coefficient of variation of control means, for two separate series of experiments are presented in Table 12.6. A similar analysis was done for the datasets of Vetulani et al[15] and is presented in Table 12.5. The coefficient of variation for the grand control mean (mean of the individual replication means) was 6.8% for

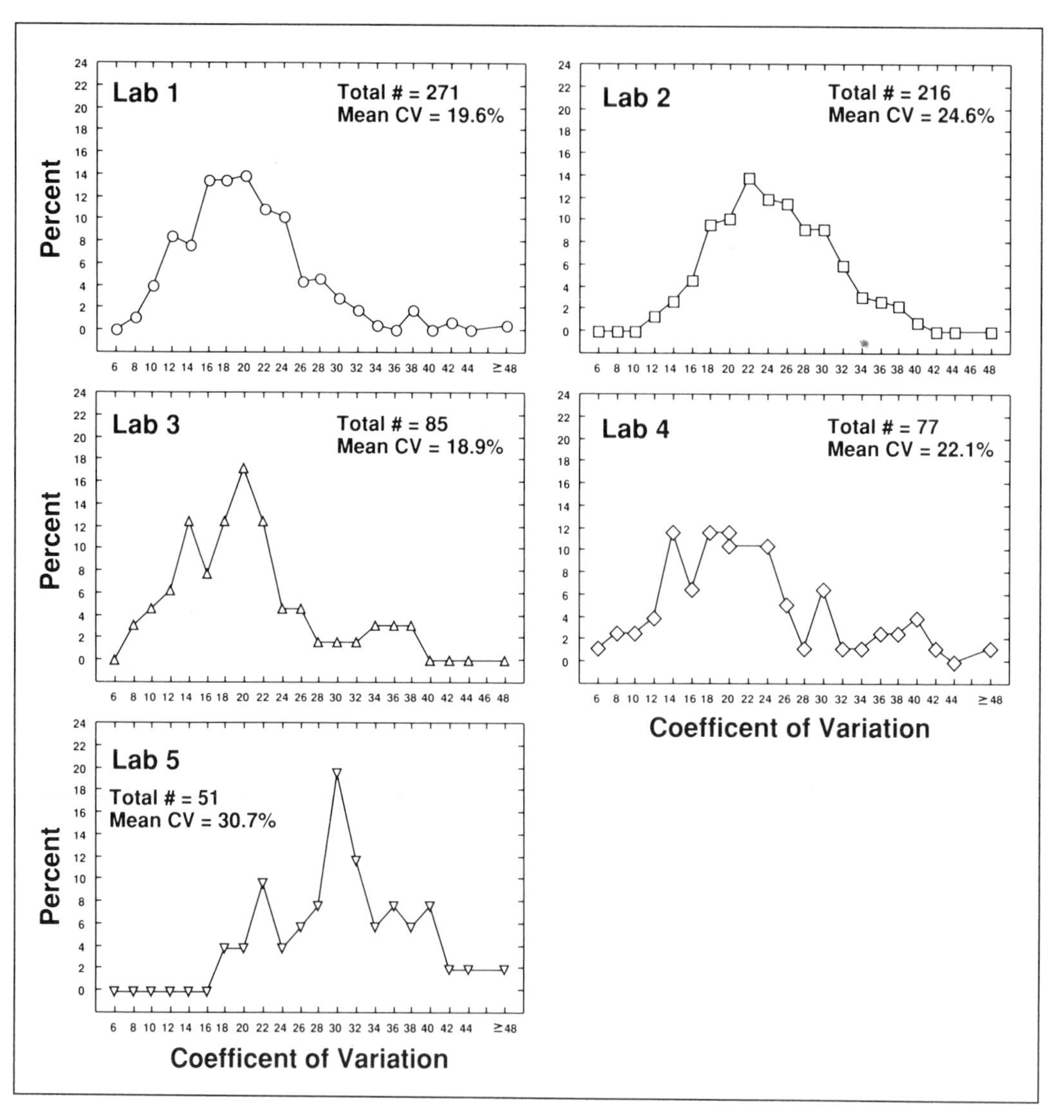

*Fig. 12.3. The distribution of the between-subject control coefficients of variation (CV) as a percentage of the total number of historical control values for Labs 1-5. The CV was determined as the [(standard deviation/mean)*100] for each group of control animals tested. Total # = the total number of control values. Mean CV = the mean for all CVs. Types of photocell devices are as follows: Lab1 - Figure-Eight Maze (circular); Lab2 - Woodard Photoactometer (square); Lab 3 - Motron (triangle); Lab 4 - Figure-Eight Maze (diamond); Lab 5 - Custom made (inverted triangle). From Crofton et al.[31]*

Table 12.5. Coefficients of variation for motor activity data

Group	Number per Group	Control Mean	SD	CV
Naive Test I	19	15.18	2.64	17.4%
II	*19*	*14.84*	*2.56*	*17.2*
III	*18*	*17.27*	*4.96*	*28.7*
IV	*18*	*16.07*	*2.76*	*17.2*
Grand Means		*15.82*	*3.23*	*20.1%*
		*(1.08, 6.8%)**		
Second Test I	*20*	*13.44*	*3.22*	*23.9%*
II	*19*	*13.28*	*3.20*	*24.1*
III	*20*	*13.96*	*2.23*	*15.9*
IV	*19*	*14.63*	*5.80*	*39.6*
Grand Means		*13.83*	*3.61*	*25.9%*
		*(0.61, 4.4%)**		

Data adapted from Vetulani et al.[15] Data were collected from groups of mice individually tested for 15 minutes in a rectangular shaped photocell device. Grand control mean = mean of control groups. SD = standard deviation of the mean. CV = (SD/mean)*100%. *represent the SD and CV for the grand mean of the individual replications (I-IV).

the first set of data and 4.4% for the second set of data. When compared to the data presented in Figure 12.3, these results indicate that variablity of control means across replications is consistently less than the variability between control subjects in any single experiment.

Crofton et al[31] have provided additional data on the reproducibility of control means of motor activity across replications. Figure 12.4 shows that mean control values were relatively stable across time. This is especially apparent for Laboratories 1 and 5. There was a slight drift upwards in time for Labs 2 and 3. The upward trend for Lab 3 resulted mainly from an increase in total test time from 25 to 30 minutes during 1987. Data for Lab 4 also were stable over time, except for a few relatively low values from vehicle-treated groups during the fall of

Table 12.6. Coefficients of variation for motor activity

Number of groups	Grand control mean	SD	CV
18	130	11	9%
19	*132*	*19*	*15%*

Data adapted from Dews.[4] Number of groups = groups of five mice tested for 15 minutes immediately following saline injection using a rectangular photocell device. Grand control mean = mean of control groups from two separate series of experiments. SD = standard deivation of the mean. CV = (SD/mean)*100%. The lower CV for the first series of experiments is expected, as data were presented as nine means of two groups of five mice each (Dews, personal communication).

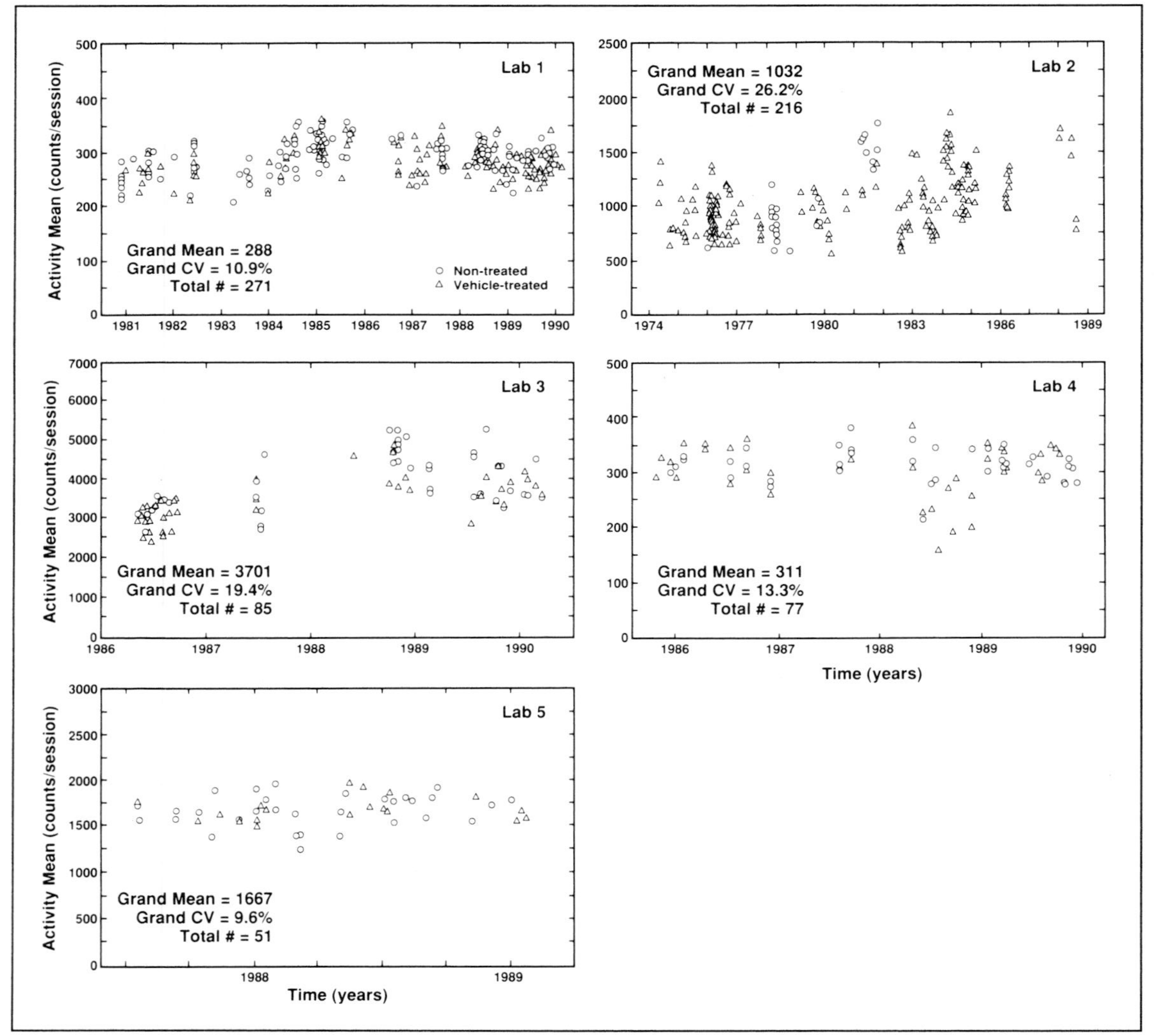

Fig. 12.4. Plots of non-treated and vehicle-treated control group means across time. Note the differences in the x- and y-axes between the plots. Grand Mean = mean of all individual control values. CV = the coefficient of variation for the Grand Mean. N = total number of individual control values. Device types are defined in Figure 12.3. (From Crofton et al).[31]

1988. The mean and CV for the control values combined across time for each individual laboratory are also presented (Fig. 12.2). The overall mean CV for replication over time was 15.9% (i.e., mean across all laboratories). The fact that control data remained so stable within laboratories over time is important information that might be used to differentiate between the actual effects of chemicals on motor activity and 'apparent' effects due to atypical control values. More importantly, for comparisons of between-laboratory and/or between-device differences (see next section) this reliability did not appear to be device- or laboratory-dependent.

Another, and possibly more important, approach to determining the reliability of motor activity measures collected within a laboratory is the direct replication of experimental results. In pharmacology and toxicology this can easily translate into the replication of dosage-effect data. Dews[4] first presented data on the replicability of a drug effect on motor activity. Motor activity was monitored in eleven groups of five mice injected with 1.25 mg/kg of methamphetamine. The overall mean CV for the replicates was 27% (grand mean ± SD = 325 ± 89). Another example of the within-laboratory replicability of data is presented in Figure 12.5. These data represent the results of three independent determinations collected over a 9-year period for the effects of the insecticide deltamethrin on motor activity. Although there was a slight difference between the data collected in 1981 and the two data sets collected in 1989, overall the data suggest a high degree of replicability. MacPhail et al[2] also presented replicability data for the effects of scopolamine. Figure 12.6 illustrates the remarkable replication of a dosage-effect curve for the increase in motor activity produced by scopolamine when measured three years apart.

INTERLABORATORY VARIABILITY

There are numerous methods that have been used to measure motor activity in laboratory animals (Table 12.7).[53] Some of the early techniques were as simple as an animal cage hung from spring-mounted metal bars, with electric contacts that activated relays and event counters.[82] Over the past few decades there has been a plethora of devices used, largely dominated by photocell and capacitance detection systems. More recently, devices using infrared and/or Doppler-radar motion detectors have also been used (cf. ref. 47, 79). There have also been several reviews of the methods used to measure motor activity[26,39,53] as well as critiques and comparisons.[3,31,53,83,84,89] The extensive variety of motor activity devices has led to a number of comparisons of the ability to measure similar behavioral events. Indeed, as pointed out by a number of researchers, different devices may record vastly different behaviors and/or different dimensions of the same behavior pattern (cf. ref. 53,84,85), as well as result in different effects of xenobiotics (cf. ref. 34). The remaining discussion will be limited to photocell devices, interlaboratory and interdevice differences, and an examination of historical-control data and the effects of xenobiotics.

Habituation is an important endpoint in the testing of xenobiotics for effects on motor activity. The US EPA Neurotoxicity Testing Guidelines specify that test sessions must be of a duration adequate to "...allow motor activity to approach asymptotic levels by at least the last 20% of the session for non-treated control animals."[24] Contrary to traditional thought, Crofton et al[31] demonstrated that there was a great similarity in the rate of habituation within a test session in data from six laboratories (utilizing five different devices). Figure 12.7 illustrates the habituation data for each laboratory. The habituation data for all laboratories, expressed as a percent of initial interval values, are presented in Figure 12.8. Regardless of the configuration of the device the rate of habituation was generally similar (see discussion in ref. 31). These results suggest that a session of approximately 30 to 60 minutes may be necessary to adequately study toxicant effects on the habituation of motor activity. One exception to this may be the

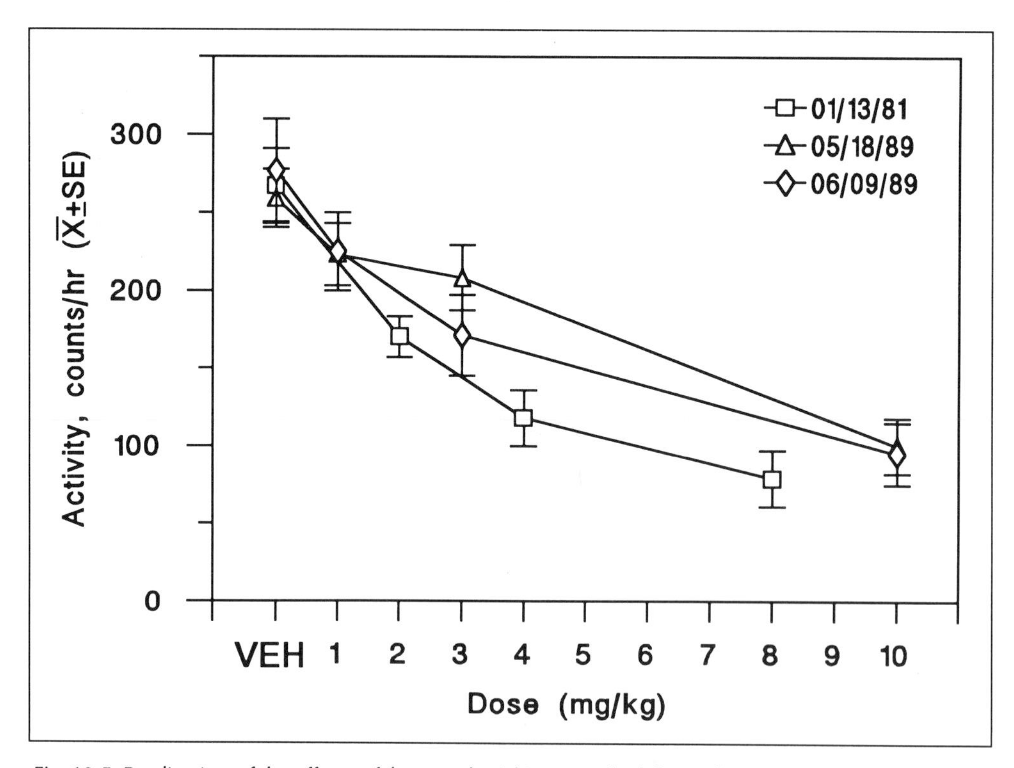

Fig. 12.5. Replication of the effects of the pyrethroid insecticide deltamethrin on motor activity. Motor activity was monitored for 1 hour using figure-eight mazes. Rats (n = ~9/group) were administered either an oral dosage of deltamethrin or corn-oil vehicle (VEH) and tested for one hour in figure-eight mazes beginning 2 hours after treatment. Each symbol represents the mean (± SE). (Data from Crofton and Reiter[99] and Crofton et al.[100])

device used in Lab 6 which appeared to require a slightly longer period of time (e.g., 70-80 min). These results are consistent with a previous report that habituation rates were similar for four different types of activity devices, including jiggle cages, photocell cages, a circular open field, and running wheels.[83] Taken together, these data suggest that these diverse devices measure the same process or construct (i.e. habituation).

Another important indicator of the reliability of a test method is the replication of treatment effects in different laboratories. Crofton et al[31] compared the dosage-effect functions for the acute effects of nine chemicals tested in six laboratories. Figure 12.9 illustrates the data for four chemicals that decreased motor activity. In every case, when the data were expressed as a percent of the vehicle control, the effects of these compounds were qualitatively similar across laboratories and devices. Consistent with previous reports, decreases in activity similar to those obtained in our experiments were observed after

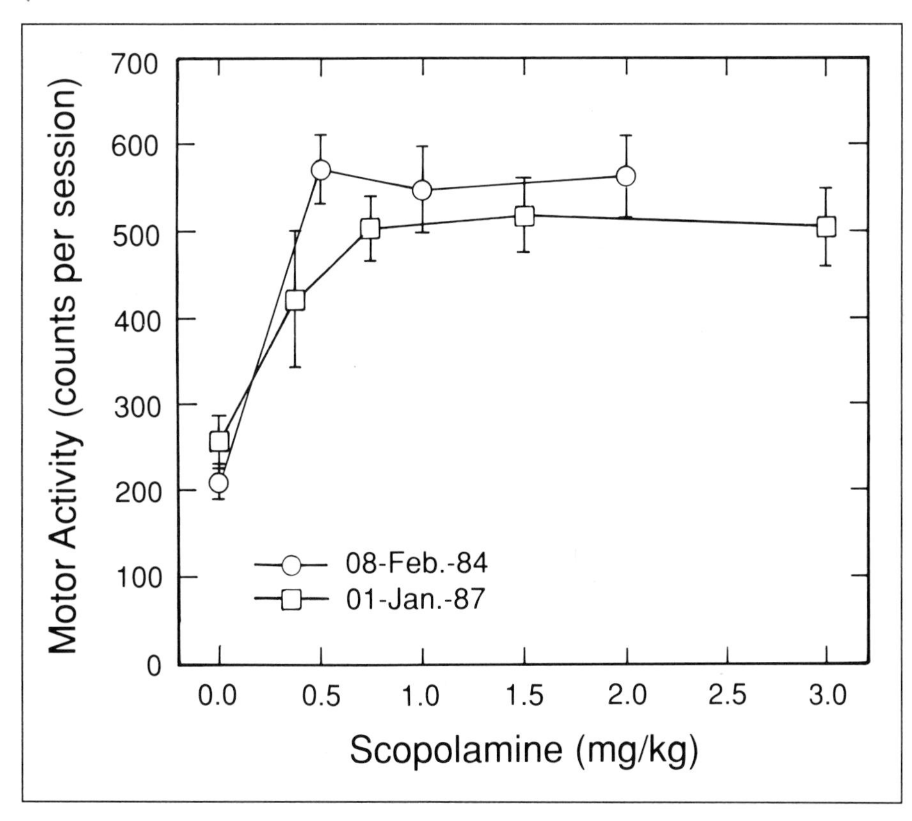

Fig. 12.6. Reproducibility of scopolamine effects on motor activity. Rats (n = 8/group) were administered either a dosage of scopolamine hydrobromide or saline vehicle (0.0 mg/kg) and tested for one hour in figure-eight mazes beginning 20 minutes after treatment. Each symbol represents the mean (± SE). (Reproduced from MacPhail et al).[2]

chlorpromazine,[86,87,88] physostigmine,[89] and carbaryl.[90] There are no previous reports of the effects of endosulfan on motor activity.

In a comparison of the ED50 (effective dosage 50%) and LOEL (lowest observed effect level) values for the different chemicals, Crofton et al[31] concluded that there was a high degree of replication between laboratories. The ratio of the maximum/minimum ED50s was less than 5.0 for all chemicals, and in most cases the ratio was less than 4. The ratio for LOEL estimates was less than 6.0. Some quantitative differences were to be expected considering the numerous differences in experimental (e.g., vehicle, route of administration, chemical purity, ambi-

Table 12.7. Categories of the different types of automated motor activity devices with selected references

Device Type	References
A. Photocell	
1. Simple environment	
Square/Rectangular	
horizontal	4,54
vertical	55
multivariate	56,57
rack-mounted home cage	58,59
Circular	60,61
2. Complex environments	
Figure-eight maze	62,63
Battig maze	64
Residential maze	65
Radial-arm maze	66
B. Mechanical Measurements	
1. Stabilimeters	
Jiggle cage	46
Tilt cage	67,68
Force platform	69,70
Piezoelectric plate	71
Phonocartridge	72
Accelerometer	73,74
Electrothermomechanical film	75
2. Running Wheels	76,77
C. Field Detectors	
Ultrasonic	78
Infrared	79,80
Doppler Radar	47
Capacitance	81

Adapted and modified from Reiter and MacPhail.[53]

ent noise levels) and organismic variables (e.g., age and strain of rat) that existed between the laboratories. Variables such as these have been shown to be important influences on the effects of chemicals on motor activity.[1,5,48,91,92]

Comparison of the variability of motor activity measures with other endpoints is made difficult by the extreme scarcity of available data. The differences in ED50s between laboratories for the effects of chemicals

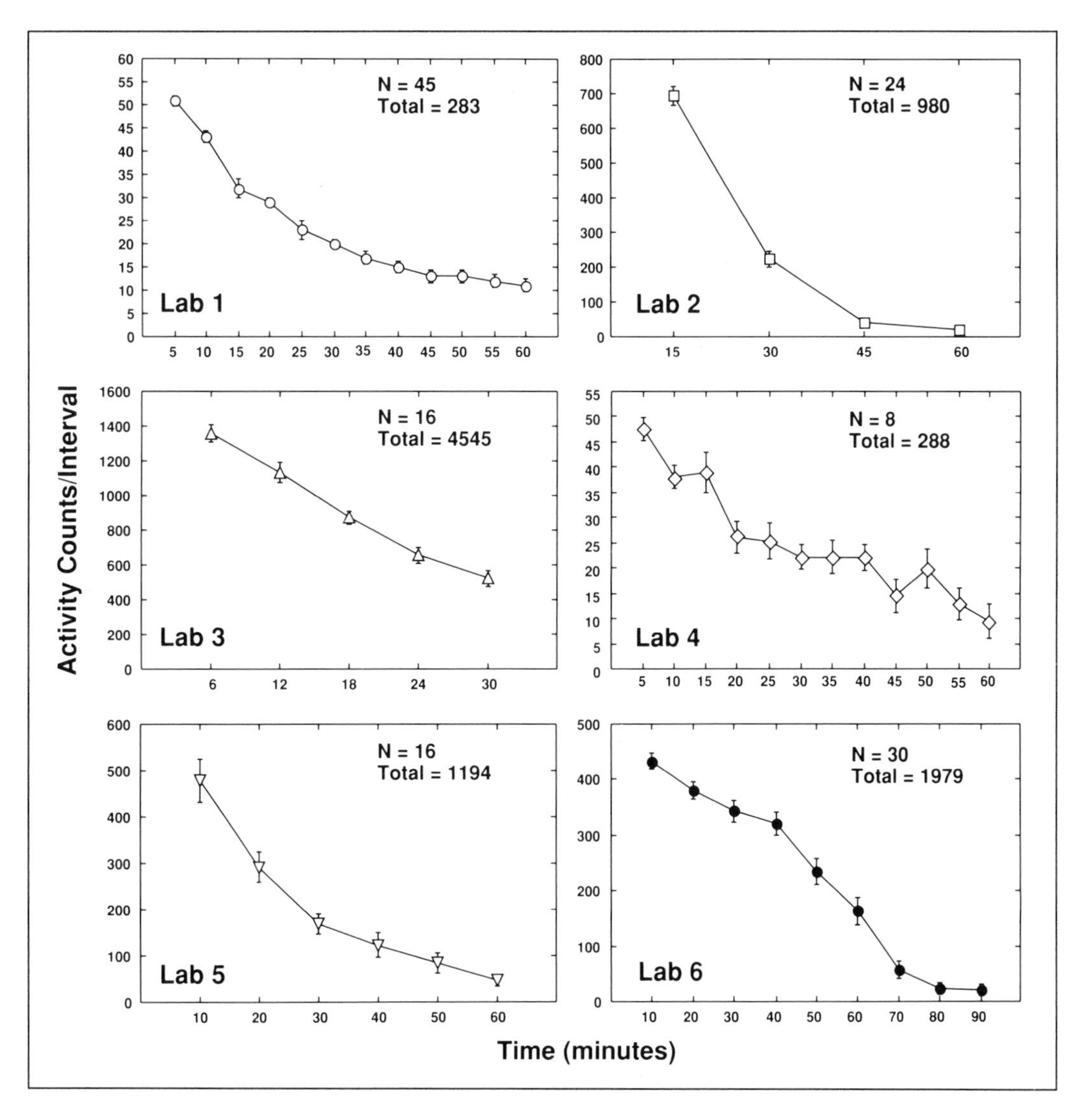

Fig. 12.7. Habituation plots for Labs 1-6. Data are expressed as the mean (± SE) motor activity data across the test session from six different laboratories. Note differences in both the x- and y-axes between plots. N = number of animals. Total = average total number of photocell interruptions for a test session. Device types are defined in Figure 12.3. Lab 6 - SDI Photocell (cage-rack mounted). (Data from Crofton et al.)[31]

on motor activity are, however, lower than the variability between laboratories obtained for LD50 estimates. In a study authorized by the Commission of the European Communities (under non-standardized test conditions), ratios of maximum to minimum LD50 values ranged from 3.6 to 11.9 with a mean of 7.0 for 5 chemicals.[93,94] In a follow-up study that employed more standardized test conditions, the range of ratios for these same 5 chemicals was from 2.4 to 8.4 with a mean of 4.4 (EPA/CEC,1979 as cited in ref. 94). The above-described interlaboratory motor activity comparison of behavioral data for 9 compounds, tested under non-standardized conditions, yielded lower ratios. The mean for the behavioral ED50s from the present study was 2.8. The mean for the behavioral LOELs was 3.6. It remains to be determined to what extent these ratios for motor activity tests could be decreased further by standardizing several of the key variables outlined in the previous sections.

An issue that has been addressed by a number of authors concerns the device-specific effects of experimental treatments. Krsiak et al[84] and Ljundberg[85] provided data on differences in drug effects in different activity test devices. The results of these studies (see refs. 5, 53 for detailed discussions) suggest it is important to understand the rela-

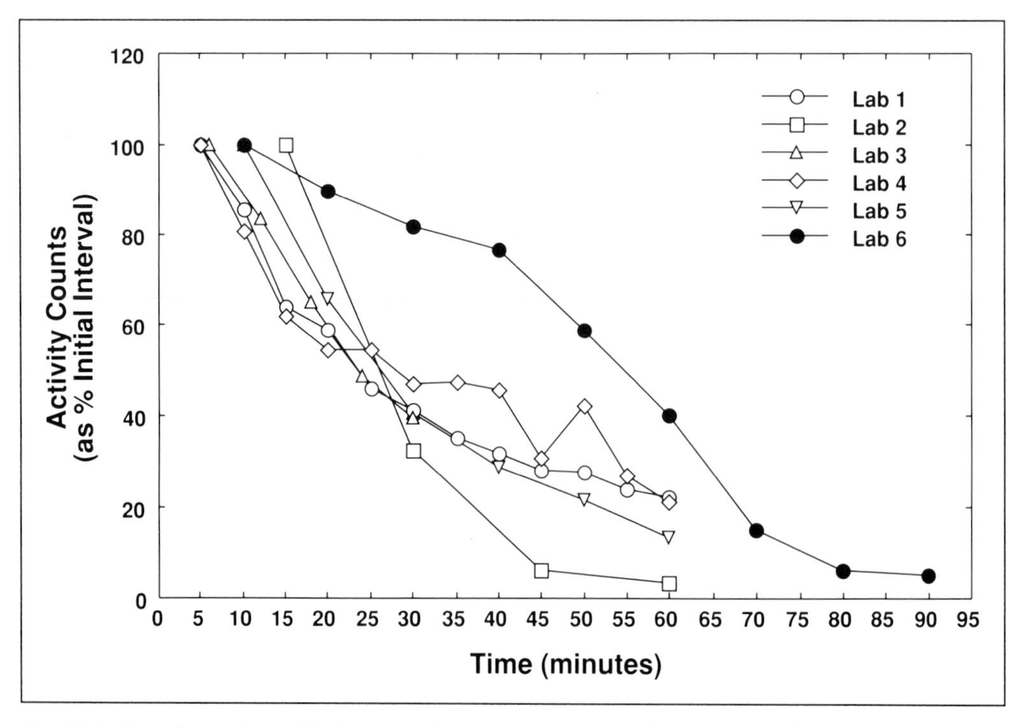

Fig. 12.8. Data from Figure 12.7 re-plotted as a percentage of the activity in the initial test interval. (Data from Crofton et al.[31])

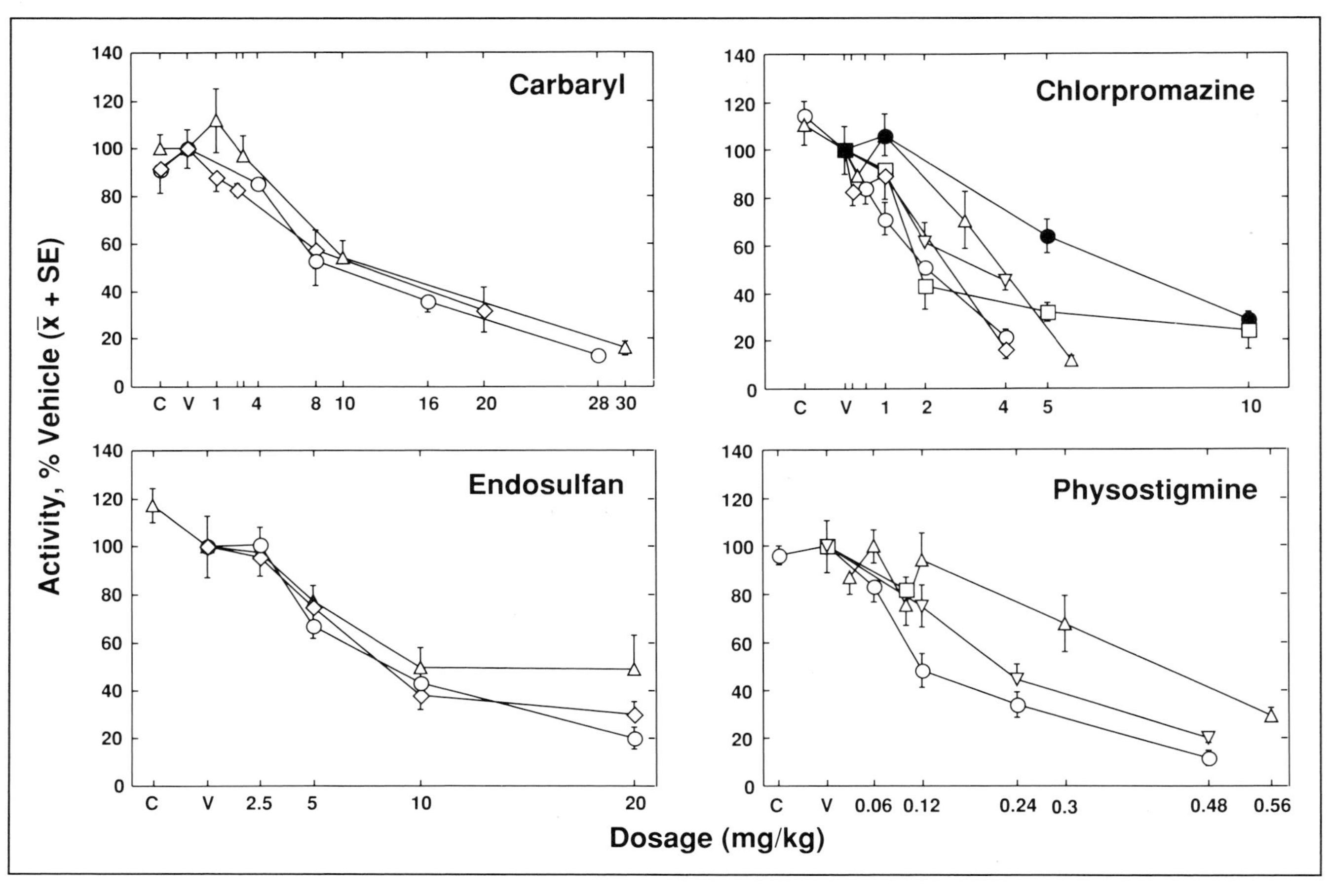

Fig. 12.9. Effects of carbaryl, chlorpromazine, endosulfan and physostigmine on motor activity. Data are plotted as the percentage of the vehicle control mean (± SE) for each laboratory. Control means (total counts), respectively, are as follows: (A) carbaryl - 330, 3418 and 354, for Labs 1, 3, and 5; (B) chlorpromazine - 311, 897, 3372, 293, 1762 and 857 for Labs 1-6; (C) endosulfan - 226, 2856 and 323, for Labs 1, 3 and 4; (D) physostigmine - 296, 897, 3918 and 1486, for Labs 1, 2, 3 and 5. Key to symbols is the same as Figure 12.7. (Data from Crofton et al.[31])

tionship between the effects of a chemical on behavior and the actual behaviors measured by the test method. For example, Ljundberg[85] reported that slow movements were recorded as increased activity in a capacitance device, but decreased activity in a photocell device. Recently, Crofton et al[31] reported interlaboratory comparative data on the effects of cypermethrin, a Type II pyrethroid insecticide (Fig. 12.10). Two independent laboratories using photocell devices (figure-eight maze) produced remarkably similar dosage-dependent decreases in activity. However, results from another photocell device (Motron) showed increased activity at the highest dosage. The authors attributed this difference to the spacing and the orientation of photocells in the two devices. The Motron, with closely spaced and vertically oriented photodetectors (i.e., a single overhead light source illuminated photodetectors in the bottom of the cage to detect horizontally directed activity), records both ambulatory and non-ambulatory activity (e.g., tremors and fine motor movements). Figure-eight mazes, on the other hand, have widely spaced photobeams (~30 cm apart) that record mainly ambulatory activities. High doses of Type II pyrethroids are known to induce various non-ambulatory activities, such as coarse tremors and choreoathetoid movements (for review see refs. 95, 96). Consistent with the data from Lab 3, Mitchell et al[97] reported increases in non-ambulatory activity in mice exposed to fenvalerate, another Type II pyrethroid, while ambulatory activity was not affected.

In some cases, the relationship between photobeam placement and device configuration may be complex. For example, in contrast to the non-ambulatory pyrethroid-induced behaviors which increased activity counts in the Motron, testing of other compounds (e.g., *d*-amphetamine and triadimefon) in that device revealed 'inverted-U' shaped dose-effect functions, suggesting that not all non-ambulatory behaviors are well recorded in this device.[31] Differences in the detection of small and large movements have been previously reported for both photocell-based[84] and toggle-box[98] activity systems. Regardless of these differences, the data presented here demonstrate that photocell-based devices are capable of reliably detecting drug- and toxicant-induced alterations in motor activity. Detailed characterization of the nature of these alterations, and of the relative contribution of ambulatory and non-ambulatory activities, may require further testing.

The results of this interlaboratory comparison indicate a good agreement both within and between laboratories in terms of the variability in motor activity data. This consistency is especially remarkable in light of the fact that no attempt was made to standardize many of the significant test factors such as age, strain, or testing protocol (see refs. 1, 5, 6). The only explicit restriction was that data had to be collected using automated photocell-based units with animals naive to the apparatus.

Several investigators have reported that motor activity measurements generate high, and by implication, unacceptable levels of vari-

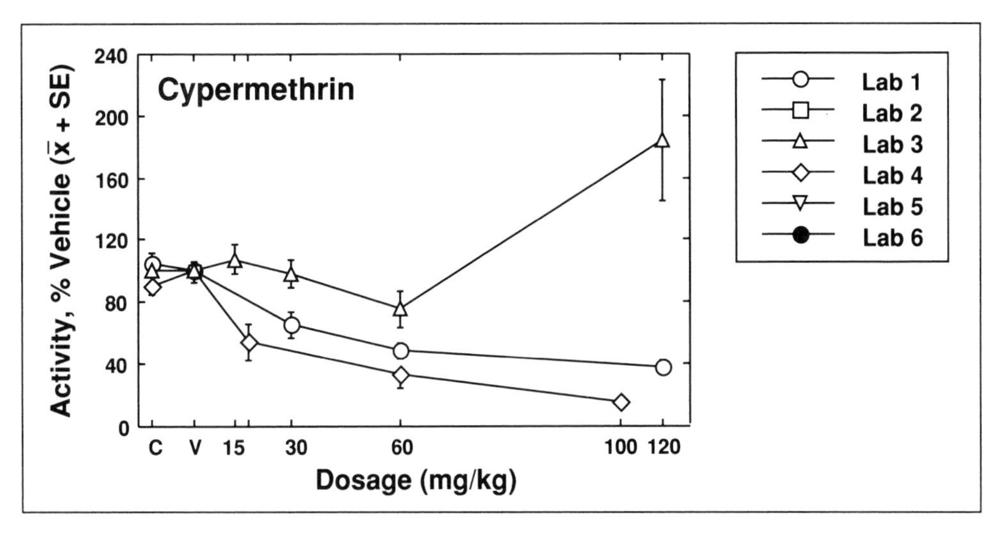

Fig. 12.10. Effects of cypermethrin on motor activity. Data are plotted as the percentage of the vehicle control mean (± SE) for each laboratory. Control means, respectively, are as follows: 321, 3572 and 342, for Labs 1, 3 and 4. Key to symbols is the same as Figure 12.7. (Data from Crofton et al.[31])

ability.[27-30] Our results contrast with the conclusions of these investigators. It is important to note, however, that variability is a joint function of biological fluctuation and experimental error. In those instances where substantial variability has been found, it may be that a greater attention to experimental design and execution would have reduced the contribution of experimental error to overall variability. Nevertheless, it is important to understand both the range and sources of variability in any procedure, or in any endpoint, especially when that procedure or endpoint is likely to be used in a regulatory context and in several different laboratories. Although the present results do not allow an objective definition of "acceptable" variability that can be applied across all testing situations, they do indicate that at the levels of variability found in the different laboratories qualitatively similar effects of chemicals on motor activity can be obtained. Discussions of intra- and interlaboratory variability would be greatly facilitated by historical variability estimates from other laboratories for other types of neurotoxicological procedures (e.g., morphological, biochemical, and neurophysiological). We strongly encourage others who have years of experience with these techniques to carry out and publish similar types of retrospective analyses.

In summary, this review demonstrates that motor activity measurements taken in different laboratories under disparate testing conditions can be reliable, reproducible, and sensitive to a variety of chemical agents. Regardless of geometric and mechanical differences that result in different baselines of activity, these devices yield generally similar levels of both within- and between-experiment control variability. The relatively low levels of within- and between-experiment variability, as well as the overall comparability between laboratories, argue that the expectation of inherently large variability in motor activity measurements[27-30] is not well founded. Moreover, the results of testing a variety of pharmacological and pesticidal chemicals indicate that these devices are capable of detecting chemical-induced alterations in motor function that in almost all cases are qualitatively and quantitatively similar across laboratories. The data presented here suggest that the specifics of device design may not be the most important variable in motor activity testing. Rather, well-defined standardized testing conditions within a laboratory appear to be of paramount importance in reducing within- and between-experiment error. Finally, we thoroughly encourage similar retrospective analyses for other tests of nervous system function likely to be routinely used to assess the neurotoxic potential of chemicals.

References

1. Reiter LW, MacPhail RC. Factors influencing motor activity measurements in neurotoxicology. In: Mitchell CL, ed. Nervous System Toxicology. New York: Raven Press, Inc., 1982:45-65.
2. MacPhail RC, Peele DB, Crofton KM. Motor activity and screening for neurotoxicity. J Amer Coll Toxicol 1989; 8:117-125.
3. Maurissen JPJ, Mattsson JL. Critical assessment of motor activity as a screen for neurotoxicity. Toxicol Indust Hlth 1989; 5:195-202.
4. Dews PB. The measurement of the influence of drugs on voluntary activity in mice. Brit J Pharmacol 1953; 8:46-48.
5. Dourish CT. Effects of drugs on spontaneous activity. In: Greenshaw EJ, Dourish CT, ed. Experimental Psychopharmacology. The Humana Press, Clifton,NJ, 1987:153-211.
6. Geyer MA. Approaches to the characterization of drug effects on locomotor activity in rodents. In: Adler MW, Cowan A, ed. Modern Methods in Pharmacology, Vol. 6. Testing and Evaluation of Drugs of Abuse. New York: Wiley-Liss, Inc. 1990:81-99.
7. Norton S. Hyperactive behavior of rats after lesions of the globus pallidus. Brain Res. Bull. 1976: 1:193-202.
8. Sanberg PR. ed. Locomotor behavior:Neuropharmacological substrates of motor activation. Pharmacol Biochem Behav 1986; 25:229-300.
9. Teitelbaum H, Milner P. Activity changes following partial hippocampal lesions in rats. J Comp Physiol Psychol 1963; 56:284-289.
10. Tilson H. Behavioral indices of neurotoxicity: What can be measured? Neurotoxicol Teratol 1987; 9:427-443.
11. Tryon W.W. Behavioral Assessment in Behavioral Medicine. NY: Springer Publishing, 1985.
12. Buelke-Sam J, Kimmel CA. Adams J et al. Collaborative behavioral teratology study: Results Neurobehav Toxicol Teratol 1985; 7:591-624.

13. MacPhail RC. Observational batteries and motor activity. Zbl Bakt Hyg B 1985; 185:21-27.
14. Pryor GT, Uyeno ET, Tilson HA et al. Assessment of chemicals using a battery of neurobehavioral tests: A comparative study. Neurobehav Teratol Toxicol 1983; 5:91-117.
15. Vetulani J, Marona-Lewicka D, Michaluk J et al. Stability and variability of locomotor responses of laboratory rodents. I. Native exploratory and basal locomotor activity of albino-Swiss mice. Pol J Pharmacol Pharm 1987; 39:273-282.
16. Vetulani J, Marona-Lewicka D, Michaluk J et al. Stability and variability of locomotor responses of laboratory rodents. II. Native exploratory and basal locomotor activity of Wistar rats. Pol J Pharmacol Pharm 1987; 39:283-293.
17. NAS/NRC. Principles for Evaluating Chemicals in the Environment. Washington, DC: National Academy of Sciences Press, 1975.
18. NAS/NRC. Principles and Procedures for Evaluating the Toxicity of Household Substances. Washington, DC: National Academy of Sciences Press Pub No 1138, 1977.
19. NAS/NRC. Toxicity Testing: Strategies to Determine Needs and Priorities. Washington, DC: National Academy of Sciences Press, 1984.
20. NAS/NRC. Principles for Evaluating Chemicals in the Environment. Washington, DC: National Academy of Sciences, 1987.
21. OECD/EPA. OECD Ad Hoc Meeting on Neurotoxicity Testing: Draft Summary Report, US Environmental Protection Agency, Washington, DC, 1990.
22. WHO. Environmental Health Criteria 60: Assessment of Neurotoxicity Associated with Exposure to Chemicals. World Health Organization, Geneva, 1986.
23. Leukroth RW, ed. Predicting Neurotoxicity and Behavioral Dysfunction from Preclinical Toxicological Data. Neurotox Teratol 1987; 9:395-471.
24. NTIS. Pesticide Assessment Guidelines, Subdivision F, Hazard Evaluation: Human and Domestic Animals. Addendum 10:Neurotoxicity, Series 81,82,83. US EPA 540/09-91-123. National Technical Information Service, PB 91-154617, 1991.
25. Gerber GJ, O'Shaughnessy D. Comparison of the behavioral effects of neurotoxic and systemically toxic agents: How discriminatory are behavioral tests of neurotoxicity? Neurobehav Toxicol Teratol 1986; 8:703-710
26. Rafales LS. Assessment of locomotor activity. In: Annau Z, ed. Neurobehavioral Toxicology. Baltimore: John Hopkins University Press, 1986:54-68.
27. CMA. Comments on proposed test rule for glycol ethers by the Chemical Manufacturers Association. (see Fed. Regist. 1987; 53(38):5935-5936).
28. Maurissen JPJ. Letter to the Editor. Toxicology 1989; 58:97-99.
29. Nolan GA. An industrial developmental toxicologist's view of behavioral teratology and possible guidelines. Neurobehav Toxicol Teratol 1985; 7:653-657.

30. Schaeppi U. Letter to the Editor: Comments on the number of experimental rats needed to test for motor activity. Toxicology 1989; 58:100-101.
31. Crofton KM, Howard JL, Moser VC et al. Interlaboratory comparison of motor activity experiments: Implications for neurotoxicological assessments. Neurotoxicol Teratol 1991; 13:599-609.
32. Rusak B, Zucker I. Biological rhythms and animal behavior. Annu Rev Psychol 1975; 27:137-171.
33. Wolfe G, Bousquet W, Schnell R. Circadian variations in response to amphetamine and chlorpromazine in the rat. Commun Pharmacol 1977;1:29-37.
34. Reiter LW. Use of activity measures in behavioral toxicology. Environ Hlth Perspect 1978; 26:9-20.
35. MacPhail RC, Crofton KM, Reiter LW. The use of environmental challenges in behavioral toxicology. Fed Proc 1983; 42:62-66.
36. Crofton KM, MacPhail RC. The effects of time of day on motor activity levels in the rat. 1994; Unpublished data.
37. Bushnell PJ. Behavioral effects of acute p-xylene inhalation in rats: Autoshaping, motor activity, and reversal learning. Neurotoxicol Teratol 1989; 10:569-577.
38. Crofton KM, Dean KF, Hamrick RC et al. The effects of 2,4-dithiobiuret on sensory and motor function in the rat. Fundam. Appl. Toxicol. 1991; 16:469-481.
39. Kulig B. Evaluating the effects of chemicals on adaptive functioning. Comp Biochem Physiol 1991; 100C:263-268.
40. Schulze GE, Boysen BG. A neurotoxicity screening battery of use in safety evaluation: Effects of acrylamide and 3,3-iminodipropionitrile. Fundam Appl Toxicol 1991; 16:602-615.
41. Llorens J, Crofton KM, Tilson HA et al. Characterization of disulfoton-induced behavioral and neurochemical effects following repeated exposure. Fundam Appl Toxicol 1993; 20:163-169.
42. Moser VC, Boyes WK. Prolonged neurobehavioral and visual effects of short-term exposure to 3,3-iminodipropionitrile. Fundam Appl Toxicol 1992; 21:277-290.
43. Tilson HA, Rech RC. Conditioned drug effects and absence of tolerance to *d*-amphetamine-induced motor activity. Pharmacol Biochem Behav 1973; 1:149-153.
44. Crofton KM. Lack of effect of multiple test chambers on the motor activity of rats, 1994 (unpublished data).
45. Crofton KM, Boncek VM, MacPhail R.C. Evidence for aminergic involvement in triadimefon-induced hyperactivity. Psychopharmacology 1989; 97:326-330.
46. Richter CP. A behavioristic study of the activity of the rat. Comp Physiol Monogr 1922; 1:1-55.
47. Gordon CJ, Fogelson L. Comparison of rats of the Fischer 344 and Long-Evans strains in the autonomic thermoregulatory response to trimethyltin administration. J Toxicol Environ Hlth 1991; 32:141-152.

48. Kallman MJ. Superior colliculus involvement in the locomotor effects of ambient noise and the stimulants. Physiol. Behav. 1983; 30:431-435.
49. McLearn GE. Strain differences in activity in mice: Influence of illumination. J Comp Physiol Psychol 1960; 53:142-143.
50. McReynolds WE, Weir MW, DeFries JC. Open-field behavior in mice:Effect of test illumination. Psychon Sci 1967; 9:277-278
51. Watzman N, Barry H, Kinnard WJ et al. Influence of chlorpromazine on spontaneous activity of mice under various parametric conditions. Arch Int Pharmacodyn 1967; 165:352-368.
52. Cohen J. Statistical Power Analysis for the Behavioral Sciences. Revised Edition. Hillsdale: Lawrence Erlbaum Assoc., 1987:8.
53. Reiter LW, MacPhail RC. Motor Activity: A survey of methods with potential use in toxicity testing. Neurobehav Toxicol 1979; 1:(suppl.1)53-66.
54. Seigel PS. A simple electronic device for the measurement of gross bodily activity of small animals. J Psychol 1964; 21:227-236.
55. Schnitzer SB, Ross S. Effects of physiological saline injections on locomotor activity in C57Bl/6 mice. Psychol Rep 1960; 6:351-354.
56. Geyer MA, Russo PV, Masten VL. Multivariate assessment of locomotor behavior: Pharmacological and behavioral analyses. Pharmacol Biochem Behav 1968; 25:277-288.
57. Ossenkopp K-P, Macrae LK, Teskey GC. Automated multivariate measurement of spontaneous motor activity in mice: Time course and reliabilities of the behavioral measurements. Pharmacol Biochem Behav 1987; 27:565-568.
58. Evans HL, Bushnell PJ, Taylor JD et al. A system for assessing the toxicity of chemicals by continuous monitoring of home cage behaviors. Fundam Appl Toxicol 1986; 721-732.
59. Oskarsson A, Ljundberg T, Stahle L et al. Behavioral and neurochemical effects after combined perinatal treatment of rats with lead and disulfiram. Neurobehav Toxicol Teratol 1986; 8:591-599.
60. Davis WM, Babbini M, Pong SF et al. Motility of mice after amphetamine: Effects of strain, aggregation and illumination. Pharmacol Biochem Behav 1974; 2:803-809.
61. Hollister AS, Breese GR, Mueller RA. Role of monoamine neural systems in l-dihydroxyphenylalanine-stimulated activity. J Pharmacol Exp Therap 1979; 208:37-43
62. Norton S, Culver B, Mullenix P. Measurement of the effects of drugs on activity of permanent groups of rats. Psychopharmacol Commun 1975; 1:131-138.
63. Reiter LW, Anderson GE, Laskey JW et al. Developmental and behavioral changes in the rat during chronic exposure to lead. Environ Hlth Perspect 1975; 12:119-123.
64. Battig K, Driscoll K, Schlatter J et al. Effects of nicotine on the exploratory locomotion patterns of female Roman high- and low-avoidance rats. Pharmacol Biochem Behav 1976; 4:435-439.
65. Elsner J, Looser R, Zbinden G. Quantitative analysis of rat behavior patterns in a residential maze. Neurobehav Toxicol 1979: 1(suppl.1):163-174.

66. Miller DB, Eckerman DA, Krigman MR et al. Chronic neonatal organotin exposure alters radial arm maze performance in adult rats. Neurobehav Toxicol Teratol 1982; 4:185-190
67. Bousfield WA, Mote FA. The construction of a tilting activity cage. J Exper Psychol 1943; 32:450-451.
68. Campbell BA, Teghtsoonian R, Williams RA. Activity, weight loss and survival time of food deprived rats as a function of age. J Comp Physiol Psychol 1961; 54:216-219.
69. Denenberg VH, Gartner J, Myers M. Absolute measurement of open field activity in mice. Physiol Behav 1975; 15:505-509.
70. Segal,D.S. and Mandell,A.J. Long term administration of d-amphetamine: Progressive augmentation of motor activity and stereotypy. Pharmacol Biochem Behav 1974; 2:249-255.
71. Lilienthal H, Winneke G, Brockhaus A et al. Pre- and post-natal lead exposure in monkeys: Effects on activity and learning set formation. Neurobehav Toxicol Teratol 1986; 8:265-272
72. Caul WF, Fernandez K, Michaelis RC. Effects of prenatal ethanol exposure on heart rate, activity, and response suppression. Neurobehav Toxicol Teratol 1983; 5:461-464.
73. Plonsky M, Reily EP. Head-dipping behaviors in rats exposed to alcohol as a function of age at testing. Neurobehav Teratol Toxicol 1983; 5:309-314.
74. Czech DA, Hoium E. Some aspects of feeding and locomotor activity in adult rats exposed to tetraethyllead. Neurobehav Teratol Toxicol 1984; 6:357-361.
75. Raisanen L, Pohjanvirta R, Unkila M, Tumisto J. A new method for the measurement of spontaneous motor activity of laboratory animals. Pharmacol Toxicol 1992; 70:230-231
76. Stewart CC. Variations in daily activity produced by alcohol and by changes in barometric pressure and diet, with a description of recording methods. Amer J Physiol 1898; 1:40-56.
77. Skinner BF. The measurement of spontaneous activity. J Gen Psychol 1933; 9:3-24.
78. Peacock LJ, Williams M. An ultrasonic device for recording activity. Am J Physiol 1962; 75:648-652.
79. Tamborini P, Sigg H, Zbinden,G. Quantitative analysis of rat activity in the home cage by infrared monitoring. Application to the acute toxicity testing of acetanilide and phenylmercuric acetate. Arch Toxicol 1989; 63:85-96.
80. Foss JA, Lochry EA. The assessment of motor activity in neonatal and adult rodents using passive infrared sensors. Abstract presented at the 12th Annual Meeting of the American College of Toxicology, Savannah, GA, 1991.
81. Svensson TH, Thieme G. An investigation of a new instrument to measure motor activity of small animals. Psychopharmacology 1969; 14:157-163.

82. Chappel CI, Grant GA, Archibald S et al. An apparatus for testing the effect of drugs on spontaneous activity of the rat. J Amer Pharmaceut Assoc 1957; 66:497-500.
83. Tapp JT, Zimmerman RS, D'Encarnacao PS. Intercorrelational analysis of some common measures of rat activity. Psychol Rep 1968; 23:1047-1050.
84. Krsiak M, Steinberg H, Stolerman IP. Uses and limitations of photocell activity cages for assessing effects of drugs. Psychopharmacologia 1970; 17:258-274.
85. Ljungberg T. Reliability of two activity boxes commonly used to assess drug-induced behavioral changes. Pharmacol Biochem Behav 1978; 8:483-489.
86. Fitzgerald RE, Berres M, Schaeppi U. Validation of a photobeam system for assessment of motor activity in rats. Toxicology 1988; 49:433-439.
87. Reiter LW. Chemical exposures and animal activity: Utility of the figure-eight maze. In: Hayes AW, Schnell RC, Miya TS, eds. Developments in the Science and Practice of Toxicology. NY: Elsevier, 1983:73-84.
88. Schreur PJK, Nichols NF. Two automated locomotor activity tests for dopamine autoreceptor agonists. Pharmacol Biochem Behav 1986; 25:255-261.
89. Vives F, Mora F. Effects of agonists and antagonists of cholinergic receptors on self-stimulation of the medial prefrontal cortex of the rat. Gen Pharmacol 1986; 17:63-67.
90. Ruppert PH, Cook LL, Dean KF et al. Acute behavioral toxicity of carbaryl and propoxur in adult rats. Pharmacol Biochem Behav 1983; 18:579-584.
91. Crabbe JC. Genetic differences in locomotor activation in mice. Pharmacol Biochem Behav 1986; 25:289-292.
92. Vetulani J, Marona-Lewicka D, Michaluk J et al. Stability and variability of locomotor responses of laboratory rodents. III. Effect of environmental factors and lack of catecholamine receptor correlates. Pol J Pharmacol Pharm 1988; 40:273-280.
93. Hunter WJ, Lingk W, Recht P. Intercomparison study of the determination of single administration toxicity in rats. J Ass Off Anal Chem 1979; 62:864-873.
94. Zbinden G, Flury-Roversi M. Significance of the LD50-test for the toxicological evaluation of chemical substances. Arch Toxicol 1981; 47:77-99.
95. Casida JE, Gammon DW, Glickman AH et al. Mechanism of selective action of pyrethroid insecticides. Ann Rev Pharmacol Toxicol 1985; 24:413-438.
96. Narahashi T. Neuronal target sites of insecticides. In: Hollingworth RM, Green MB, eds. Sites of Action for Neurotoxic Pesticides, American Chemical Society Symposium Series No. 356, Washington, DC. 1987:226-250.
97. Mitchell JA, Wilson MC, Kallman MJ. Behavioral effects of Pydrin and Ambush in male mice. Neurotoxicol Teratol1988; 10:113-119.
98. Vetulani J, D'Udine B, Sansone M. A toggle-floor box: The reliability of

crossings in the evaluation of drug-induced locomotor changes in mice. Pol J Pharmacol Pharm 1988; 40:33-36

99. Crofton KM, Reiter LW. Effects of two pyrethroids on motor activity and the acoustic startle response in the rat. Toxicol Appl Pharmacol 1984; 75:318-328, 1984.
100. Crofton KM, Somerholter L, Gilbert ME. Vehicle and route dependent effects of deltamethrin on motor function in the rat. Neurotoxicol Teratol 1995; 17:489-495.

CHAPTER 13

Multivariate Analyses of Locomotor and Investigatory Behavior in Rodents

Mark A. Geyer and Martin P. Paulus

MEASUREMENT CONSIDERATIONS

A variety of instrumentally or operationally defined measures of motor activity have been used to assess the behavioral effects of drugs or other manipulations, whether as strict measures of locomotor activity or as measures of more context-dependent constructs such as arousal, curiosity, emotionality, or exploration. In psychopharmacology, measures of activity are often used as bioassays of drug effects or to establish macroscopic characteristics for drug classes. For example, psychoactive drugs are defined as "stimulants" or "depressants" largely on the basis of their effects on gross measures of the motor activity of rodents.

Motor Behavior Versus Locomotor Behavior

It is important to recognize that what is often called spontaneous or general motor activity does not constitute a unitary class of behavior. Rather, depending upon the nature of the recording technique, many different behavioral actions contribute to the measure obtained. If suitable criteria are utilized, each of these actions could be defined as a response and measured and studied in its own right.[1] Thus, the macroscopic measure of behavior called motor activity actually consists of assemblies of microscopic responses. Hence, attempts to indis-

---

Measuring Movement and Locomotion: From Invertebrates to Humans, edited by Klaus-Peter Ossenkopp, Martin Kavaliers and Paul R. Sanberg.

criminately detect any movement of the animal and to combine all these responses into one category called motor activity constitute a gross oversimplification of the behavior of the organism. While such coarse measures of motor activity have some value as assays of drug effects, they provide little or no information about the behavior of the animal or the nature of a drug-induced change in that behavior.

Such considerations have led most investigators to rely on measures of locomotor rather than motor behavior. Locomotor activity can be operationally defined as movement from place to place and is virtually always one of the behavioral responses that provides a major contribution to any measure of general motor activity. It is, however, a somewhat more specific measure because the observational or automated monitoring of the behavior is limited to units reflective specifically of movements of the animal of some minimal distance or from one place to another. Such units are often called "crossovers" or "crossings" and require ambulation by the animal. By design, such measures are insensitive to movements related to sniffing, grooming, eating, drinking, tremor, or breathing. As the field has advanced, many investigators have begun to measure locomotor responses concurrently with other behaviors, such as rearings, object contacts, holepokes, or patterns of behavior (e.g. circling) in order to enhance their ability to characterize drug effects and to interpret their results.

ADVANTAGES OF MULTIVARIATE ASSESSMENTS

The Value of Multiple Concurrent Measures

Critical reviews of activity measures invariably emphasize the value of obtaining multiple measures of activity concurrently.[2-4] In part, such recommendations stem from the interrelatedness of different behaviors. Even behaviors that are in some sense independent, such as sleeping and grooming, are related in a measurement sense because they compete with one another for expression. To address such issues and to draw valid conclusions about the direct effects of an experimental manipulation generally requires the use of concurrent measures of different behaviors. For example, a reduction in rearing behavior could result from either motor ataxia or a selective increase in horizontal locomotion rather than a direct effect on rearing per se. Such possibilities can only be distinguished when both behaviors are measured simultaneously. In order to draw conclusions about any one aspect of activity, other contributions to the measured behavior must be excluded, controlled, or monitored. The major advantage provided by the use of multiple concurrent measures of behavior is the potential assessment of the validity of the investigator's hypothetical constructs. At the simplest level, multivariate characterizations of behavior enable one to clarify interpretations that could be disputed because of the possibility of an intervening variable.

Identification of Response Competition

It is always advisable to supplement the automatic recording of multiple aspects of locomotor and/or investigatory behavior with direct observations. Because different behavioral actions are often mutually exclusive and therefore compete with each other for expression, adequate characterizations of a drug effect can require the use of a clearly defined inventory of behavior. Such an inventory should include behaviors exclusively elicited by the drug as well as behaviors normally exhibited by the test animal in the given situation. In some instances, a valid interpretation of the data provided by the automated device will depend upon the use of observational techniques and the adequacy of the behavioral inventory. For example, with a device that selectively detects ambulatory movements, the dose-effect curve of amphetamine in rats first increases and then decreases. The decrease in locomotion at higher doses parallels the appearance of stereotyped behaviors which interfere with the manifestation of locomotor activity. Hence, it is apparent that interpretation with regard to possible underlying mechanisms requires concurrent measures of both locomotion and stereotypy. For example, animals pretreated with an inhibitor of catecholamine biosynthesis before receiving a moderate dose of amphetamine exhibit more locomotion than without the pretreatment.[5] Interpretation solely on the basis of locomotor measures would lead to the invalid conclusion that the pretreatment potentiated the mechanisms underlying amphetamine-induced locomotion. In fact, the same result (increased locomotion) would be obtained with a lower dose of amphetamine, one which did not elicit stereotypy. Hence, the more appropriate interpretation is that the synthesis inhibitor reduced the effectiveness of amphetamine.[5]

Exploration Versus Activation

More complex considerations are relevant in the use of locomotor activity measures as indicators of constructs such as arousal or exploration. The challenge has been to distinguish between activity related to an animal's internal level of arousal and activity elicited by external stimuli. Berlyne[6] has developed the most explicit theoretical description of the factors influencing exploratory behavior. He has argued that the concept of exploration is necessary to explain the observations that rats often act to increase their exposure to novelty, e.g. by spontaneous alternation, spending more time exploring unfamiliar areas of a chamber and avoiding familiar areas. Most theorists have concluded that the amount of exploratory behavior is directly related to the novelty and complexity of stimuli in the environment, and, in reciprocity with the process of habituation, inversely proportional to the organism's prior experience with those stimuli.[7-9]

Because typical activity measures are influenced by many factors, behavioral scientists have begun to use holeboards to provide specific measures of investigatory responding. A holeboard is simply a test chamber with holes into which burrowing animals such as rats frequently poke their noses. Thus, the holes serve as specific stimuli which elicit easily measured inspective responses. The complexity and/or novelty of these stimuli can be manipulated by placing various objects within the holes. Holepoke measures exhibit good test-retest reliability and appear to be valid as measures of investigation, e.g. dishabituation of the response is elicited by the addition of novel objects to specific holes.[10,11] It is important to emphasize that, just as measures of locomotion in the absence of specific measures of investigatory behavior are difficult to interpret in terms of exploratory behavior, inferences based solely on measures of holepoking or head-dipping are very questionable unless treatment effects on general levels of activity are assessed simultaneously. Only when measures of locomotion and holepokes are combined can the general arousing or sedating effects of a manipulation be discriminated from more specific effects on responsiveness to discrete exteroceptive stimuli. For example, while both amphetamine and apomorphine increase locomotor activity, amphetamine increases and apomorphine decreases the frequency of holepokes.[12,13] Such observations indicate that measures of holepoking should not be used without concurrent measures of locomotor activity.

Behavioral Profile Analyses

The crucial aspects discussed above are embedded in the suggestions made in several reviews of methodological issues relevant to the assessment of motor activity.[3,13,14] The fundamental conclusion of virtually all such reviews is that it is highly advantageous to assess multiple aspects of exploratory and locomotor activity simultaneously. The multivariate assessment of unconditioned behavior provides the investigator with the opportunity to assess the validity of hypothetical constructs, to make more confident comparisons with other results in the literature, to examine the generality and/or specificity of an observed effect, to identify the contribution of response competition, and to detect artifacts. In the context of characterizing the behavioral effects of psychoactive drugs by themselves and especially in their interactions with other drugs or experimental manipulations, the availability of multiple measures enables the development and use of behavioral profiles. For example, some groups[15] have developed locomotor activity chambers which provide a multitude of simultaneously recorded variables in order to characterize the profiles of changes induced by different drugs or other neurobiological manipulations.

Similarly, motivated by the careful analysis of behavioral sequences by Norton,[16] other groups[17] are differentiating between different categories of behavior to describe the effects of substances and lesions. Potentially, such uses of behavioral profiles can provide a considerable increase in the specificity of one's characterization of the effects of an experimental manipulation.

AN EXAMPLE: THE BEHAVIORAL PATTERN MONITOR

The Behavioral Pattern Monitor (BPM) was designed to combine the features of activity and holeboard chambers and to measure individual response frequencies and durations.[11,18,19] Each chamber consists of a large (30.5 by 60 cm) black Plexiglas box containing 3 floor and 7 wall holes equipped with infrared beams and a wall touch-plate for the detection of rearings. The chamber is criss-crossed with infrared beams which are sampled by a microcomputer using readily available software and hardware (San Diego Instruments, San Diego, CA). Each of the eight chambers is enclosed in an electrically shielded and ventilated wooden box. For daytime studies, each chamber is illuminated from above by a 7.5 Watt lamp. Wide-angle lenses permit observation of the entire chamber without disturbing the animal. Each chamber is also equipped with an external push-button to record the time of a manipulation (e.g. injection). The computer records the sequences of holepokes, rearings, and the current position of the animal determined by the status of beam breaks with a temporal resolution of 55 msec and a spatial resolution of 3.8 cm. A variety of descriptors are obtained from the raw data, including the total number of photobeam breaks, crossovers from one 15 cm square to another, or more qualitative descriptors such as entries into and time spent in the center or the corners. Because the record of all the raw data is permanent, it may be used for computer reconstructions of the pattern of movements on paper or on a video display or for the calculation of descriptive statistics reflective of treatment-induced differences in these patterns (see below). The inclusion of an attached home cage and a connecting door which may be opened remotely enables the design of free exploration experiments with the BPM system (see refs. 18, 20). Further, behind each hole is located a black cylinder into which objects or lights may be placed. Hence, the novelty and/or complexity of specific holes may be manipulated to elicit specific inspective responses or responses to novelty.[11] A variety of experiments have clearly demonstrated the utility of this system in the study of locomotor and investigatory behavior.

CHARACTERIZING THE SPECIFICITY OF DRUG ACTION

A fundamental issue in the characterization of drug effects on behavior is specificity. In the present context, an illustrative example is provided by the category of drugs labeled stimulants. In sharp contrast to the advances in precision and specificity so apparent in most areas of neurosciences and pharmacology, much of the behavioral psychopharmacology literature continues to rely on measures of behavioral activity that cannot differentiate between drugs such as amphetamine and caffeine or between apomorphine and cocaine. That is, if one collects only a single measure of locomotor activity, drugs as different as amphetamine, apomorphine, scopolamine, caffeine, 3, 4-methylenedioxy-N-methylamphetamine (MDMA or Ecstasy), and nicotine are often indistinguishable. Hence, to examine the value of the multivariate behavioral assessment provided by the BPM system, the effects of various stimulant drugs have been compared in systematic dose-response studies.[19,21-23] The goal was to determine whether the development of profiles of locomotor and investigatory behaviors would enable distinctions to be made which are not possible with standard measures of the amount of activity.

In the studies summarized here and elsewhere,[24] naive male rats were tested only once during their initial exposure to the BPM chambers. Each experiment involving a stimulant drug included 4 or 5 groups of 8-12 animals each. Test sessions were conducted during the dark phase of the animals' light/dark cycle and lasted 60 min. Subcutaneous injections of saline or one of several doses of the test drug were given 10 min prior to the introduction of the animal to the chamber. The following doses (in mg/kg) of each drug were tested: Amphetamine, 0.25, 0.5, 1.0, and 2.0; scopolamine, 0.125, 0.25, 0.5, and 2.0; caffeine, 2.5, 5.0, 10.0, 15.0, and 20.0; apomorphine, 0.1, 0.5, 1.0, and 2.0; nicotine, 0.0625, 0.125, 0.25, and 0.5; MDMA, 1.25, 2.5, 5.0, and 10.0; and lisuride, 0.005, 0.015, 0.03, and 0.06. These experiments are detailed in the original reports of these studies.[21,23,25] For each experiment, repeated-measures and mixed-design analyses of variance were performed for selected variables. Dunnett's tests were used to compare each treatment group with the control group. All statistical comparisons reported here were derived from comparisons of the particular dose group with the corresponding control group, although some figures depict only the results from the most typical control group.

All the above-listed drugs elicited dose-related increases in either total photobeam breaks or crossovers, which are defined as movements from one 15 cm square to another. The effects of a representative dose of each drug on crossovers during the first and second halves of the hour-long test session are shown in Figure 13.1. Clearly, all of the drugs can be classified as stimulants on the basis of their shared ability to increase such measures of locomotor activity. Even the simplest of multivariate assessments, however, began to differentiate these drugs from one another. Many drugs have differential effects on entries into central areas that are unrelated to differences in overall levels of activity. Scopolamine, apomorphine, and MDMA shared a common effect in that animals tended not to enter the center of the chamber, as shown in Figure 13.2. These three drugs produce characteristic patterns of hyperactivity in which the animals rarely move away from the walls. On the other hand, the increase in center entries produced by caffeine is in direct proportion to the effects of the drug on total movements. Such observations demonstrate that the separate measurement of central versus peripheral movements is of considerable value both in the detection of the behavioral effects of drugs and in the differentiation of the effects of drugs that would otherwise seem similar. The dopamine agonist lisuride, which is a structural relative of LSD and has important effects on serotonergic systems,[25] also increased entries into the center to about the same extent that it increased crossovers. Thus, its effects contrast with those of LSD, which markedly and preferentially decreases center entries.[26] In contrast, amphetamine was the only drug that produced a preferential increase in center entries.

The BPM also provides explicit measures of exploratory or investigatory behavior, namely holepokes and rearings. In all cases, each drug had similar effects on both these behaviors. That these two responses reflect a common underlying dimension of behavior is further supported by factor analyses of large numbers of control animals.[27] The effects of the representative doses of the drugs on holepokes are summarized in Figure 13.3. Scopolamine markedly increased both holepokes and rearings, while apomorphine virtually abolished and MDMA reduced both behaviors. Lisuride also significantly decreased both holepokes

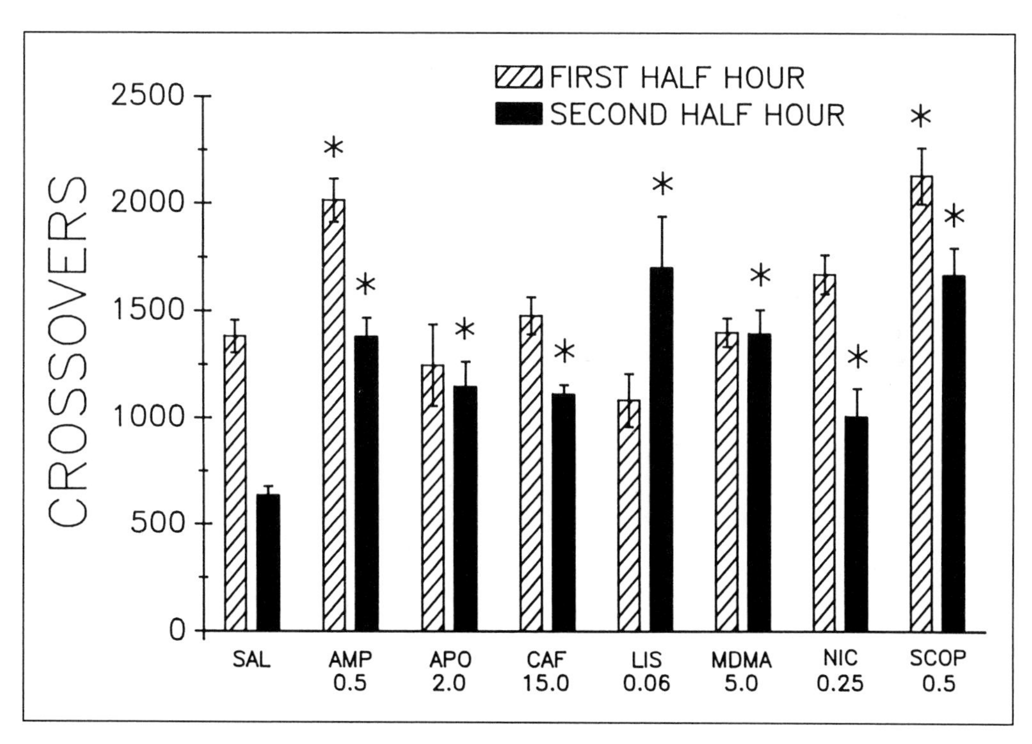

Fig. 13.1. Effects of stimulants on crossovers. The effects of the selected doses of the various stimulant drugs on crossovers are shown as group (N = 10-12) means ± SEM for successive halves of the hour-long test sessions. At these doses (shown in mg/kg), each drug significantly increased locomotor activity during the last half of the test session. The control values shown are the median values from the separate control groups used for each stimulant study. Statistical comparisons were based on each particular control group. APO = apomorphine; AMP = d*-amphetamine; CAF = caffeine; LIS = lisuride; MDMA = methylenedioxymethamphetamine; NIC = nicotine; SCOP = scopolamine; * = significantly different from corresponding control, $p < 0.05$*

and rearings, despite increasing crossovers and center entries. Although caffeine and nicotine produced similar increases in crossovers and at least tended to increase center entries, caffeine increased and nicotine decreased both holepokes and rearings. Thus, although at the doses selected for comparison all these drugs produce roughly comparable increases in the *amount* of locomotor activity, they are readily discriminated by using a rather simple form of multivariate or profile analysis. Just as these drugs may be differentiated biochemically on the basis of binding or other neurochemical effects or pharmacologically by virtue of their differential sensitivities to receptor antagonists or synthesis inhibitors, so may they be differentiated at a behavioral level using only a single test paradigm.

UTILITY OF ANALYSES OF SPATIAL AND TEMPORAL PATTERNS OF ACTIVITY

Patterns of Locomotor Activity

A relatively new and sensitive approach to the study of drug effects on locomotor and exploratory behavior is based on the examina-

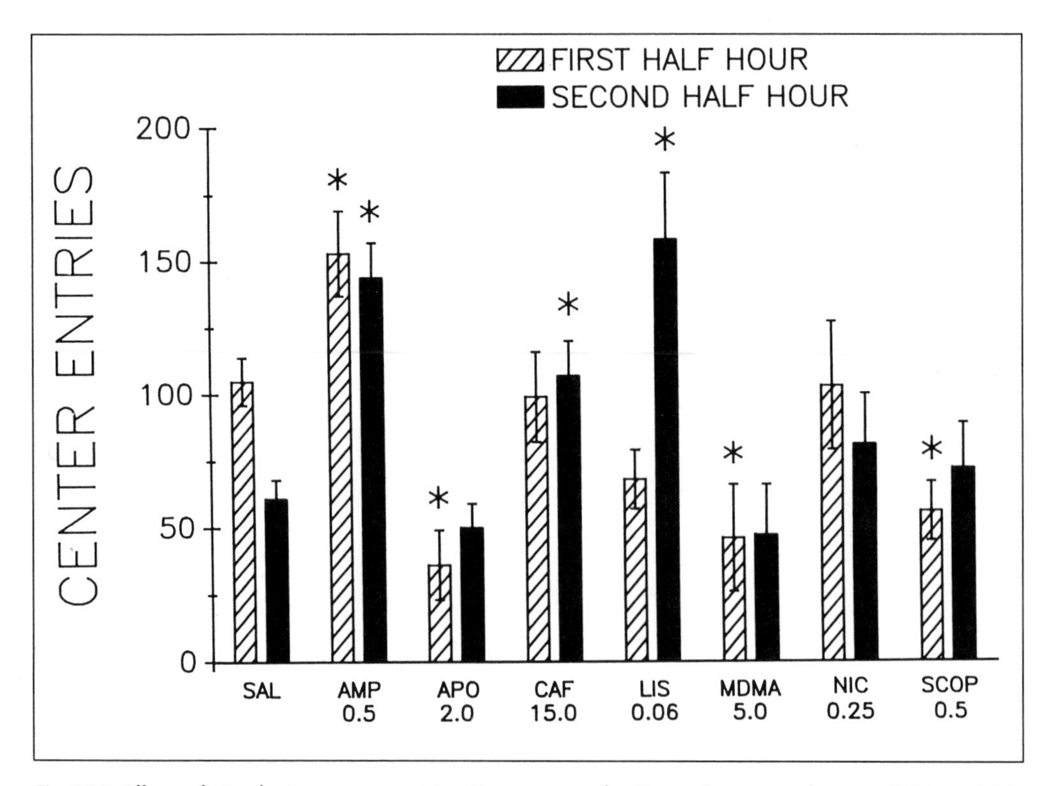

*Fig. 13.2. Effects of stimulants on center entries. Group means for Center Entries are shown as in Figure 13.1. The center region is illustrated in Figure 13.6. * = significantly different from corresponding control, $p < 0.05$.*

tion of the patterns of locomotion as the animal explores the chamber by plotting the sequence of movements. Lat[14] first noted that relatively high doses of amphetamine (e.g. 5.0 mg/kg) often induce perseverative spatial patterns of locomotion. Subsequently, Schiorring[28] used tracings of locomotor movements to demonstrate the repetitive or stereotyped nature of the spatial patterns of locomotion exhibited by rats treated with high doses of amphetamine and tested in a large open field. As indicated above, the BPM system permanently stores all the movement patterns of the animal together with the duration of each investigatory response or pause in a particular x-y position. One of the most instructive uses of these data, with regard to gaining an understanding of the structured manner in which a rat explores its environment, has been the generation of reconstructed visual images of the sequences of holepokes, rearings, and locomotor movements on the computer terminal. The flexibility with which one can speed up or slow down this display and the degree to which the displayed information is abstracted greatly facilitate the appreciation of treatment-induced differences in the animals' behavior. The ability to replay an hour of movements in less than a minute helps one to recognize and remember perseverative patterns.

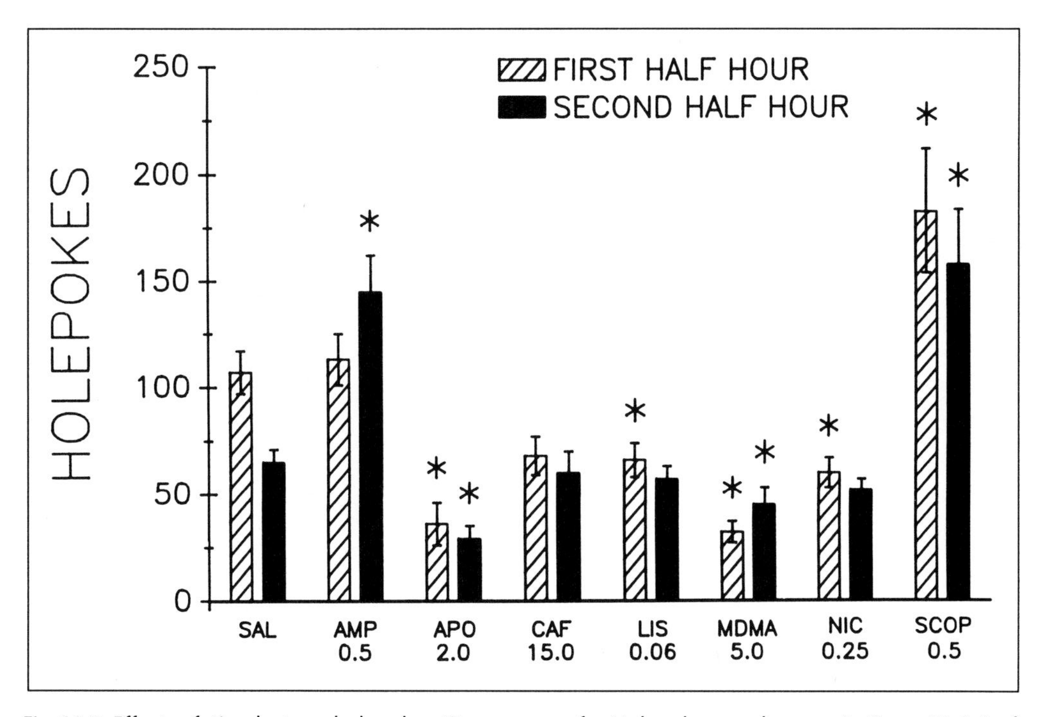

*Fig. 13.3. Effects of stimulants on holepokes. Group means for Holepokes are shown as in Figure 13.1. Each chamber contains three floor and seven wall holes. * = significantly different from corresponding control, $p < 0.05$.*

Analyses of spatial patterns of locomotion reveal remarkably consistent structures in the behavior of untreated rats. As expected, there are general tendencies, which are consistent for virtually all untreated animals, to avoid the center region and to stay near a corner of the chamber. The structure of the movement patterns themselves was most easily identified by observation of the video displays of the movements when animals were tested in a free exploration paradigm in which the animal could move freely between a home cage and the larger BPM chamber. Most animals remain for extended periods in the home cage and make excursions to various parts of the larger chamber and back following progressively more fixed routes over time. Typically, the outward part of an excursion is more frequently interrupted by investigatory holepoking and rearing than is the return part of the excursion. When tested in the more typical forced exploration situation, the behavior is similar except that each animal selects a particular corner as its home area. In some environments and after some drug treatments, multiple home bases may be identifiable.[29] Each rat, however, clearly develops its own particular spatial pattern of movements, which is predictable across time within a session and between sessions.

Drug Effects on Spatial Patterns of Locomotion

The consistency in the locomotor patterns of untreated rats has led to the study of drug-induced changes in these patterns per se. For example, the stimulant drugs discussed above in the context of multivariate assessments have also been examined in terms of their influences on spatial patterns of locomotion.[21,23] Even at doses producing comparable increases in the *amount* of locomotor activity, some stimulant drugs are readily distinguishable from others by virtue of qualitative aspects of the animals' locomotor patterns. Some drugs, such as low doses of amphetamine, disrupt the normal structure by producing highly varied patterns of directional changes, as illustrated for an individual animal in Figure 13.4. Other stimulant drugs essentially replace the normal patterns of locomotion with new, even more highly structured patterns. For example, both apomorphine and scopolamine induce movement patterns which are highly predictable and somewhat characteristic of each drug. Most animals treated with apomorphine run around the perimeter of the chamber consistently in one direction for most of the session, as shown in Figure 13.5. Although scopolamine-treated animals also rotate around the perimeter of the chamber, they frequently change directions and pause en route to investigate the holes and rear against the wall, responses only rarely seen with apomorphine-treated rats.[19]

Intermediate combinations have also been noted. For example, doses of 5 or 10 mg/kg of the serotonin-releasing compound MDMA cause animals to rotate around the chamber, changing directions occasionally as with scopolamine, but without holepoking or rearing as with apomorphine. It also appears that stimulants such as caffeine and nicotine

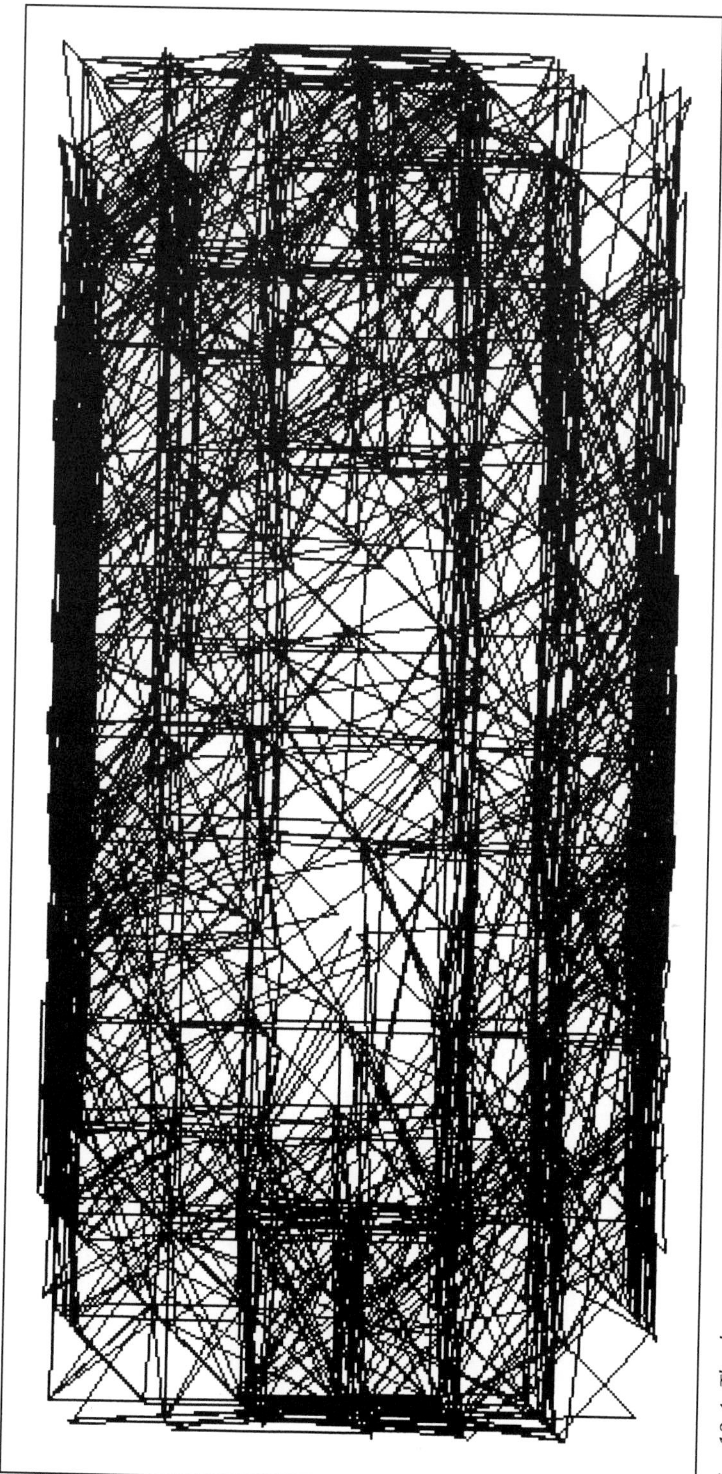

Fig. 13.4. *The locomotor pattern induced by amphetamine. Shown here are the movement patterns exhibited by a representative animal given* amphetamine and tested for one hour in the Behavioral Pattern Monitor. To avoid exact retracings of the same lines, ±40% variability has been added to successive x-y positions.

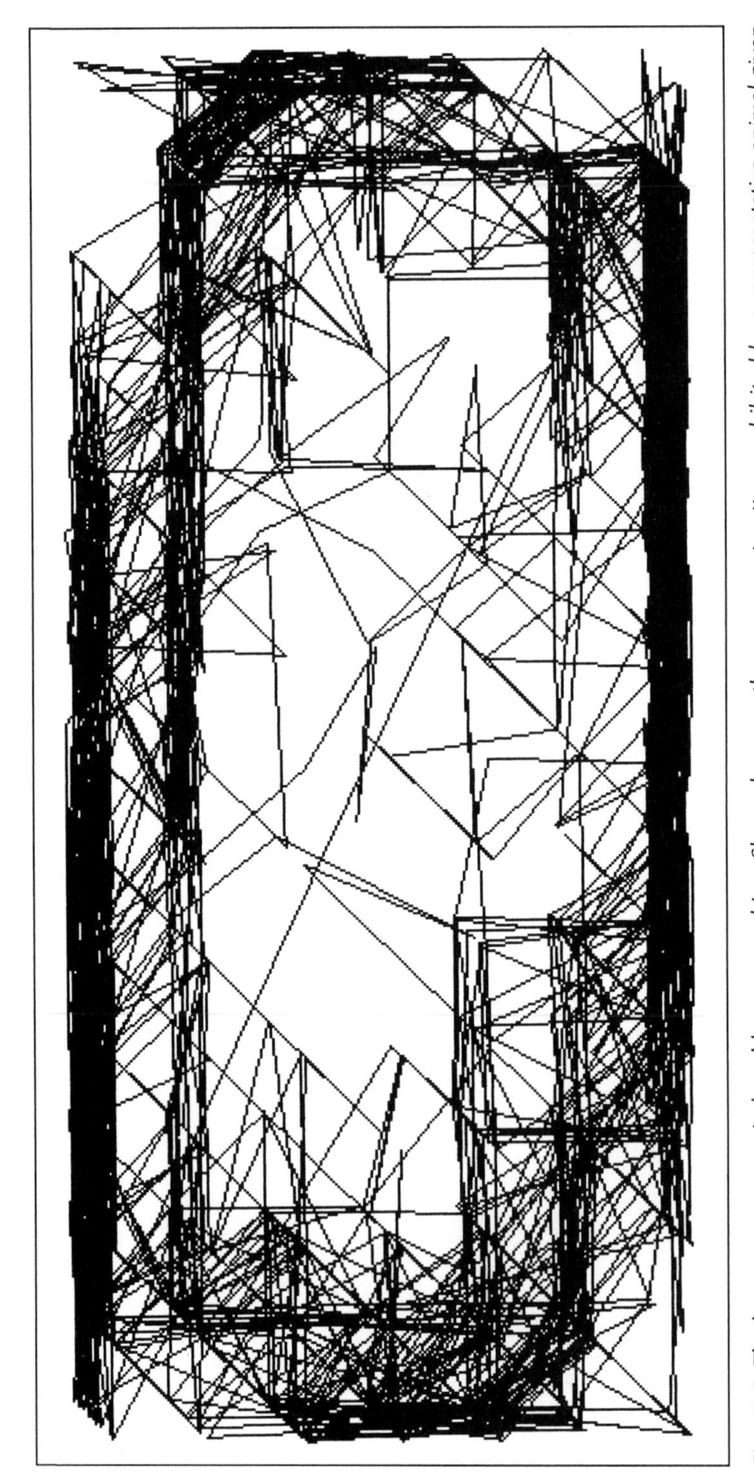

Fig. 13.5. The locomotor pattern induced by apomorphine. Shown here are the movement patterns exhibited by a representative animal given apomorphine and tested for one hour in the Behavioral Pattern Monitor. To avoid exact retracings of the same lines, ±40% variability has been added to successive x-y positions.

do not disrupt the normal structure of the animals' spatial patterns of locomotion. With these drug treatments, it is evident that each animal adopts a preference for a particular home area and establishes preferred excursion routes which are no less predictable than are those of controls. That is, the structure of their locomotor patterns is largely similar to those exhibited by untreated or saline control animals. These drugs increase activity primarily by reducing the duration of each visit in the home corner. Accordingly, the strongest differences between caffeine or nicotine versus saline controls occur after 20-30 minutes, when the control animals begin to pause for longer periods of time in their self-selected home corner.

Measures of Perseverative Patterns of Locomotion

Despite the recent advent of automated devices which can record such patterns, the statistical description and analysis of the resulting data have posed a difficult problem. Statistical assessments of behavioral sequences have been explored most extensively by ethologists, some approaches having been relevant to the characterization of locomotor movement patterns.[30-32] We have had some success with a measure called the Spatial CV.[19,21] In our first attempts to use this metric to statistically describe and evaluate the sequences of position changes, the data were reduced into transitions between any of five arbitrarily defined areas: the two ends; the center; and the two long walls (see Fig. 13.6). Subsequent applications of this approach have involved the calculations of transitions between any of nine areas.[21,23] In either case, transitions between the five or nine areas can be displayed in an appropriate matrix with 16 or 40 permissible cells (see Fig. 13.6). Relative transition frequencies are then calculated as percent of total, and the Spatial Coefficient of Variation (CV) is derived from this set of numbers. To the extent that an animal preferentially repeated certain transitions, the Spatial CV increases. A more uniform or random distribution of these spatial transitions produces a low Spatial CV.

Figure 13.7 illustrates the differential effects of the various stimulant drugs on the CV5 statistic. As expected from the observations of different patterns described above, the effects of the drugs on the CV5 were independent of their effects on the amount of activity. The drugs that were noted by observation to produce perseverative or stereotyped patterns of locomotor hyperactivity—scopolamine, MDMA, and especially apomorphine—all significantly increased the CV5. Conversely, amphetamine, which increased the frequency of directional changes and produced an unpredictable pattern of locomotion at the doses tested, significantly decreased the CV5. Nicotine and caffeine had minimal effects on this measure of the degree of structure or predictability in the spatial pattern of locomotion. Although lisuride was observed to produce repetitive rotational movements, these predictable patterns were limited to the early part of the test session and tended to form oval patterns centered on the diagonal of the chamber.[25] Hence, because this particular pattern did not conform to the arbitrary Cartesian coordinate system used in the calculation of the CV5, the statistical measure was inconsistent with the observed behavior. Such an example reflects the need to constantly compare the results of abstracted descriptive statistics with the object being measured, in this case, locomotor patterns. Discussed elsewhere[33] are some newer measures that do not suf-

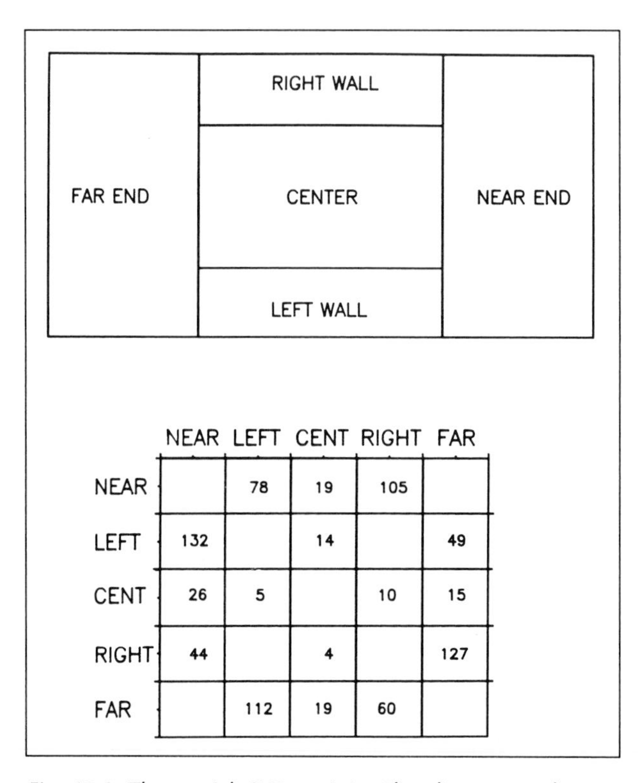

	NEAR	LEFT	CENT	RIGHT	FAR
NEAR		78	19	105	
LEFT	132		14		49
CENT	26	5		10	15
RIGHT	44		4		127
FAR		112	19	60	

Fig. 13.6. The spatial CV5 statistic. The diagram at the top represents the five regions into which the chamber is divided by the analysis program for the assessment of the CV5 and for the definition of center entries. To calculate the CV5, transitions of the rat from one region to another are cumulated as illustrated in the matrix. This particular matrix comes from an animal treated with scopolamine, which makes animals run around the periphery of the chamber in both directions. Hence, the numbers in this matrix include several large numbers and many small numbers because this animal tended to exhibit the same movement pattern consistently. Accordingly, the standard deviation or coefficient of variation–CV5–of this set of numbers is relatively high, i.e. 0.890. An animal that distributed its movements more randomly or uniformly throughout the chamber would produce a matrix filled with more similar numbers and therefore a low CV5. Thus, the CV5 statistic increases to the extent that an animal repeats certain spatial movement patterns to the exclusion of others.

fer from the weakness inherent in any arbitrary definitions of responses, such as those used to derive the CV5 measure, and therefore more accurately describe the behavioral changes induced by lisuride. Despite such occasional limitations of the Spatial CV measures, the results depicted in Figure 13.7 reveal that they provide additional information that is not evident in any other measure and that is independent of drug-induced changes in the amount of activity.

The distribution of the transitions between the five or nine areas can also be used to assess the degree to which an individual animal exhibits the same spatial pattern of movement from one part of a session to another or from one day to another. To assess the degree of consistency, Pearson's correlation coefficients can be calculated on the 16 or 40 pairs of values from the transition matrices. For example, because animals typically follow the same paths in both the first and second halves of a given test session, highly significant correlations are obtained routinely between the corresponding sets of transition frequencies.[21] Furthermore, some drug treatments significantly disrupt these correlations.[18,26] Such novel measures allow one to address questions that might otherwise be intractable to study. For example, consider the conditioned hyperactivity engendered by repeatedly testing rats in a distinctive environment after injections of amphetamine.[34] As typical of classical conditioning paradigms, the conditioned behavior is evidenced

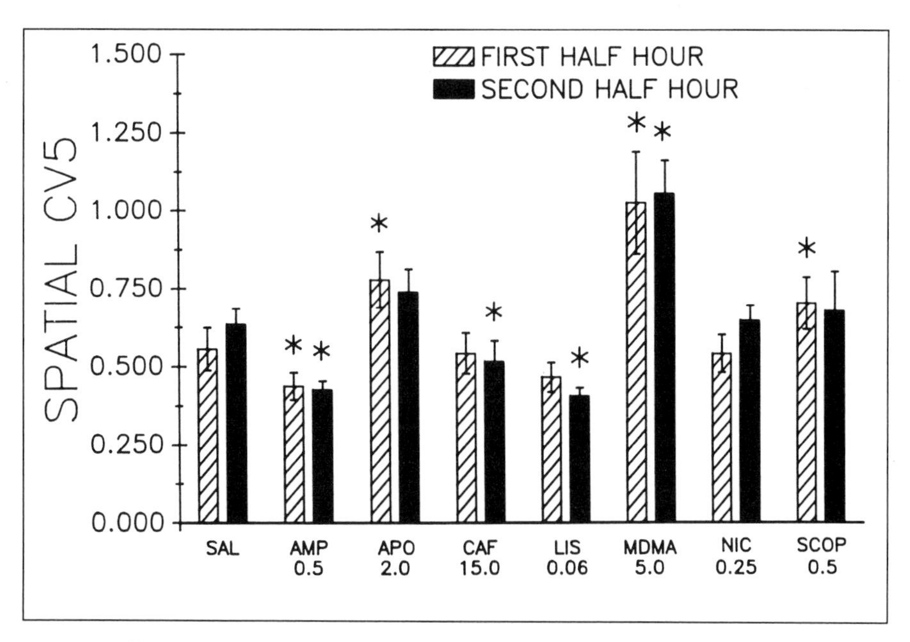

*Fig. 13.7. Effects of stimulants on the spatial CV5. Group means for CV5, or the Coefficient of Variation, are shown as in Figure 13.1. The Spatial CV5 is defined in Figure 13.6. An increase in the Spatial CV5 reflects a more repetitive pattern of movements. * = significantly different from corresponding control, $p < 0.05$.*

by increased activity in a nondrug (i.e. nonUCS) test session relative to rats that have received unpaired presentations of the drug and the test environment (i.e. the CS). Does this increased activity reflect a conditioned response or might it be due to the effects of dishabituation produced by exposing the rat to the test environment in the nondrug state instead of the previous drug state? In the former case, the pattern of each animal's activity (i.e. the topography of the CR) should be similar to the activity exhibited by that animal under drug. In the latter case, the pattern of activity should be more like the activity exhibited by the animal when first introduced to the chamber before conditioning. When the correlations between each animal's patterns of movements, as described by the transition matrices, were calculated, the patterns were more similar to the behavior under drug than to the behavior elicited by the novel environment.[35] Hence, one could conclude that the increased activity on the test day represented a conditioned response rather than a dishabituation response. It should be noted that measures of the amount rather than the pattern of activity could not have supported such a conclusion.

While descriptive statistics such as the Spatial CV have proven useful, much more work in this area is warranted. The combination of multivariate assessments and pattern analyses provided by systems such as the BPM promises to enhance the study of drug effects on locomotor activity in much the same way as the switch from whole-brain to regional analyses of brain chemistry revolutionized our understanding of drug effects on neurotransmitters. The advent of new technologies such as video tracking systems and the associated computer-based pattern analyses should have considerable impact in this area. Further, the application of methods used for the analysis of nonlinear dynamical systems is certain to supply a variety of additional measures which have enormous potential to quantify and characterize the effects of drugs on such a complex, dynamic, and metastable behavioral system as unconditioned motor activity (see refs. 21,33).

Acknowledgments

This work was supported by a grant from the National Institute on Drug Abuse (NIDA) (RO1-DA02925). M.A. Geyer was supported by a Research Scientist Award from the National Institute of Mental Health (KO5-MH01223). Much of work summarized here was reviewed similarly in a NIDA Technical Review (Geyer and Paulus, 1992).

References

1. Skinner BF. The measurement of spontaneous activity. J Gen Psychol 1933;9:3-24.
2. Geyer MA. Approaches to the characterization of drug effects on locomotor activity in rodents. In: Adler MW, Cowan A, eds. Testing and Evaluation of Drugs of Abuse. New York: Wiley-Liss, Inc, 1990: 81-99.

3. Reiter LW, MacPhail RC. Motor activity: A survey of methods with potential use in toxicity testing. In: Geller I, Stebbins WC, Wayner MJ, eds. Test Methods for Definition of Effects of Toxic Substances on Behavior and Neuromotor Function. Vol 1. Suppl 1. New York: Ankho International Inc, 1979: 53-66.
4. Robbins TW. A critique of methods available for the measurement of spontaneous motor activity. In: Iversen LL, Iversen SD, eds. Handbook of Psychopharmacology Vol 7, 1979: 37-82.
5. Segal DS. Behavioral and neurochemical correlates of repeated d-amphetamine administration. In: Mandell AJ, ed. Advances in Biochemical Psychopharmacology. New York: Raven Press, 1975: 247-261.
6. Berlyne DE. Curiosity and exploration. Science 1966; 153:25-33.
7. Kumar R. Psychoactive drugs, exploratory behaviour and fear. Nature London 1968; 218:665-667.
8. McReynolds P. Exploratory behavior: A theoretical interpretation. Psychol Reports 1962; 11:311-318.
9. Montgomery KC. The relation between fear induced by novel stimulation and exploratory behavior. J Comp Physiol Psychol 1955; 48:254-260.
10. File SE, Wardill AG. Validity of head-dipping as a measure of exploration in a modified holeboard. Psychopharmacologia 1975; 44:53-50.
11. Flicker C, Geyer MA. Behavior during hippocampal microinfusions: I. Norepinephrine and diversive exploration. Brain Res Rev 1982; 4:79-103.
12. Geyer MA, Light RK, Rose GJ, Peterson LR, Horwitt DD, Adams LH, Hawkins RL. A characteristic effect of hallucinogens on investigatory responding in rats. Psychopharmacol 1979; 65:35-40.
13. Ljungberg T, Ungerstedt U. Automatic registration of behavior related to dopamine and noradrenaline transmission. Eur J Pharmacol 1976; 36:181-188.
14. Lat J. The spontaneous exploratory reactions as a tool for psychopharmacological studies. A contribution towards a theory of contradictory results in psychopharmacology. In: Mikhelson MY, Longo VG, Votava Z, eds. Pharmacology of Conditioning, Learning and Retention. Oxford: Pergamon Press, 1965: 47-66.
15. Sanberg PR, Zoloty SA, Willis R et al. Digiscan activity: Automated measurement of thigmotactic and stereotypic behavior in Rats. Pharmacol Biochem Behav 1987; 27:569-572.
16. Norton S. On the discontinuous nature of behavior. J Theoret Biol 1968; 21:229-243.
17. Teitelbaum P, Szechtman H, Sirkin DW et al. Dimensions of movement, movement subsystems and local reflexes in the dopaminergic system underlying exploratory locomotion. In: Spiegelstein MY, Levy A, eds. Behavioral Models and the Analysis of Drug Action. Proceedings of the 27th OHOLO Conference, Amsterdam: Elsevier Scientific Publishing Company, 1982: 357-385.

18. Adams LH, Geyer MA. LSD-induced alterations of locomotor patterns and exploration in rats. Psychopharmacol 1982; 77:179-185.
19. Geyer MA. Variational and probabilistic aspects of exploratory behavior in space: Four stimulant styles. Psychopharm Bull 1982; 18:48-51.
20. Welker WI. Free versus forced exploration of a novel situation by rats. Psychol Rep 1957; 3:95-108.
21. Geyer MA, Russo PV, Masten VL. Multivariate assessment of locomotor behavior: Pharmacological and behavioral analyses. Pharmacol Biochem Behav 1986; 25:277-288.
22. Geyer MA, Russo PV, Segal DS, Kuczenski R. Effects of apomorphine and amphetamine on patterns of locomotor and investigatory behavior in rats. Pharmacol Biochem Behav 1987; 28:393-399.
23. Gold LH, Koob GF, Geyer MA. Stimulant and hallucinogenic behavioral profiles of 3,4-methylenedioxymethamphetamine (MDMA) and N-ethyl-3,4-methylenedioxyamphetamine (MDE) in rats. J Pharmacol Exp Ther 1988; 247:547-555.
24. Geyer MA, Paulus, MP. Multivariate and nonlinear approaches to characterizing drug effects on the locomotor and investigatory behavior of rats. Neurobiological Approaches to Brain-Behavior Interaction, NIDA Research Monograph Series 1992; 124:203-235.
25. Adams LH, Geyer MA. Patterns of exploration in rats distinguished lisuride from lysergic acid diethylamide. Pharmacol Biochem & Behav 1985; 23:461-468.
26. Adams LH, Geyer MA. A proposed animal model for hallucinogens based on LSD's effects on patterns of exploration in rats. Behav Neurosci 1985; 5:881-900.
27. Paulus MP, Geyer MA. Three independent factors characterize spontaneous rat motor activity. Behav Brain Res 1993; 53:11-20.
28. Schiorring E. An open field study of stereotyped locomotor activity in amphetamine treated rats. Psychopharmacol 1979; 66:281-287.
29. Eilam D, Golani I, Szechtman H. D2-agonist quinpirole induces perseveration of routes and hyperactivity but no perseveration of movements. Brain Res 1989; 26:255-267.
30. Bekoff M. Quantitative studies of three areas of classical ethology: Social dominance, behavioral taxonomy, and behaviorial variability. In: Hazlett BA, ed. Quantitative Methods in the Study of Animal Behavior. New York: Academic Press, 1977: 1-47.
31. Berg CJ. Development and evolution of behavior in mollusks, with emphasis on changes in stereotypy. In: Burghardt GM, Bekoff M, eds. The Development of Behavior: Comparative and Evolutionary Aspects. New York: Garland, 1978: 3-17.
32. Elsner J, Looser R, Zbinden G. Quantitative analysis of rat behavior patterns in a residential maze. In: Geller I, Stebbins WC, Wayner MJ, eds. Test Methods for Definition of Effects of Toxic Substances on Behavior and Neuromotor Function, Vol 1, Suppl 1. New York: Ankho International Inc, 1979: 163-174.

33. Paulus MP, Geyer MA. Assessing the organization of motor behavior: New approaches based on the behavior of complex physical systems. (this volume).
34. Tilson HA, Rech RC. Conditioned drug effects and absence of tolerance to d-amphetamine-induced motor activity. Pharmacol Biochem Behav 1973; 1:149-153.
35. Gold LH, Koob GF, Geyer MA. Spatial pattern analysis reveals similarities between amphetamine conditioned and unconditioned locomotion. Behav Pharmacol 1990; 1:209-220.

CHAPTER 14

Assessing the Organization of Motor Behavior: New Approaches Based on the Behavior of Complex Physical Systems

Martin P. Paulus and Mark A. Geyer

The present chapter describes our initial attempts to develop a comprehensive and quantitative framework for the experimental analysis of unconditioned motor behavior in analogy to the treatment of complex systems in physics and nonlinear dynamics. This framework connects microscopically measured behavioral elements with macroscopically defined behavioral patterns. Simple and extended scaling measures extract information about the average spatial, temporal, or sequential organization of movements as well as the fluctuation between spatially, temporally, or sequentially distinct subsets of behavioral patterns. The statistical evaluation of drug-induced differences in behavioral organization enables a detailed and neurobiologically meaningful analysis of the neurotransmitter-specific modulation of behavior.

Unconditioned motor activity paradigms elicit a wide range of behaviors from the behavioral repertoire of the animal. Although these paradigms typically are used only to measure the amount of activity as a reflection of the overall level of arousal,[1,2] the actual behavior of the animal in such situations reflects a complex and organized sequence of events. Traditional univariate or multivariate analyses of unconditioned motor behavior are based on the assumption that this behavior consists

Measuring Movement and Locomotion: From Invertebrates to Humans, edited by Klaus-Peter Ossenkopp, Martin Kavaliers and Paul R. Sanberg.

of clearly distinguishable and discrete behavioral elements[3] and therefore only quantify the frequencies and durations of these elements or categories of behavior.[4] These approaches fail to describe the sequential aspects of the organization of the behavior exhibited by an animal exploring an environment. Indeed, throughout the literature on behavioral analysis, the study of patterns of behavior is still in its infancy. Until very recently, there have been no detailed quantitative methods that relate the observation of individual motor acts or microscopic behavioral events to sequences of motor acts or macroscopic patterns of behavior. The approach described below reflects an attempt to apply the new tools of theoretical physics and statistical mechanics to the study of patterns and sequences of behavior.

TRADITIONAL APPROACHES USING DISCRETE RESPONSE CATEGORIES

The approach outlined in this chapter attempts to solve several fundamental problems associated with traditional approaches to the analysis of behavior in unconditioned motor activity paradigms. First, in traditional analyses, the only response categories assessed are those defined by the experimenter based on arbitrary definitions. For instance, amphetamine and related psychomotor stimulants are known to disrupt normal behavioral responses, fragment behavioral sequences, and introduce new elements into the normal repertoire.[5-8] Hence, drug-specific categorical rating scales (e.g. amphetamine stereotypy) have evolved, reflecting the fact that the arbitrary definitions of responses appropriate for normal behavior are inappropriate for drug-induced behavior. The situation is complicated even further by the fact that rating scales designed for one drug (e.g. amphetamine) are often inappropriate for another drug (e.g. MDMA)[9] or even for the original drug in combination with a putative antagonist. This fundamental problem constrains the ability of traditional measures to support inferences about the relationship of drug effects to the normal behavioral repertoire of the animal.

Second, the traditional approaches are insufficient in quantifying the sequential arrangement of behavioral elements. While several investigators have acknowledged that behavior consists of elements that are arranged purposefully in sequence,[3-10] evaluation techniques based on these approaches have not evolved beyond descriptively categorizing and enumerating pre-defined behavioral sequences. While this approach has some utility, it is tantamount to simply defining a new behavioral response using more complicated criteria. Hence, it does not overcome the fundamental weakness of experimenter-defined responses.

Most of the quantitative analyses of sequences of behavior are rooted in the theory of Markov processes[11] or involve run statistics or time-series analyses. Hence, they remain based upon arbitrary definitions of discrete responses. Although these approaches have confirmed that sequences of motor acts are not independent random events but show varying degrees of interdependency, they have demonstrated only limited utility, particularly in the characterization of drug effects.

Third, in traditional approaches, the temporal and spatial resolutions used to define the measures are chosen arbitrarily. These choices are based frequently on the qualitative separation of temporal and spatial scales. As recent quantitative studies indicate,[12] however, there appear to be no distinct separations of behaviors into discrete temporal scales. Instead, "pauses" and "behavioral actions" are found on all time scales.

Fourth, the neurobiological systems governing the organization of behavior may not correspond to the a priori categories of behavioral responses defined and studied by the experimenter. For example, it is common to define some criterion distance an animal must move to score a "movement," such as the distance between photocells, or the 15 cm movements we have called "crossovers" or "crossings."[13] Although experimentally useful, such arbitrary measures bear no correspondence to any particular response of the animal and are not related specifically to any underlying neural substrate. Instead, the influences of different neural systems subserving behavioral organization are likely to be associated with adaptive rearrangements of particular behavioral elements.

Recent developments in nonlinear dynamics, the physics of complex systems, and the thermodynamic formalism for the ergotic theory of dynamical systems provide a framework for a quantitative analysis of behavioral organization[14,15] that may overcome some of these problems. The common goal of these approaches is to analyze macroscopic phenomena resulting from the interaction of many degrees of freedom[16,17] and the complicated behavior resulting from nonlinear dynamical systems with few degrees of freedom.[18-20] In general, the measures provided by these approaches quantify the relationships between individual behavioral elements and the overall behavior observed along a continuum. Thus, the state or "phase" of the animal's behavior is described quantitatively by measures which are analogous to thermodynamic potentials. Qualitative transitions between different behavioral states result in changes of the functions which are analogous to phase transitions in thermodynamics and statistical mechanics. Experimental manipulations can be conceptualized as parameter-induced changes of the measures, which are analogous to response functions describing a controlled perturbation in thermodynamic systems. Using this analogy to thermodynamics, the behavior of the organism is treated as a complex system of interacting elements, which is arguably appropriate given the many factors influencing the moment-to-moment behavior of an animal exploring its environment. This approach acknowledges that the key to the quantitative analysis of behavioral organization is the assessment of the interdependencies between behavioral elements.

QUANTITATIVE ASSESSMENT OF BEHAVIOR AND BEHAVIORAL ORGANIZATION

It has long been recognized in behavioral analysis that behavior consists of purposefully organized sequences of acts that can be observed by the motor output of the animal.[21] Accordingly, behavioral organization can be defined as the selection, ordering, and sequencing of behavioral elements in response to external or internal stimuli to form flexible, yet stable, macroscopic patterns of behavior. The present approach to the quantitative assessment of behavioral organization is based on extensive investigations of unconditioned motor activity using the Behavioral Pattern Monitor (BPM).[13] The BPM is based on a commercially available system (San Diego Instruments, San Diego, CA) and collects, with high temporal and spatial resolution, information about the locomotor movements and investigatory responses (rearings and holepokes) of rats in a 30.5 by 61 cm chamber. As discussed elsewhere, we have long used the multivariate profile of locomotor and investigatory behaviors provided by the BPM to elucidate the behavioral characteristics and neuropharmacological mechanisms of psychoactive drugs.[22-24] At the same time, new approaches have been developed that enable us to better quantify the drug-induced changes we observe in this complex behavior. Specifically, similar to ensembles in statistical mechanics of physical systems, movement sequences of a rat in the BPM having specific spatio-temporal properties provide the central building blocks for a quantitative description of behavior. Measures obtained from these ensembles, such as the dynamical entropy and the scaling exponents described below, are used to quantify the dynamical and geometrical organization of behavioral sequences.

Complexity Measures of Behavior

Entropy measures

One of the several approaches we have explored involves the quantitative analysis of the complexity of the animal's behavior. The notion of complexity is applied typically to systems that are made up of complicated or interrelated elements. Quantitatively, statistical complexity is associated with the amount of computation or computational effort required to reproduce a given output.[25] To assess quantitatively the sequential organization of rat motor behavior in the BPM, we adapted and used measures of complexity based on the ergotic theory of dynamical systems.[26] The dynamical entropy analysis of unconditioned rat motor behavior is based on the idea that the recorded behavioral sequences, i.e. the behavioral events exhibited by the rat in the BPM, reflect the evolution of a dynamical system. In particular, the behavioral events are not evaluated with respect to their rate of occurrence, as in traditional measures of the amount of activity, but with respect to the evolution of initially similar behavioral event sequences. The behavior of the rat is thought to be complex if one cannot predict subsequent event sequences in the BPM from the preceding events. The biological significance of this approach is that it measures how the sequential organization of behavioral events is affected by drugs and other manipulations of the central nervous system.

In our initial assessments,[26] the topological dynamical entropy was calculated to assess the degree of association of all possible event sequences, while the metric dynamical entropy assessed the association of the likely event sequences. We applied these measures to a comparison of 3,4-methylenedioxymethamphetamine (MDMA or Ecstasy) and *d*-amphetamine, because our extensive behavioral observations had indicated that these drugs produced hyperactive states dominated by qualitatively different spatio-temporal patterns of locomotion across a wide range of doses.[9] As predicted, the entropy measures quantified the fact that the effect of MDMA on the sequential organization of behavior was clearly different from the effect of d-amphetamine, despite the similar levels of hyperactivity produced by the two drugs. Furthermore, the behavioral effects of MDMA were characterized by striking individual differences. Some animals in the higher dose groups showed topological entropy values in the range of the saline controls, whereas other animals exhibited low topological entropy values associated with a greater decrease in the metric entropy. These results emphasized that different animals can exhibit quantitatively different behavioral states that coexist within the treatment regimen of MDMA. More generally, these findings confirmed that the entropy measures of complexity were effective in capturing the qualitative differences in drug-induced patterns of behavior that were so readily appreciated by human observers but were not reflected in traditional measures.

The extension of entropy measures

Although these entropy measures provided new insights into drug-induced changes in the behavioral repertoire of the animal, these measures provide only an assessment of the average complexity, and thus fail to quantify the fluctuations or variations of complexity of different movement sequences. The average dynamical entropy was sensitive predominantly to overall behavioral changes of the organism. Hence, we extended the evaluation of the dynamical characteristics of movements by calculating the fluctuation spectrum of local dynamical entropies, the $S(h)$ function (which is also called $S(\alpha)$ in earlier work[27]).

Specifically, we have applied the thermodynamic entropy formalism[14] to cocaine-perturbed unconditioned behavior. Previously, the $S(h)$ function has been used to describe generic non-linear systems such as hyperbolic saddle attractors and repellers.[19,28] The $S(h)$ describes the topological entropy of the animal's movement sequences and may be visualized as the number of local branching rates on successive levels of a complex tree.

The quantitative characterization of the detailed structure of this tree can capture the dynamical "fingerprint" of the animal's behavior. The main results of our studies showed that: (1) rat movements were characterized by event sequences with widely differing dynamical characteristics; (2) the dynamically different event sequences were affected differentially by cocaine treatment; and (3) the microcanonical evaluation of the *S(h)* function indicated that the behavioral sequences seem to be generated by two distinct processes having different and characteristic local dynamical entropies (h_l and h_h). These processes are analogous to different phases in the thermodynamic description and extend naturally to typical inferences regarding different "categories" of behavior. At low doses (10 or 20 mg/kg), cocaine increased the contribution of high local dynamical entropies, indicative of relatively unpredictable behavioral sequences. At the highest dose (40 mg/kg), cocaine induced large variations between rats. Based on the *S(h)* function, the animals could be differentiated into a subgroup with predominantly low entropy sequences and another subgroup in which the sequences resembled the dynamical structure of saline control animals. The application of the dynamical entropy analysis within the framework of large fluctuation statistics showed that unconditioned motor behavior consists of dynamically distinct event sequences that are affected differentially by drugs.

Temporal and geometrical characteristics of unconditioned motor behavior: α and d

The assessment of behavioral organization can be approached from both sequential and hierarchical points of view. Sequentially, behavior can be thought of as consisting of the consecutive arrangement of behavioral elements, as in the case of the complexity measures above. Accordingly, the evaluation should quantify the sequence length-independent properties of the behavioral organization. The dynamical entropy, h, was developed to quantify the sequential properties of behavioral organization. From the hierarchical point of view, behavior can be thought of as consisting of behavioral elements that are organized to form behavioral components on successively larger spatial or temporal scales. Accordingly, the evaluation should quantify the scale-invariant properties of the behavioral organization. As described below, the spatial and temporal scaling exponents, d and α, quantify the hierarchical properties of behavioral organization.

Scaling measures

To complement the entropy measures assessing the sequential organization of behavioral elements, we introduced scaling measures describing both the geometrical structure of movement patterns and the temporal durations of behavioral elements to characterize hierarchical aspects of behavioral organization. The approach is based on the scaling characteristics of a variable of interest that are obtained from the recording device without a priori definitions of categorical events.[12,29] This hierarchical approach relates measures that quantify characteristics of behavioral elements on different spatial and temporal resolutions to macroscopic behavioral patterns. In general, scaling measures are based on the concept of dimensionality in the field of fractal geometry[12,30-33] and the emergence of scaling phenomena near second-order phase transitions.[17,34] In both contexts, quantitative characteristics of the system on a smaller spatio-temporal scale can be related to its characteristics on larger scales. In general, this relationship is expressed in the following functional equation

$$[Measure]_{spatio\text{-}temporal\ scale\ A} \approx [spatio\text{-}temporal\ scale\ A]^{scaling\ exponent}[Measure]_{spatio\text{-}temporal\ scale\ B}$$

That is, the value of a measure on one spatio-temporal scale can be related via the scaling exponent to another scale. Functions that obey this relationship are said to be scaling. This property is crucial in statistical mechanical systems near phase transitions, i.e. complex systems that exhibit large fluctuations. In these systems, properties on a large spatio-temporal scale are related to the characteristics of the system on a small scale. In addition, differences in scaling behavior of these systems enable distinctions to be made of different classes of complex systems. Transferring these results to behavioral systems leads to the basic assumption that a single measure will not describe the results adequately. Rather, a function which relates the quantity of interest to its variation depending on intervening variables may provide a more complete description. In other words, insights about the system may be gained by observing a quantity of interest (like locomotor activity) on different levels of observational perspective. Moreover, these functions link the microscopic behavioral variables, e.g. smallest resolvable movements, to macroscopic behavioral patterns, e.g. exploratory behavioral strategies.

The temporal scaling exponent

Specifically, we have defined two global scaling measures from our BPM data: (1) the temporal scaling exponent, α, quantifies the power law distribution of "dwell times" or event durations, characterizing the temporal structure of the animal's behavior; (2) the spatial scaling exponent, d, quantifies the geometrical structure of consecutive movements in the BPM chamber. In most cases, responses are defined as movements without considering how long it takes to observe a response. The temporal scaling approach can be formulated by considering a measuring instrument that records the position of the animal in the box with different time resolutions.

Specifically, the temporal scaling exponent, α, is defined via:

$$[Number\ of\ events]_t \approx t^{-\alpha}\ [Number\ of\ events]_{l_{(t=1)}}$$

Basically, the number of observations within a given time resolution depends on the time and a characteristic temporal scaling exponent, alpha or α. More simply stated, the number of responses having a certain duration decays with a power law behavior. The interpretation of α may be facilitated by an example. An animal treated with a stimulant drug like amphetamine will exhibit many fast locomotor responses due to the increased amount of activity. Conversely, slow responses will be correspondingly infrequent when compared to control animals. Such an effect will result in a rapid decay of the number of events observed with increasing event durations; thus a larger temporal scaling exponent α will be obtained. A rat exhibiting less locomotor activity in the BPM when compared to controls will exhibit relatively more slow responses, thereby slowing the decay of the number of the events across increasing event durations and yielding a smaller α. Thus, the temporal scaling exponent, α, is used to describe comprehensively the ratios of fast versus slow movements of the rats based on the observation that the distribution of event durations follows a simple power law relationship. From a theoretical point of view it is interesting to note that power law relationships frequently signify long range correlations and hierarchical organization. Thus, the empirical observation of a power law distribution for dwell times may indicate a temporally complex organization involving different time scales.

The spatial scaling exponent

Similarly, the assessment of the geometrical characteristics of unconditioned motor behavior in animals is based on the path length, i.e. the Euclidean distance traveled after *n* steps. Thus, the spatial scaling exponent, *d*, is defined via

$$[Path\ length]_n \approx n^{2-d}\ [Path\ length]_{l\ (l=1)}$$

This measure describes how rough or convoluted is the spatial path taken by the rat and is based on the fact that the observed distance of a non-straight line depends upon the length of the ruler used to calculate the distance. The scaling exponent *d* is computed by fitting the slope of the line of log(L) (the measured path length) versus log(l) (the ruler length) with a least square procedure. The physical interpretation of the exponent *d* can be appreciated by considering an example of a path observed in the BPM chamber, which is schematically given in Figure 14.1. In the first case, successive observations result in locations of the rat in the box that are connected by straight lines. The function $L(l)$ results in a linear dependence on l, thus giving the simplest result, namely that the scaling exponent for a straight line is 1. In the second case, consider a path that is very irregular and covers only a moderate distance after many successive observations. In this case, the average distance measured will be smaller with a lower resolution instrument than with a high resolution instrument, resulting in

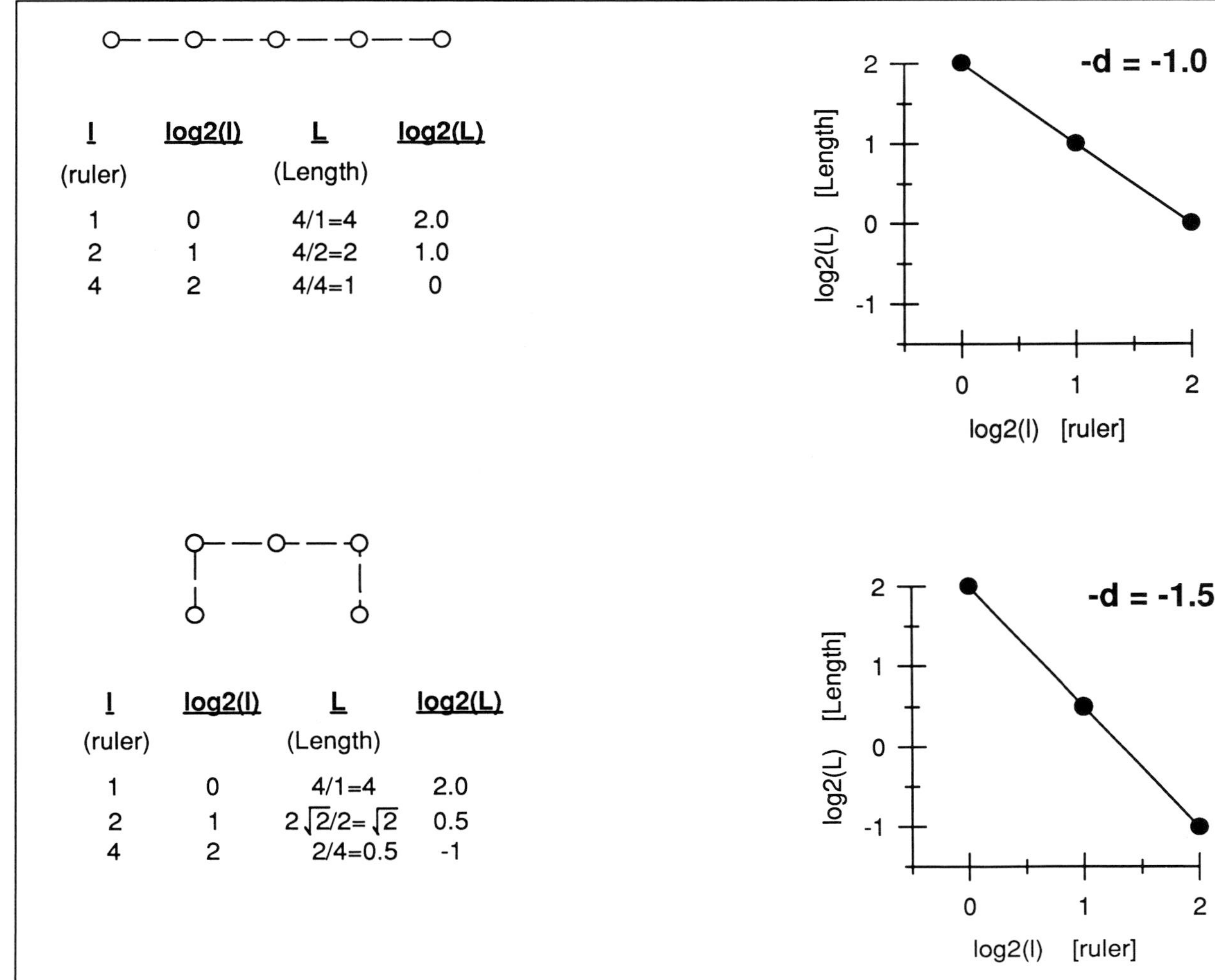

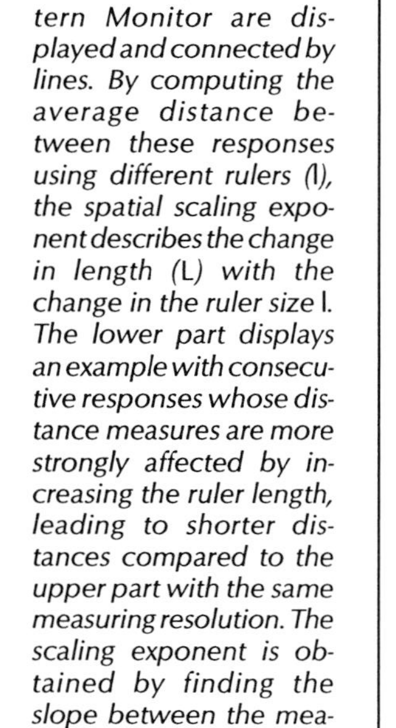

Fig. 14.1. Calculation of the spatial scaling exponent d. On the left, two different patterns of four consecutive movements within the Behavioral Pattern Monitor are displayed and connected by lines. By computing the average distance between these responses using different rulers (l), the spatial scaling exponent describes the change in length (L) with the change in the ruler size l. The lower part displays an example with consecutive responses whose distance measures are more strongly affected by increasing the ruler length, leading to shorter distances compared to the upper part with the same measuring resolution. The scaling exponent is obtained by finding the slope between the measuring resolution and the average distance computed.

a stronger decay of the average distance than with the straight path and therefore in a higher *d* exponent. The spatial scaling exponent, *d*, consequently characterizes how path lengths depend on the resolution of the instrument and allows one to quantify different qualitative geometrical features of the locomotor behavior.

The introduction of the spatial scaling exponent, *d*, was motivated by observations that stimulant drugs that produced similar changes in the amount of motor activity produced different geometrical patterns of activity.[13,35] For example, we have shown that a variety of drugs that stimulate motor activity via different neurotransmitter systems, produce different spatio-temporal patterns of locomotor behavior.[5,13,24,36] As predicted, both d and α were affected sensitively and differentially by these various stimulant drugs, providing quantitative confirmations of the previous visual observations of qualitative differences in the drug effects.[12] In addition, scaling measures helped to overcome some of the problems associated with the use and interpretation of traditional measures of locomotor activity. For example, the distance between photobeams in an activity monitor serves as an intervening variable when locomotor activity is assessed by counting the number of photobeam interruptions. Changes in this variable can lead to qualitatively and quantitatively different results for the same treatment.[12,38] The spatial scaling exponent essentially summarizes the geometrical information contained in movements observed with different resolutions that corresponds experimentally to varying the distance between photobeams.

Application of scaling exponents to distinguish drug effects

After developing the scaling measures, we assessed their utility by testing the general hypothesis that the spatial and temporal scaling exponents can capture emergent behavioral states induced by psychostimulants adequately, sensitively, and dose-dependently. The effects of drugs on these exponents were assessed by locating the different substances in a $(d - \alpha)$ plane constructed from these exponents.[12] That is, to summarize both the spatial and temporal effects of a drug on motor activity in the BPM, a plane can be constructed that consists of two axes. The first, the d axis, describes changes in the spatial composition of the movements; the second, the α axis, displays the overall level of activity. The units used for the $d - \alpha$ plane are z-scores based on the standard deviation of the control group, with the origin being the mean for the control group. The utility of the $d - \alpha$ plane is particularly evident when drugs are compared that increase motor activity but act presumably via different pharmacological mechanisms or neurotransmitter systems. Accordingly, we compared the effects of a variety of psychostimulant drugs in order to address hypotheses regarding the behavioral processes affected by these drugs.[12,36,38] The spatial scaling exponent, *d*, quantitatively differentiated behavioral effects of drugs that had been separated previously only using qualitative descriptions. Several behavioral response categories emerged from comparisons of the locations of different drugs in the d - α plane. Scopolamine, MDMA, lisuride, and high doses of apomorphine increased α while decreasing d, whereas amphetamine, nicotine, and caffeine produced an increased α with no change or an increase in d. The increases in α produced by all these drugs simply confirmed in a more sensitive and dose-related manner the fact that these drugs are called stimulants largely because they increase photocell counts in such studies.[1] Across all the drugs compared, the sensitivity of α proved to be much greater than either crossovers or total beam breaks as a measure of changes in the amount of activity. Such results indicate that α is an important indicator that enables us to distinguish even small changes in activity. More importantly, the inclusion of the geometrical characteristics of movements using d in addition to changes in α was able to separate this broad class of "stimulants" into subgroups that are known to differ in their mechanisms of action, as well as their psychological effects in humans. Thus, measures of patterns of behavior can complement traditional measures of unconditioned motor behavior and facilitate the identification and objective study of neurobiological mechanisms of drug action.

In other studies, we have used the scaling exponents to better characterize the behavioral effects of methylenedioxy-substituted phenethylamines, which are complex compounds both pharmacologically and behaviorally.[9,38,39] These drugs affect both dopamine and serotonin systems and have psychoactive effects distinct from classical hallucinogens and psychomotor stimulants.[40-44] The application of scaling and entropy measures facilitated the differentiation of the behavioral effects induced by MDMA-like drugs, which had previously been classified as "stimulants," from the behavioral effects of amphetamine-like drugs. Briefly, we discovered that the profound locomotor activation produced by MDMA and related drugs is not due primarily to dopamine release, but to serotonin release.[39-41,45,46] Specifically, MDMA-induced hyperactivity was blocked by selective serotonin uptake blockers or by the serotonin synthesis inhibitor parachlorophenylalanine, but not by the catecholamine synthesis inhibitor α-methyltyrosine. The use of scaling measures enabled us to further differentiate the effects of MDMA from those of either amphetamine-like psychostimulants or classical hallucinogens. Comparisons of the behavioral effects of MDMA across both repeated tests and repeated administrations of the drug confirmed that the spatial scaling exponent, d, was affected differently from the more traditional measures. For example, the MDMA-induced decrease in entries into the center of the BPM exhibited tolerance, in contrast to the decreases in d produced by MDMA. Hence, the effects of MDMA on the geometry of the animal's movements, as reflected by d, could be dissociated from the rotational behavior characteristically induced by MDMA. Overall, d proved to be the most sensitive of our various measures of the effects of serotonin releasers on the spatial structure of the locomotor paths exhibited by the animals. As detailed elsewhere,[39] the combination of new and old measures assessing the behavioral effects of these drugs yields more information than can be obtained by reliance on any one set of measures.

Based on structure-activity considerations, several methylenedioxy-substituted phenethylamines were tested in the BPM and evaluated using the d - α plane.[38] The results enabled us not only to discriminate the behavioral effects of these compounds from those of hallucinogens or psychostimulants, but also to relate the behavioral effects to specific biochemical characteristics of these substances. The discriminative power of the d - α plane is remarkable considering that the detection of behavioral differences between these compounds previously required much more elaborate and time-consuming procedures such as drug-discrimination tests. With this approach, behavioral effects of drugs can be characterized and quantified in a single test session using a procedure that does not require repeated administrations of the drug to the animals. Thus, the effects of chronic versus acute exposures to the drugs can now be assessed reliably.

THE EXTENSION OF THE SCALING APPROACH

Geometrically, behavioral patterns can be defined as particular combinations of event sequences observed within a collection of behavioral events. The scaling approach yielding d and α characterizes quantitatively the overall geometrical and temporal structure of behavioral events independent of the spatio-temporal resolution with which the events were measured. While this approach enabled us to distinguish pharmacological agents such as *d*-amphetamine from scopolamine even at doses that produce comparable levels of hyperactivity, it provided no information about the contributions of different geometrical movement patterns to the overall observed behavior. In analogy to and based on a similar rationale as the development of the generalized entropy function, $S(h)$, the geometrical characterization using the spatial scaling exponent, d, was extended to assess the relative contributions of event subsequences having different geometrical characteristics. The spectrum of local spatial scaling exponents, $f(d)$, quantifies the respective contributions of different local spatial scaling exponents, d_i. This function provides an assessment of behavioral events that is also independent of the measuring resolution. The differences between behavioral events are not categorized a priori, but emerge from the evaluation of the local scaling exponents.

The extended scaling assumption is based on the idea that the local scaling relationship between the variable of interest and the experimental parameter is characterized by a range of scaling exponents, d_i, rather than only an average scaling exponent, d. The term local refers to a spatially or temporally limiting condition, i.e. the geometrical characteristics are calculated for circumscribed event segments corresponding to consecutive movements of the animal, as illustrated graphically elsewhere.[12,38] Specifically, the path length of a movement segment, *i*, is characterized by the local spatial scaling exponent, d_i via:

$$[Path\ length_i]_n \approx n^{2-d_i}\ [Pathlength_i]_{l\ (l=1)}$$

The relative contributions of different local spatial scaling exponents are quantified by a scaling function ($[\#d_i]$) that describes the frequency of the local exponents as a function of the changing spatiotemporal scale. Specifically, the fluctuation spectrum of local spatial scaling exponents, *f(d)*, is defined by

$$[\#d_i]_n \approx n^{f(d_i)}[\#d_i]_{l\ (l=1)}$$

Although the scaling function is related monotonically to the occurrence frequency of movement sequences with different geometrical characteristics, the contributions of different local scaling exponents are independent of the measuring resolution (for further details see ref. 47).

This idea reflects the fact that animals display a variety of different movement sequences, presumably representing different behaviors. Here, the motor activity of rats in the BPM is conceptualized as movements that occur on different scales. These movements may involve small local movements characterized by consecutive photobeam breaks within the same region of the chamber, such as those produced during small head movements, grooming, rearing, holepoking, or focal perseverative behaviors such as biting or gnawing. Alternatively, the animal may exhibit some long, distance-covering movements that serve to bring it into contact with different parts of the chamber. Such movements appear as straight paths without interruption by local movements and often reflect the frequently observed traverses along the walls. During a test session, a normal rat will exhibit both local and distance-covering movements, as well as intermediates which represent combinations of these movements. The *f(d)* function provides information regarding the differential effects of a manipulation on geometrically defined subsets of the motor activity. In contrast to the counting of behavioral responses defined a priori by an experimenter, this approach quantifies the relative contributions of movements having different geometrical characteristics.

A detailed quantitative assessment of drug effects on the path structure is obtained from the comparisons of ($\bar{d}$) and the $\overline{f(d)}$ functions relative to the control group. The statistical significances of drug effects are expressed by conservative z-transformations, as detailed elsewhere.[47] The z-transformed curves, $f_{z,A}(d)$ are called local pattern differences and signify alterations in the contributions of specific d_is relative to controls. While these functions evaluate local differences, overall changes in the path structure are assessed by z-transformed differences in the spatial scaling exponents, d_z. Therefore, the z-transformed *d*-differences and the local pattern differences yield different information quantifying the overall and local effects on the geometrical path structure, respectively.

Differential drug effects revealed by the spectrum of local spatial scaling exponents

In a previous study, changes in the average spatial scaling exponent, *d*, indicated significant differences between the effects of cocaine and *d*-amphetamine on the hierarchical aspect of behavioral organization.[29] Thus, several studies were conducted based on the general hypothesis that indirect dopaminergic agonists such as *d*-amphetamine or cocaine produce distinctive changes in behavioral organization despite having similar effects on motor activity levels. Specifically, we investigated the effects of d-amphetamine, cocaine, GBR 12909, and nomifensine on the behavioral organization of unconditioned motor behavior. While these drugs have many similarities both in their mechanisms of action and in their effects on our multivariate behavioral profiles, they nevertheless differ in their relative potencies as dopaminergic agents and have additional effects on serotonergic and noradrenergic systems. Because we had found dramatic differences in the geometrical structure of movements for dopaminergic versus serotonergic drugs,[38,39,41] we hypothesized that the differential neurochemical effects of these substances should be detectable as distinctive changes of the geometrical characteristics of the movement sequences. The extension of the spatial scaling exponent, the fluctuation spectrum of local spatial scaling exponents, *f(d)*,[47] was used to test this hypothesis.

The detailed assessment of the geometrical path patterns (see ref. 29) induced by amphetamine, cocaine, GBR 12909, and nomifensine revealed drug-specific effects on geometrically distinct behavioral subsets. The average spatial scaling exponent, *d*, was not altered significantly compared to controls and did not differ between low doses of these drugs. Nevertheless, the contribution of local path patterns with different geometrical characteristics was affected significantly by these substances. Consequently, differences between controls and these drugs as well as between these compounds became evident with the *f(d)* analysis. The *f(d)* functions were affected differentially and dose-dependently by *d*-amphetamine, cocaine, GBR 12909, and nomifensine. Specifically, at lower doses, all four drugs reduced the fluctuation range of local path patterns such that highly local movements and/or straight movements contributed significantly less to the overall path pattern. This reduced range of the fluctuation spectrum indicated that rats treated with < 2 mg/kg *d*-amphetamine, < 20 mg/kg cocaine, < 20 mg/kg GBR 12909, or < 10 mg/kg nomifensine engaged predominantly in meandering movements with local scaling exponents between 1.3 and 1.7. The reduction of the fluctuation range of the local path patterns induced by the four stimulants was accompanied dynamically by a reduced path predictability indicated by an increase of the dynamical entropy, *h*. The tendency for *d*-amphetamine, GBR 12909, and nomifensine to increase the dynamical entropy quantified an aspect of unconditioned motor behavior that has been described in other behavioral paradigms as a "randomization of responses." Thus, the mutual generic behavioral change induced by low doses of indirect dopamine agonists is characterized by a reduced variety of path patterns combined with an increased variability in the sequential association of movement sequences. At higher doses, both GBR 12909 and nomifensine shifted the overall geometrical characteristics of the paths towards local or circumscribed movement sequences. In contrast, while *d*-amphetamine up to 4 mg/kg did not change the overall geometrical characteristics of the paths, 40 mg/kg cocaine strongly decreased the average scaling exponent, *d*. That is, cocaine-treated rats exhibited straight or directed movements, as illustrated in Figure 14.2. The reduced contribution of low local d_i values ($d_i < 1.4$) associated with low doses of *d*-amphetamine and cocaine was attenuated or reversed at higher doses. As with cocaine, animals treated with 4 mg/kg *d*-amphetamine also engaged more frequently in straight or directed movements. Overall, using the *f(d)* function, the behavioral effects on motor activity of GBR 12909 and nomifensine were distinguished clearly from those of cocaine and *d*-amphetamine, which is consistent with neuropharmacological differences in the mechanisms influenced by these drugs. The changes within the spectrum of local spatial scaling exponents indicated that the "recruitment" of straight movement sequences versus local movements can be affected independently.

INDEPENDENT FACTORS GOVERNING MOTOR BEHAVIOR

A comprehensive description of behavioral states should be based on a set of linearly independent measures. The results of the drug studies demonstrated that the dynamical entropy, the spatial scaling exponent, and the temporal scaling exponent, could be influenced independently. Nevertheless, we had no evidence that these measures corresponded to inherently independent dimensions of rat motor behavior.

To examine the hypothesis that sequential and hierarchical behavioral organization are independent of the amount of motor activity, we analyzed a large group of drug-naive animals pooled from various experiments. Specifically, the correlation matrix for activity measures, (counts and α), the spatial scaling exponent, *d*, the dynamical entropy, *h*, and measures of exploratory behavior (*% rears/counts* and *% pokes/counts*) were subjected to a factor analysis.[48] The factor analysis retrieved three factors explaining 77% of the total variance generated by these measures. The first factor loaded on the counts measure

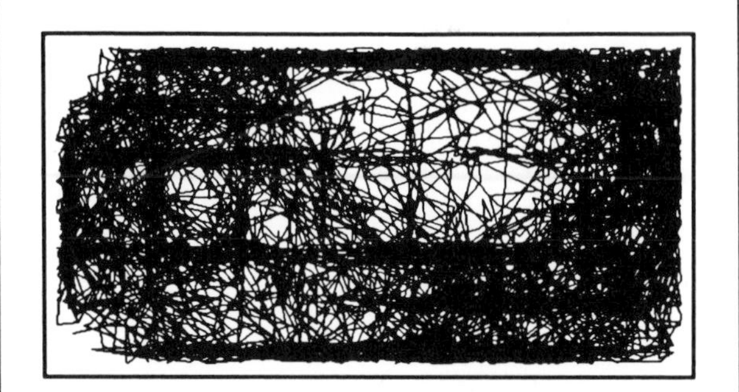

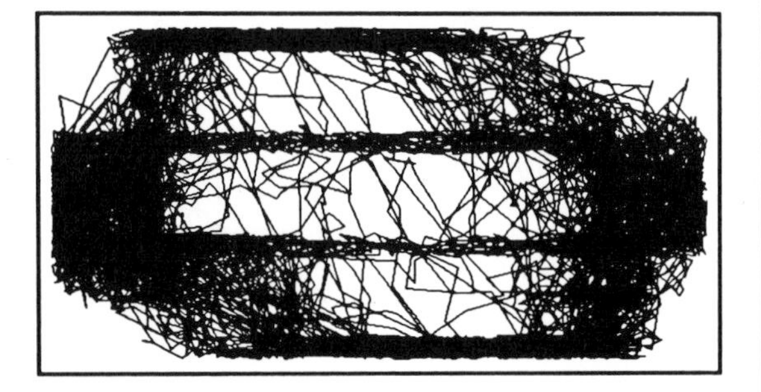

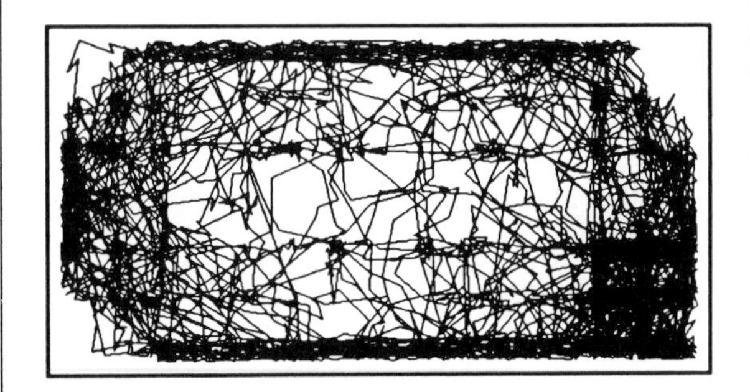

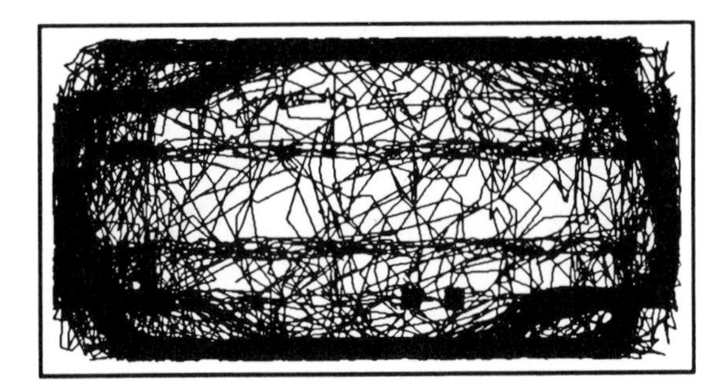

Fig. 14.2. Examples of spatial patterns of movements in the Behavioral Pattern Monitor. Individual rats were monitored for one hour after (top to bottom): 0.5 mg/kg d-amphetamine; 4.0 mg/kg d-amphetamine; 5.0 mg/kg cocaine; or 40.0 mg/kg cocaine. After low doses of amphetamine, rats typically move throughout the chamber. After high doses of amphetamine, more straight movements are observed both along the walls and through the center. Highly circumscribed movements are also seen at the ends of the chamber. After low doses of cocaine, the path patterns are similar to those exhibited by control animals, including the demarcation of a home area (e.g. lower right corner for this rat) coupled with distributed movements primarily close to the walls. After high doses of cocaine, the patterns become more dominated by long straight movements, with occasional local activity near the ends of the chamber.

Available Free Titles

Please check three titles in order of preference.
Your request will be filled based on availability. Thank you.

- ❒ Water Channels
  Alan Verkman, University of California-San Francisco
- ❒ The Na,K-ATPase: Structure-Function Relationship
  J.-D. Horisberger, University of Lausanne
- ❒ Intrathymic Development of T Cells
  J. Nikolic-Zugic, Memorial Sloan-Kettering Cancer Center
- ❒ Cyclic GMP
  Thomas Lincoln, University of Alabama
- ❒ Primordial VRM System and the Evolution of Vertebrate Immunity
  John Stewart, Institut Pasteur-Paris
- ❒ Thyroid Hormone Regulation of Gene Expression
  Graham R. Williams, University of Birmingham
- ❒ Mechanisms of Immunological Self Tolerance
  Guido Kroemer, CNRS Génétique Moléculaire et Biologie du Développement-Villejuif
- ❒ The Costimulatory Pathway for T Cell Responses
  Yang Liu, New York University
- ❒ Molecular Genetics of Drosophila Oogenesis
  Paul F. Lasko, McGill University
- ❒ Mechanism of Steroid Hormone Regulation of Gene Transcription
  M.-J. Tsai & Bert W. O'Malley, Baylor University
- ❒ Liver Gene Expression
  François Tronche & Moshe Yaniv, Institut Pasteur-Paris
- ❒ RNA Polymerase III Transcription
  R.J. White, University of Cambridge
- ❒ src Family of Tyrosine Kinases in Leukocytes
  Tomas Mustelin, La Jolla Institute
- ❒ MHC Antigens and NK Cells
  Rafael Solana & Jose Peña, University of Córdoba
- ❒ Kinetic Modeling of Gene Expression
  James L. Hargrove, University of Georgia
- ❒ PCR and the Analysis of the T Cell Receptor Repertoire
  Jorge Oksenberg, Michael Panzara & Lawrence Steinman, Stanford University
- ❒ Myointimal Hyperplasia
  Philip Dobrin, Loyola University
- ❒ Transgenic Mice as an In Vivo Model of Self-Reactivity
  David Ferrick & Lisa DiMolfetto-Landon, University of California-Davis and Pamela Ohashi, Ontario Cancer Institute
- ❒ Cytogenetics of Bone and Soft Tissue Tumors
  Avery A. Sandberg, Genetrix & Julia A. Bridge, University of Nebraska
- ❒ The Th1-Th2 Paradigm and Transplantation
  Robin Lowry, Emory University
- ❒ Phagocyte Production and Function Following Thermal Injury
  Verlyn Peterson & Daniel R. Ambruso, University of Colorado
- ❒ Human T Lymphocyte Activation Deficiencies
  José Regueiro, Carlos Rodríguez-Gallego and Antonio Arnaiz-Villena, Hospital 12 de Octubre-Madrid
- ❒ Monoclonal Antibody in Detection and Treatment of Colon Cancer
  Edward W. Martin, Jr., Ohio State University
- ❒ Enteric Physiology of the Transplanted Intestine
  Michael Sarr & Nadey S. Hakim, Mayo Clinic
- ❒ Artificial Chordae in Mitral Valve Surgery
  Claudio Zussa, S. Maria dei Battuti Hospital-Treviso
- ❒ Injury and Tumor Implantation
  Satya Murthy & Edward Scanlon, Northwestern University
- ❒ Support of the Acutely Failing Liver
  A.A. Demetriou, Cedars-Sinai
- ❒ Reactive Metabolites of Oxygen and Nitrogen in Biology and Medicine
  Matthew Grisham, Louisiana State-Shreveport
- ❒ Biology of Lung Cancer
  Adi Gazdar & Paul Carbone, Southwestern Medical Center
- ❒ Quantitative Measurement of Venous Incompetence
  Paul S. van Bemmelen, Southern Illinois University and John J. Bergan, Scripps Memorial Hospital
- ❒ Adhesion Molecules in Organ Transplants
  Gustav Steinhoff, University of Kiel
- ❒ Purging in Bone Marrow Transplantation
  Subhash C. Gulati, Memorial Sloan-Kettering Cancer Center
- ❒ Trauma 2000: Strategies for the New Millennium
  David J. Dries & Richard L. Gamelli, Loyola University

and the temporal scaling exponent, α, with a slight contribution by the dynamical entropy, h. This factor can be identified readily as describing the "amount of activity" of the animals in the BPM chamber. The second factor loaded on the spatial scaling exponent, d, the dynamical entropy, h, and to a minor extent on the *% pokes/counts* measure. Since this factor involved mostly the measures that assess dynamical and geometrical characteristics of behavioral organization, it may be called "sequential response organization." The third factor included both *% rears/counts* and *% pokes/counts* and is therefore easily conceptualized as the "exploratory activity" of the animals in the BPM chamber. These three factors have proven to be remarkably stable across many subgroups of over 500 control animals tested over a decade.

Therefore, spontaneous or unconditioned motor behavior is characterized by at least three independent factors that may be modulated differentially by various neurotransmitters and their interactions. The effects of pharmacological manipulations on these factors can be obtained by transforming the experimental results using the factor score matrix. Based on the assumption that differential effects on independent factors of unconditioned motor behavior are mediated by distinct neurobiological substrates, future experiments will be designed to identify these substrates. Alternatively, differential changes of variables that normally co-vary within one factor may reflect a de-coupling of concomitant behavioral responses, which may be interpreted as a response disintegration.

IDENTIFYING AND MEASURING BEHAVIORAL PHASE TRANSITIONS

One important reason to use the analogy with statistical mechanics is to adapt the notion of a phase transition to behavior. Physically, a phase transition is characterized by a qualitative change of the state of the system from one phase into another. Behavioral phase transitions refer to qualitative changes in the behavioral subsets characterizing the behavioral topography. Although much more work remains to be done in this area, we have already obtained evidence that these approaches to behavioral analysis will lead to the identification and quantitation of phase transitions in behavior.

Coexisting Dynamical States in Cocaine-induced Behavioral Activation

The assessment of the sequential organization of behavior using the generalized entropy formalism described above revealed the coexistence of behavioral event sequences having different dynamical characteristics. Specifically, cocaine changed dose-dependently the fluctuation spectrum of local dynamical entropies, $S(h)$, from a small concavity to a marked discontinuity.[29] This change of $S(h)$ is analogous to the development of a phase transition in the framework of statistical mechanics. Behaviorally, this conclusion would imply that, in the saline-treated animals, large fluctuations between different entropic states are possible, whereas in the cocaine-treated animals, transitions are confined more rigidly to one or the other subset (h_l, h_h), leading to an overall lack of entropically varied responsiveness. The fact that $h - S(h) \neq 0$, i.e. that not all possible paths have the same dynamical entropy, which can be also interpreted as a finite escape rate, suggests that the different entropic phases $(h_l h_h)$ correspond dynamically to competing local "repellers." Thus, the dynamical characteristics of a subset of sequences of behavioral events can be conceptualized as generated by a local repeller with h_l that eventually is mapped into another interval which itself behaves locally like a repeller with h_h and corresponds to behavioral sequences that are very unpredictable. Consequently, the resulting behavioral sequences may result from local repellers whose insets overlap but may not necessarily form an underlying attractor. Consequently, the fluctuation spectra of ergodic measures derived from the probability distributions may depend crucially on the escape rate, which may result in an order parameter description of the system. Thus, the "ease" with which a local repeller is mapped into the inset of another repeller with different entropic characteristics may be an important mechanism by which the animal can adjust its behavioral sequences to the environmental and internal demands.

Phase Transitions in the d - α Plane

Conceptually, a behavioral state can be defined by a specific set of the macroscopic parameters that govern the function describing the system. Accordingly, one can conceptualize a phase transition as a change of state within the parameter space produced by a change in a control parameter. For example, the dose of a drug can serve as a control parameter. We hypothesized that this change of state could be smooth, i.e., a small change of the control parameter leads to a small change in the state, or discontinuous, i.e., a small change will result in a sudden change of state. As an example of a smooth change, the changes in the amount of locomotion produced by some drugs are continuous and monotonically related to dose over a wide range. With drugs such as amphetamine, however, the behavior changes suddenly from locomotor activity to focused stereotypies as the dose increases. We assume that the identification of such transitions is important for the specification of the underlying neurobiological substrates. Hence, we predicted that some drugs would yield behavioral phase transitions at critical dose-ranges, reflected as discontinuities in the dose-response functions. We have observed such rapid transitions in several experiments. For example, activity-related and geometrical phase transitions can be observed readily in the d - α plane as "jumps" from one location in the plane to another. Biphasic dose response curves were obtained for apomorphine and lisuride along the "activity dimension" in the

8. Nickolson VJ. Detailed analysis of the effects of apomorphine and d-amphetamine on spontaneous locomotor behaviour of rats as measured in a TV-based automated open-field system. Eur J Pharm 1981; 72:45-56.
9. Gold LH, Koob GF, Geyer MA. Stimulant and hallucinogenic behavioral profiles of 3,4-methylenedioxymethamphetamine and N-ethyl-3,4-methylenedioxyamphetamine in rats. J Pharmacol Exp Ther 1988; 247:547-555.
10. Teitelbaum P, Szechtman H, Sirkin DW et al. Dimensions of movement, movement subsystems and local reflexes in the dopaminergic systems underlying exploratory locomotion. In: MY Spiegelstein, A Levy, eds. Behavioral Models and the Analysis of Drug Action. Amsterdam, Oxford, New York: Elsevier, 1982: 357-385.
11. Bakan P. Response Tendencies in attempts to generate random binary sequences. Am J Psychol 1960; 73:127-31.
12. Paulus MP, Geyer MA. A temporal and spatial scaling hypothesis for the behavioral effects of psychostimulants. Psychopharmacology 1991; 104:6-16.
13. Geyer MA, Russo PV, Masten VL. Multivariate assessment of locomotor behavior: pharmacological and behavioral analyses. Pharmacol Biochem Behav 1986; 25:277-288.
14. Ruelle D. Statistical Mechanics, Thermodynamic Formalism. Reading, MA: Addison-Weseley, 1978.
15. Ruelle D. Chaotic Evolution and Strange Attractors: The Statistical Analysis of Time Series for Deterministic Nonlinear Systems. New York: Cambridge University Press, 1989.
16. Chandler D. Introduction to Modern Statistical Mechanics. New York: Oxford University Press, 1987.
17. Stanley HE. Introduction to Phase Transitions and Critical Phenomena. New York: Oxford University Press, 1987.
18. Badii R. Conservation laws and thermodynamic formalism for dissipative dynamical systems. Rivista Del Nuova Cimento 1989; 12:1-72.
19. Bohr T, Rand D. The entropy function for characteristic exponents. Physica 1987; 25D, 387-398.
20. Bohr T, Jensen M. Order parameter, symmetry breaking, and phase transitions in the description of multifractal sets. Phys Rev 1987; A 36:4904-4915.
21. Fabre JHC. Souvenirs Entomologiques, etudes sur l'instinct et les Moeurs des insects, Vol 1. Paris: Librairie Delagrave, 1943.
22. Adams LM, Geyer MA. LSD-induced alterations in locomotor patterns and exploration in rats. Psychopharmacol 1982; 77:179-185.
23. Flicker C, Geyer MA. Behavior during hippocampal microinfusions: I. Norepinephrine and diversive exploration. Brain Res Rev 1982; 4:79-103.
24. Geyer MA. Variational and probabilistic aspects of exploratory behavior in space: Four stimulant styles. Psychopharmacol Bull 1982; 18:48-51.
25. Crutchfield JP, Young K. Inferring statistical complexity. Phys Rev Lett 1989; 63:105-108.

26. Paulus MP, Geyer MA, Gold LH, Mandell AJ. Application of entropy measures derived from the ergodic theory of dynamical systems to rat locomotor behavior. Proc National Acad Sci, USA, 1990; 87:723-727.
27. Paulus MP, Geyer MA, Mandell AJ. Statistical mechanics of a neurobiological dynamical system: The spectrum of local entropies (S (α)) applied to cocaine-perturbed behavior. Physica A 1991; 174:567-577.
28. Halsey TC, Jensen MH, Kadanoff LP, Procaccia I, Shraiman BI. Fractal measures and their singularities: The characterization of strange sets. Phys Rev A 1986; 33:1141-1151.
29. Paulus MP, Callaway CW, Geyer MA. Quantitative assessment of the microstructure of rat behavior: II. Distinctive effects of dopamine releasers and reuptake inhibitors. Psychopharmacol 1993; 113:187-198.
30. Feder J. Fractals. New York: Plenum Press, 1988.
31. Higushi T. Approach to an irregular time series on the basis of fractal theory. Physica D 1988; 31:277-283.
32. Mandelbrot B. Fractals: Form, Chance and Dimension. San Francisco: Freeman, 1977.
33. Meyer-Kress G. Dimensions and Entropies in Chaotic Systems: Quantification of Complex Behavior. Berlin: Springer, 1986.
34. Wilson KG. Problems in physics with many scales of length. Sci American 1985; 158-179.
35. Adams LM, Geyer MA. Patterns of exploration in rats distinguish lisuride from lysergic acid diethylamide. Pharmacol Biochem Behav 1985; 23:461-468.
36. Geyer MA, Paulus MP. Multivariate and nonlinear approaches to characterizing drug effects on the locomotor and investigatory behavior of rats. Neurobiological Approaches to Brain-Behavior Interaction. NIDA Research Monograph Series 1992; 124:203-235.
37. Geyer MA. Approaches to the characterization of drug effects on locomotor activity in rodents. In: MW Adler, A Cowan, eds. Testing and Evaluation of Drugs of Abuse. New York: Wiley-Liss, Inc., 1990: 81-99.
38. Paulus MP, Geyer MA. The effects of MDMA and other methylenedioxy substituted phenylalkylamines on the structure of rat locomotor activity. Neuropsychopharmacol 1992; 7:15-31.
39. Callaway CW, Nichols DE, Paulus MP et al. Serotonin release is responsible for the locomotor hyperactivity in rats induced by derivatives of amphetamine related to MDMA. In: Fozard JR, Saxena PR, eds. Serotonin: Molecular Biology, Receptors and Functional Effects. Basel: Birkhauser, 1991: 491-505.
40. Callaway CW, Geyer MA. Tolerance and cross-tolerance to the activating effects of 3,4-methylenedioxymethamphetamine and a serotonin $5HT_{1B}$ agonist. J Pharm Exp Ther 1992; 263:318-326.
41. Callaway CW, Wing LL, Geyer MA. Serotonin release contributes to the locomotor stimulant effects of 3,4-methylenedioxymethamphetamine (MDMA) in rats. J Pharmacol Exp Ther, 1990; 254:456-464.

42. Glennon RA. Stimulus properties of hallucinogenic phenalkylamines and related designer drugs: formulation of structure-activity relationships. NIDA Research Monograph 1989; 94:43-67.
43. Johnson MP, Hoffman AJ, Nichols DE. Effects of the enantiomers of MDA, MDMA and related analogues on [3H]serotonin and [3H]dopamine release from superfused rat brain slices. Eur J Pharmacol 1986; 132:269-276.
44. Nichols DE. Differences between the mechanism of action of MDMA, MBDB, and the classic hallucinogens. Identification of a new therapeutic class: Entactogens. J Psychoactive Drugs 1986; 18:305-313.
45. Callaway CW, Rempel N, Peng RY, Geyer MA. Serotonin 5-HT\d1\u-like receptors mediate hyperactivity in rats induced by 3,4-methylenedioxymethamphetamine. Neuropsychopharm 1992; 7:113-127.
46. Rempel N, Callaway CW, Geyer MA. Serotonin\d1B\u receptor activation mimics behavioral effects of presynaptic serotonin release. Neuropsychopharmacol 1992; 8:201-212.
47. Paulus MP, Geyer MA. Quantitative assessment of the microstructure of rat behavior: I. *f(d),* the extension of the scaling hypothesis. Psychopharmacol 1993a; 113:177-186.
48. Paulus MP, Geyer MA. Three independent factors characterize spontaneous rat motor activity. Behav Brain Res 1993b; 53:11-20.

APPENDIX A

APPENDIX TO CHAPTER 5

Warren O. Eaton, Nancy A. McKeen and Kimberly J. Saudino

SAS PROGRAM FOR INPUTTING DATA FROM FIGURE 5.2 AND CALCULATING SUMMARY VALUES

A. SAS Program Steps

```
DATA ACTO;
 * -- Input statement uses SAS time and date formats. Numerical
      suffixes on variable names correspond to limbs, viz., 1—
      right arm, 2—left arm, 3—right leg, and 4—left leg.;
 INPUT ID 1 @3 BEGIN DATETIME13. @16 (ACTNO1-ACTNO4)(3.)
      @28 (STRT1-STRT4)(TIME9.)/ @2 (OFFMIN1-OFFMIN4)(3.) @15
              END DATETIME13.
      @28 (STOP1-STOP4)(TIME9.);
TOTMIN = (END-BEGIN)/60; * Total mins between placement and final
      removal is calculated;
 * -- Variable arrays are defined for iterative calculations —;
      ARRAY AU (LIMB) AU1-AU4; * Total actometer units
              between BEGIN & END;
      ARRAY STOP (LIMB) STOP1-STOP4; * Final actometer
              readings;
      ARRAY STRT (LIMB) STRT1-STRT4; * Initial actometer
              readings;
      ARRAY MIN (LIMB) MIN1-MIN4; * Total mins actometer worn
              on a limb;
      ARRAY OFFMIN (LIMB) OFFMIN1-OFFMIN4; * Total mins off |
              for each limb;
      ARRAY AU_RATE (LIMB) AU_RATE1-AU_RATE4; * Actometer
              units per 30 mins;
      ARRAY AU_LOG (LIMB) AU_LOG1-AU_LOG4; * Common log of units
              per 30 mins;
 * -- Identical calculations are completed for all 4 limbs. —;
      DO LIMB = 1 TO 4; DROP LIMB; * Counter variable not
              retained for output;
       AU = (STOP - STRT); * Raw activity units calculated;
       MIN = TOTMIN - OFFMIN; * Mins acto worn calculated;
       AU_RATE = (AU/MIN) * 30; * Actometer units per 30 mins
              calculated;
```

```
        AU_LOG = LOG10(AU_RATE); * Log of AU_RATE calculated;
       END;
 * -- Summary actometer scores are calculated —;
       AL_RATE = MEAN(OF AU_RATE1-AU_RATE4);
       AL_LOG = MEAN(OF AU_LOG1-AU_LOG4);
 LABEL BEGIN  = 'Actometer attachment in real time'
          ACTNO1 = 'Right arm actometer #'
          STRT2    = 'Left arm actometer reading at BEGIN'
          STOP3    = 'Right leg actometer reading at END'
          OFFMIN4 = 'Total mins actometer off left leg'
          END   = 'Final actometer removal in real time'
          TOTMIN = 'Mins real time between attachment and final
              removal'
          AL_RATE = 'Untransformed mean actometer units per 30
              mins'
          AL_LOG = 'Common log of mean actometer units per 30
              mins';
* Raw data entered in 2 lines following 'CARDS' ; CARDS;
1 06MAR95:14:10 27 15 09 36 01:43:43 04:46:28 05:46:32 04:18:43
 15 15 26 22 08MAR95:14:14 02:57:57 05:37:29 06:34:07 05:15:19
;
PROC PRINT;
 FORMAT BEGIN END DATETIME13. STRT1-STRT4 STOP1-STOP4 TIME9. AU1-
      AU4 MIN1-MIN4 OFFMIN1-OFFMIN4 4. AL_RATE AU_RATE1-AU_RATE4
      5.1 AL_LOG AU_LOG1-AU_LOG4 5.3;
RUN;
```

B. Output from Preceding Program

```
OBS ID        BEGIN   ACTNO1  ACTNO2   ACTNO3 ACTNO4   STRT1    STRT2
1    106MAR95:14:10    27      15        9      36  1:43:43  4:46:28
OBS  STRT3      STRT4  OFFMIN1 OFFMIN2 OFFMIN3  OFFMIN4          END
1  5:46:32   4:18:43     15      15      26       22  08MAR95:14:14
OBS  STOP1     STOP2    STOP3    STOP4  TOTMIN      AU1     AU2     AU3
1  2:57:57  5:37:29 6:34:07 5:15:19   2884      4454   3061    2855
OBS AU4  MIN1   MIN2  MIN3   MIN4 AU_RATE1 AU_RATE2 AU_RATE3 AU_RATE4
1  3396  2869  2869 2858   2862    46.6      32.0      30.0      35.6
OBS AU_LOG1 AU_LOG2 AU_LOG3 AU_LOG4    AL_RATE  AL_LOG
1     1.668   1.505   1.477   1.551     36.0    1.550
```

APPENDIX B

APPENDIX TO CHAPTER 3

Klaus-Peter Ossenkopp and Martin Kavaliers

INDEX OF INSTRUMENTATION COMPANIES

Charnwood Dynamics
17 South Street, Barrow on Soar
Leicestershire LE128LY
England
Tel. int+44-1509-620388
FAX int+44-1509-416791

CODA-3
3D Motion Analysis

Columbus Instruments
950 North Hague Avenue
P.O. Box 44049
Columbus, OH 43204
Tel. (614) 276-0861
FAX (614) 276-0529

Activity Measurement System

Coulbourn Instruments, Inc.
7462 Penn Drive
Allentown, PA 18106
Tel. (215) 395-3771
FAX (215) 391-1333

Animal Activity Analyzer
Video Tracking Activity System

Dragonfly, R&D, Inc.
P.O. Box 1725
Silver Spring, MD 20915
Tel. (301) 424-8921

Animal Research Instrumentation

Harvard Apparatus, Inc.
22 Pleasant Street
South Natick, MA 01760
Tel. (508) 655-7000

Animal Behavior Systems

Company	Products
HVS Image Ormond Crescent, Hampton England TW12 2TH Tel. In U.S. (800) 225-9261	Activity Measurement Systems
IITC Inc. Life Science Instruments 23924 Victory Blvd. Woodland Hills, CA 91367 Tel. (818) 710-1556 FAX (818) 992-5185	Rotometry Systems
Konigsberg Instruments, Inc. 2000 Foothill Blvd. Pasadena, CA 91107 Tel. (818) 449-0016	Telemetry
Lafayette Instrument Company P.O. Box 5729 3700 Sagamore Parkway N. Lafayette, IN 47903 Tel. (800) 428-7545	Activity Wheels
Les Distributions Physiomonitor Ltee. 1470 De Coulomb, Suite 205 Boucherville, Quebec, Canada J4B 7K2 Tel. (514) 449-6140	Activity Measurement Systems
Letica S/A, Scientific Instruments Cromo 37, 08907 Hospitalet (Barcelona) Spain Tel. +34-9-33366062 FAX +34-9-33354210	Spontaneous Motor Activity Recording and Tracking
MED Associates Box 47 East Fairfield, VT 05448 Tel. (317) 447-2216 FAX (317) 447-7457	Animal Activity Monitors

Mini-Mitter Co., Inc.
P.O. Box 3386
Sunriver, OR 97707
Tel. (503) 593-8639
FAX (503) 593-5604

Animal Activity Telemetry

Nalge Company,
75 Panorama Creek Drive
Box 20365
Rochester, NY 14602
Tel. (716) 264-3893

Activity Wheels

Noldus Information Technolgy bv
Business & Technology Center
Costerweg 5,
6702 AA Wageningen
The Netherlands
Tel. +31-8370-97677
FAX +31-8370-24496

Video Tracking and Motion Analysis System

Northern Digital, Inc.
403 Albert Street
Waterloo, Ontario
Canada N2G 3V2
Tel. (519) 884-5142

3D Motion Analysis

Omnitech Electronics, Inc.
5090 Trabue Road
Columbus, OH 43228-9990
Tel. (614) 878-6644
FAX (614) 878-3560

Activity Measurement Systems
Digiscan Acitivity Monitor

Paul Fray Ltd
Flint Bridge,
Ely Road, Waterbeach
Cambridge, UK CB5 9PG
Tel. +44-223-441134
FAX +44-223-441017

Activity Measurement Systems

Peak Performance Technologies, Inc
7388 S. Revere Parkway #601
Englewood, CO 80112
Tel. (303) 799-8686
or (800) 745-7325

Activity Measurement Systems
2D & 3D Video and Computer Motion Measurement

San Diego Instruments, Inc. Suite G 9353 Activity Road San Diego, CA 92126 Tel. (619) 530-2600 FAX (619) 530-2646	Activity Measurement Systems Poly-Track Video Tracking
Stanford Software Systems P.O. Box 8068 Stanford, CA 94309-8068 Tel. (415) 854-5359	Activity Measurement Systems
TSE, Technical & Scientific Equipment GmbH Ludwigstr. 10 6380 Bad Homburg v.d.H. Germany Tel. +49-6172-26421 FAX +49-6172-26428	Video Activity System
Wildlink, Inc. 2924 98th Avenue North Brooklyn Park, MN 55444 Tel. (800) 421-8340	Satellite links for monitoring field activity

INDEX

Page numbers in italics denote figures (f) or tables (t).

G

H

I

J

K

L

M

N

O

S

T

U

V

W

X

Z